Too Loud, Too Bright,
Too Fast, Too Tight

ALSO BY SHARON HELLER

*The Vital Touch: How Intimate Contact
with Your Baby Leads to Happier, Healthier Development*

Too Loud, Too Bright, Too Fast, Too Tight

What to Do If You Are Sensory Defensive in an Overstimulating World

Sharon Heller, Ph.D.

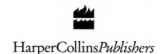

HarperCollins*Publishers*

HarperCollins books may be purchased for educational, business, or sales promotional use. For information, please write: Special Markets Department, HarperCollins Publishers Inc., 10 East 53rd Street, New York, NY 10022.

FIRST EDITION

Designed by Sarah Maya Gubkin

Printed on acid-free paper

Library of Congress Cataloging-in-Publication Data

Heller, Sharon.
    Too loud, too bright, too fast, too tight : what to do if you are sensory defensive in an overstimulating world / Sharon Heller. —1st ed.
        p.   cm.
    Includes bibliographical references and index.
    ISBN 0-06-019520-7
    1. Sensitivity (Personality trait).   I. Title.

BF698.35.S47 H45   2002
155.9'11—dc21

2001058335

02   03   04   05   06   WB/RRD   10   9   8   7   6   5   4   3   2   1

To Robert,
easy, playful, calming

It is very confusing, and very frustrating, to spend so much effort being so afraid to be touched, and working so very hard to avoid being touched, when it is touching and being touched that I need most of all.

—PAT HOLBROOK

Acknowledgments

I am enormously grateful to Moya Kinneally, Carol Kranowitz, and Steven Cool for their careful and thorough reading of the manuscript and valuable suggestions, and to Betsy Hancock, Jeannetta Burpee, Judy Kimball, Troy Mills, and Dean Howell for reading and commenting on various sections. My heartfelt thanks to friends Carolyne Singer, Hilary Leibowitz, and Mayo Viscioso for their helpful input.

I want to thank Leslie Stern, my first editor at HarperCollins, for her initial help and encouragement. Gail Winston, my managing editor, was an author's dream—thorough, committed, and efficient. Thanks to my agent, Mary Ann Naples of Creative Culture, for her ongoing support and encouragement throughout.

I greatly appreciate the many sensory-defensive people who allowed me to share their stories. Pat Holbrook, the owner of the chatline Adultsid (adults with sensory integration dysfunction), is an enormously insightful person whose articulate descriptions of her own lifelong struggle with sensory defensiveness greatly enhanced my understanding of this problem and substantially contributed to the writing of this book. I want to thank as well the other members of this chatline who shared their stories.

Lastly, I want to thank occupational therapist Patti Oetter. My therapist at the Ayres Clinic and my mentor over the last seven years, Patti has taught me much of what I know about sensory integration and the problem of sensory defensiveness. She is unusually perceptive and has an extraordinary ability to tune in to others and make one feel she's right there.

Because little has been published on sensory defensiveness, and especially in adults, much of the information in this book came from occupational therapy workshops given by Patricia and Julia Wilbarger, Patti Oetter, Nancy Lawton-Shirley, Sheila Frick, Mary Kawar, Marie Anzalone, and Steven Cool. Conversations with occupational therapists Carolyn Slutsky and Deborah Milam further advanced my knowledge.

Contents

Introduction: Too Sensitive for Your Own Good   1

Part 1 - Living Outside the Comfort Zone

Chapter 1 – Senses on the Defense   23

Chapter 2 – Sensory Processing: The Touchy Nervous
System   39

Chapter 3 – Levels of Defensiveness: From Mild to
Maddening   73

Part 2 - Secondary Effects: From Dis-Ease to Disease

Chapter 4 – Weaving a Web of Fear: Sensory
Defensiveness Across the Lifespan   93

Chapter 5 – From Anxiety to Addictions   119

Chapter 6 – The Body Erupts: The Psychosomatic
Side of Sensory Defensiveness   145

Part 3 - Your Sensory Diet

Chapter 7 – Getting Started   157

Chapter 8 – Priming the Pump   169

Chapter 9 – Sound Health   193

Chapter 10 – Seeing the Whole Picture   207

Chapter 11 – Air Control   223

Chapter 12 – A Harmonious Space   235

Part 4 - Removing Treatment Obstacles

Chapter 13 – Food for Your Nervous System   249

Chapter 14 – Breathing Lessons   265

Chapter 15 – Posturing for Inner Peace   281

Chapter 16 – Mind/Body—Only Connect!   299

Appendix A: Sensory Defensiveness Survival Kit   309

Appendix B: Defensive Reactions to Sensation   313

Notes   319

Glossary   337

Resource Guide   343

Index   361

Too Loud, Too Bright,
Too Fast, Too Tight

Introduction

Too Sensitive for Your Own Good

"Relax," people would tell Dr. H., a college professor, "stop letting everything bother you." But she couldn't and she didn't know why. The labels in her clothing, someone opening a bag of potato chips, the odor of her new car, the flashing pointer on the computer screen, the computer's hovering noise—*everything seemed to drive her crazy*.

Driving in traffic, or going to the mall, a restaurant, or even to a friend's could feel like maneuvering through a sensory minefield, and at times she needed to brace herself to go out. Her skin, ears, eyes, nose, taste buds, and teeth were all overly sensitive.

What's life like for everyone else, she wondered?

She felt old, weighted down, and vulnerable, and she had a pervasive underlying sense of terror. By turns drained and wired, by the end of the day her body was exhausted but her insides vibrated. At night she was unable to rest or concentrate but would lie awake for hours, hoping she could quiet her nerves enough to face another day. Why couldn't she shut out unwanted sensations and relax?

It wasn't for lack of trying. She took yoga, practiced deep-breathing exercises, used aromatherapy, and tried to meditate. But during yoga, the overhead lights, the whirring of the air conditioner, the rough carpet touching her feet, the body odors of others in the group, and her instructor's squeaky voice would grate on her nerves, even when she was not unduly stressed. During meditation, noises slit open her inner sanctum. If her cat brushed her arm with his whiskers, her skin crept and she had to break from the stillness to rub the spot. Moreover, whatever relaxation these activities afforded seemed short lived. She worried that this might be as good as it gets.

Fortunately, it isn't. I am Dr. H. This book is my attempt to enlighten others whose senses are also in overdrive and explain why this happens, what it means, and what they can do about it.

What made me so overreactive? Stress? Anxiety? That's part of it. But as a psychologist, I knew this explanation was incomplete. Though psychotherapy relieved my depression and crippling anxiety, I remained an artful dodger of sensation. As I aged, the sensory world seemed to invade my space more and more and created an ongoing tension that I felt helpless to control. Always there was a vague, nagging feeling that something more was wrong. But what?

And then, in 1996, while writing *The Vital Touch*, a book on mother-and-baby intimacy, I happened upon a talk by occupational therapist and counseling psychologist Patricia Wilbarger. She described children who are fussy and hard to calm, shrink from human touch, arch their back and cry when they are picked up. These children hate to be bathed and have their hair washed and throw off hats, clothes, and blankets. Many startle easily to noise or certain movements. She called their behavior *sensory defensiveness*.

Hmmm. Could sensory defensiveness explain some of my extreme excitability and need to escape into a cave?

Hoping for some answers, I called Ms. Wilbarger, who along with her daughter Julia, has made it her mission to understand, identify, and treat sensory defensiveness. Yes, she confirmed, I certainly sounded sensory-defensive. But, she reassured me, there are treatments, including one she has devised, and they work at any age.

What relief! My tendency to become easily overstimulated had a name and a framework of understanding beyond stress and anxiety. It started with how my body reacted to sensation.

Sensory defensiveness is a condition that encompasses a constellation of symptoms, including tension, anxiety, avoidance, stress, anger, and even violence, that result from aversive or defensive reactions to what most people consider nonirritating stimuli.[1] Though largely unrecognized, sensory defensiveness is not uncommon. As many as 15 percent of otherwise normal adults have a nervous system that is overly sensitive to sensation. What is interesting, ho-hum, pleasurable, or exalting for most people can be irritating, disgusting, alarming, and even painful to them.

Sensory defensives don't just feel sensitive to sensation. Along with having acute sensitivity, they feel bothered and distracted by sensation. Musicians or artists, for example, can have keen senses but are not necessarily irritated by sensation. Picasso indisputably had superior vision. Yet he read by the light of a naked bulb over his bed, a glare that would make many defensives uncomfortable. And while many people with attention deficit hyperactivity disorder (ADHD) are sensory defensive, some feel distracted but not necessarily bothered by sensation. Some people don't notice an odor in musty sheets; others notice it but are unconcerned. The sensory defensive says, "No way can I sleep in that bed!"

For most adults, this hypersensitivity is a long-standing and an unnamed problem. Their parents often recall that they were unusually sensitive during infancy—they may not have liked being cuddled, they may have startled easily to noise. They were likely overly fussy and had sleep or eating problems.

Here are many common symptoms of sensory defensiveness.

- Feeling annoyed when certain textures touch your skin
- Recoiling from light, ticklish touch or when someone, particularly a stranger, unexpectedly touches you
- Startling to loud, sudden, or piercing sounds
- Being unable to shut out constant noise
- Wincing at bright lights: becoming disorganized by excessive visual stimulation
- Grimacing at odors others don't notice
- Feeling light-headed and sick from chemicals in the environment
- Avoiding foods of a certain taste or texture
- Feeling anxious when experiencing sudden or fast movement, when bending forward or backward, or from heights, unstable surfaces, swings, or roller coasters
- Shunning crowds

If any of this rings true, you might be sensory-defensive to some degree. To find out, take the self-test in the accompanying box.

SENSORY DEFENSIVENESS SELF-TEST

Sensory Experience

Check any of these stimuli that seem to bother you more than they bother other people.

___ Smells
___ Sounds
___ Lights, contrasts, reflections, or objects close to your face
___ Eye contact
___ Touching dirt, glue, or paint
___ Walking barefoot in grass or sand
___ Tags and labels in your clothes (which you generally remove)

__ Turtleneck tops, tight-fitting clothes or belts, elastic waistbands, materials in clothes

__ The feeling of jewelry (rings, earrings, necklaces, or bracelets)

__ Certain food textures in your mouth

__ Looking down a long flight of stairs, going down an escalator, or riding in a glass elevator

__ Creams or lotions on your skin

__ Cutting your nails or washing your hair

__ Baths or showers

__ Someone touching you from behind or unexpectedly

__ Someone standing too close

__ Strangers approaching you and putting their arm around your shoulder, especially of the opposite sex

__ Crowded areas such as elevators, malls, subways, some city streets, shops, or bars

__ Shaking or holding a stranger's hand

__ Vibrations from vehicles, elevators, furnaces, air conditioners, or appliances

Check any of the following that apply to you.

__ Getting car sick

__ Getting dizzy *very* easily

__ Feeling hot or cold easily

__ Dreading to go to the dentist

__ Feeling certain parts of your body especially sensitive (often, but not always, the scalp)

__ Discomfort with being hugged when growing up, except perhaps by your mother

__ Discomfort with physical intimacy because touching bothers you

__ Problems with coordination and balance

__ Very active as a child or now

__ Feeling you must mentally prepare yourself for situations in which people are apt to touch you

__ Attempting to avoid situations in which your senses will be stressed

Mental Experience

Check any of the following that apply to you.

__ Easily frustrated

__ Pronounced mood swings

__ Inability to unwind and self-calm

__ Sleep problems: going to sleep, waking up, sleeping too little, too much

__ Feeling anxious much of the time

__ Sometimes feeling panic

__ Dislike of new situations

__ Difficulty in transitioning from one situation to another

__ Feeling thrown when lacking control or in unpredictable situations

__ Low self-esteem

__ Impulsiveness

__ Perfectionism or compulsion

How do you know if you are sensory-defensive? As the symptoms are an exaggeration of behaviors that fall within a normal human range, it's not necessarily clear. Given enough stress, anyone will feel touchy. And some withdraw from touch because of emotional wounds, not hypersensitivity to tactile stimuli.[2] Nor does a dislike of certain materials on your skin, or a stranger's touch, or crowded places necessarily mean that you are sensory-defensive. But if routine sensations bother you more than they do others, if you avoid situations that will stress your senses, and if you become anxious easily and can't easily unwind, you may very well be sensory-defensive. How sensory-defensive you are will depend on how much avoiding sensation disrupts your life, rules your choices, and creates emotional and bodily upheaval.

People with mild cases may feel irritated by many clothing textures and toss and turn at night to the sound of a dripping sink, but find that life is basically manageable. Though they may be more edgy, fastidious, and restless than most, they see themselves as garden-variety neurotics, not people with a "disorder."

People with a severe case suffer hair-raising sensitivity to barely noticeable stimuli. To them, life feels like a bed of thorny roses—an ongoing struggle to avoid getting pricked, scratched, rubbed, or brushed by anything or anyone touching their skin. A gentle hand on their shoulder can feel like a claw, and if you suddenly pat their back, they might need to exert extreme control to not spontaneously punch you.[3] Other senses will be heightened as well. Ears may feel like loud amplifiers, and the defensive flees in panic from the low-frequency waves of a looming helicopter. Eating, washing, dressing, loving, working, playing—all activities are carefully scrutinized to avoid unpleasant sensations and seek out soothing ones. Disease, tension, and frustration are their constant companions, and undue stress severely diminishes their ability to interact with the world. Life is rarely joyful.

At this level of severity, most have been diagnosed as learning disabled, ADD, autistic, developmentally delayed, schizophrenic, or severely emotionally disturbed. They generally get referred for some form of therapy. But some are just quirky, ordinary people leading otherwise normal lives and don't necessarily appear disabled: that the slightest touch makes them want to jump out of their skins may not be visible to others. These people—normally functioning adults with mild to severe sensory defensiveness—are the focus of this book.

Most of you reading this book will be unfamiliar with the condition of sensory defensiveness. The psychological literature scarcely mentions it, and the popular press limits it largely to a problem of some "out-of-sync" children.[4] Yet, the condition is as old as that familiar fairy tale "The Princess and the Pea."

In the 1960s, this condition was officially identified by A. Jean Ayres, an occupational therapist. Ayres noticed that hyperactive children often avoided touching or being touched, wearing certain types of clothing, having their hair washed, having their nails cut, or being in crowds, as well as other skin contact experiences. She believed the condition, which she called *tactile defensiveness*, caused their hyperactivity and distractibility. From this, she developed the theory of sensory integration. Her treatments for this condition included sensorimotor activities, like skin brushing and rolling under thick blankets. By the 1980s, occupational therapists began to feel that this defensive response involved not just the sense of touch but was a central tendency to react defensively to all sensations, hence the term *sensory defensiveness*.

Ayre's work was groundbreaking. For over forty years, occupational therapists have been successfully treating sensory defensiveness in special-needs populations, including the autistic. But an untold number of otherwise normal functioning adults have gone largely undiagnosed and untreated for this condition. How can people gain insight into their behavior if their problem is not identified? How can they even begin to think about solutions? With so little research done in this area, some professionals question whether sensory defensiveness is even an actual condition. Outside the field of occupational therapy, there are no hard-core scientific data to prove that it exists.

In fact, hypersensitivity has long been studied in psychology as the cause of introversion, an inborn characteristic. Numerous studies have shown that some people have a low sensory threshold; quickly reaching their saturation point, they get easily overstimulated by sensation. To avoid overstimulation, they direct their attention inward and appear restrained and inhibited.

Yet sensory defensiveness goes beyond inborn temperament. Though evidence suggests a genetic link—at least half of sufferers have a sensory-defensive parent or child—the sensory defensive population ranges in temperament from super shy to party animal.[5] In some family members the defensiveness is severe and goes beyond basic temperament. These people are born into a different universe than most.

Nor do you have to be born hypersensitive. Any trauma that disrupts the nervous system at any age can generate sensory defensiveness: prenatal insult from drugs, illness, and maternal stress; birth complications, such as asphyxia, post-birth trauma, or prematurity; head trauma; physical, sexual, or psychological abuse; chemical abuse; or post-traumatic stress disorder.[6] Severe or long-standing trauma creates toxic levels of stress that alters brain chemistry and literally rewires the brain. In some Vietnam combat vets, abused women, and victims of child abuse, the hippocampus, a structure important to memory and learning, shrinks.[7] Under extremely stressful conditions, an excess of the neurotransmitter glutamate kills cells, making the brain less able to inhibit sensory input.[8] Sexually abused girls show consistently higher-than-normal levels of the stress hormone cortisol throughout the day and exaggerate in response to stimulation.[9]

The sensory and emotional deprivation of children found in orphanages such as those in Romania starves the brain of the nourishment needed to learn from and cope with the world. The children are depressed and don't develop adequate sensorimotor, or intellectual functions. Some are so severely tactile defensive that they withdraw from human contact as if painful, in spite of loving adoptive parents.[10]

Sensory defensiveness can also result from allergies and illness such as chronic fatigue syndrome and fibromyalgia. Exposure to environmental toxins, such as air contaminants, destructive viruses, and other chemicals that enter our bodies may contribute to the problem as well. In some cases, the cause is simply unknown.

Sensory defensiveness appears to favor neither race nor ethnicity, though some evidence indicates that women suffer from it more than men. Women show greater acuity in every sense but sight and are more thin-skinned. Women's brains are bathed in different hormones than men's; most women report varying sensitivity around menstruation, pregnancy, and menopause.

Adding to the problem of sensory defensiveness are the noise, artificial lighting, chemical overkill, and crowds that lurk around every corner of modern urban life, resulting in stimulation that is too intense, frequent, fast, and long-lasting for any nervous system to assimilate. For most, this is exhausting. For the sensory defensive, it is overwhelming. Rather than open their senses to take in the world, they feel compelled to turn off their senses to expel the world.

And the problem is not just sensory overload. While modern life overloads our eyes, ears, and nose, it also robs us of organizing touch and movement. Many modern societies have experienced a breakdown of the extended family, isolation, an emphasis on self-reliance, and child care that caches babies in containers rather than carrying them.[11] All of this creates physical barriers to the human intimacy our bodies were designed for, leaving many people with skin hunger. A sedentary lifestyle minimizes energizing movements that nourish the brain. Have you been hugged today? Have you worked up a sweat?

Like the canaries in the coal mine, the sensory defensive should stand as a warning that sensory overload is dangerous for everyone. It impairs concentration, increases irritability and vulnerability to illness, decreases quality of life, and pushes everyone to levels of stress unknown before modern technology. Consciously or not, people are constantly registering sensations that offend the nervous system and take energy, resources, and effort to tune out. Very low level sounds (30 to 50 decibels) cause people to shift from deep sleep to light sleep. People working in a noisy environment show increased levels of the stress hormone epinephrine even if they don't feel particularly stressed.[12] And people working in a room permeated by the odor of burnt dust lose their appetites, even though they don't notice the smell.

Nevertheless, most get by. But what is going on in the brain of the sensory defensive that they don't—are they brain-damaged? Fortunately, this is rarely true. In most cases the brain is miswired, causing an exaggeration of the normal innate protective response to bodily harm.[13]

If a spider crawls up your arm or you smell smoke, your alarm system goes off. The sympathetic branch of the autonomic nervous system in the brain expends energy to arouse you, and stress hormones, like adrenaline, are released into the bloodstream to prepare you to flee or fight: your heart rate accelerates, your breathing quickens, your palms sweat, your legs stiffen, your hands clench, and your blood rushes from your gut to your heart and lungs (thus the sinking feeling in your stomach when you're afraid). When the threat is past, the parasympathetic branch of the autonomic nervous system kicks in and calms you back to baseline.

But the automatic pilot of the sensory defensives' nervous system is calibrated at a faster speed (breathing, heart rate). Like the fire alarm falsely tripped by boiling water, their nervous system misperceives certain harmless sensations as dangerous. They hit with a bang, and what appears as a trickle in the normal nervous system feels a torrent. Behaving as they were designed, their bodies respond as if their very survival were at stake. In preparation to defend against the primal threat, stress chemicals course through the bloodstream, causing an explosion of discomforting sensations—racing heart, knotted stomach, tight chest—and an outpouring of fear emotions from which the person does not easily recover. In self-protection, they may leave the lunch date early or snap at the waiter, unwittingly reacting out of proportion to the situation but in proportion to a brain that perceives danger.

Living at the mercy of a nervous system ready to spring at the slightest provocation, the sensory defensive are more susceptible to little stressors and conflict. They really *do* sweat the small stuff—buckets full. This constant overreaction to ordinary stressors is exhausting and leaves little for life's real problems.

To protect against the disconcerting assault of overstimulation, they are always on guard, ready to flee or fight the discomfort. Even during sleep, their body may be in a hyperalert state, and their light, restless sleep contributes to their exhaustion. Over time, chronic, unrelenting, and uncontrollable stress locks their body into a hypervigilant self-protective stance, typified by a worried look and rigid posture, and keeps their body flooded with toxic stress hormones that eventually lead to illness.

The more extreme the defensiveness, the more anxiety and stress escalate along with other psychological problems, even in emotionally healthy environments. A sensory-defensive person may feel close to someone but withdraw from his light caress because touch bothers her or she feels repulsed by the scent of his skin. Not surprisingly, research shows anxiety disorders and depression to be a common by-product of sensory defensiveness—a syndrome Patricia Wilbarger named *sensory affective disorder*.[14]

Sufferers know that their overreactivity is not normal, but they don't know why it happens. And though they feel easily overstimulated, they are generally not fully conscious of how this experience influences behavior. Take Marge. Ready to chain her kids to the wall after a day of shopping for school clothes, Marge assumed that she had PMS, or had not had enough sleep, or was in a bad mood or just plain demented. Then she stood in front of the mirror and pulled her hair off the back of her neck. Suddenly she felt a hundred times better. Better able to tolerate the commotion that her kids were making, she stopped screaming, related to them calmly, and redirected their energy.

Having learned about sensory defensiveness, Marge could associate her relief with taking the hair off her neck to result from alleviating tactile defensiveness. But most sufferers are in the dark about why they react with such intensity. Such uncertainty keeps their defensive systems set on high.

If sufferers try to share their experiences, they find that others tend to view their overreactivity as a personality flaw over which they should exert self-control. Despairing friends might advise, "Chill out," or "Don't let stress get to you." Overwrought family members might tell them to "Get over it" or "Stop being so neurotic," reinforcing the sufferer's feelings of being different and misunderstood. Feeling crazy, they deny their feelings and struggle to fit in and appear normal, draining their energy.

Psychologists and medical professionals often misdiagnose the hyper-reactivity, anxiety, and stress as psychological rather than sensory in origin and treat it as such. Says Teresa, hospitalized for depression:

> During group sessions in the hospital, I used to wear leftover fatigues from my brother's army days. The psychiatrist saw this as a defense mechanism, a way of "wearing armor" to keep people away and a denial of femininity. He never quite understood that I wore fatigues because they were so very comfortable and that wearing a dress, which moved around more on my body, made me feel uncomfortable and vulnerable.

Psychological treatment, a mind-over-matter approach, has limited effectiveness in treating defensiveness. The brain makes no distinction between a real or a perceived threat—it just reacts. Thought has no time to influence action. Psychotherapy might help sufferers feel less emotional and better about the self, but sensory terror will continue to dictate what they can do, where they can go, with whom and when. Many defensives will spend years in therapy with little decrease in their hypersensitivity or understanding of its underlying cause. Writes Natalie:

> I've been in behavioral therapy for depression, post-traumatic stress disorder, anxiety, and panic attacks for many years. I have found a lot of help for these problems with my therapist, but I remain jittery. I always felt like these labels didn't fit me entirely, that something else was wrong, but I didn't know what it was. So I chalked it up to being a little crazy inside.

Nor do psychotropic drugs like Prozac appear to make a substantial impact. As they are targeted for specific receptor sites in the nervous system, they boost the neurotransmitter serotonin and sway the emotional brain, improving mood and coping, but they don't directly influence the more primitive "survival" brain.

Few are likely to outgrow sensory defensiveness. Instead, defensives cope by developing strategies to compensate for their symptoms. They wear soft cotton clothing with the labels cut out; they shop at odd hours to avoid crowds; they exercise until they drop to calm raw nerves.

And this is only the beginning. Even when the condition is mild, coping with sensory invasion creates layers of problems that, in unsuspected ways, affect every aspect of life and prevent the person from knowing the full range of human experience. Because they need to carefully orchestrate their environment to escape irritation, the sensory defensive may appear controlling, stubborn, willful, bossy, picky, or' complaining. Wired from stress, they may seem fidgety, agitated, short-tempered, impulsive, impatient, or volatile. Needing to withdraw from stimulation, they may appear preoccupied, unfriendly, or reclusive. Such behavior compromises relationships, as loved ones get caught in the crossfire.

Defensives can be insufferable!

Do they have any choice? Not when they are in response mode. Their behavior is not a reflection of their need to control, manipulate, or drive others crazy but of *the organization of their nervous system at that moment and under those conditions*.[15] Each of us acts in accordance with the information our senses feed us. If we feel overwhelmed, our nervous systems drive us to defend against overstimulation and preserve the self. To grasp this concept requires a paradigm shift from viewing behavior as primarily psychologically motivated to seeing it as an end product of sensory processing.

What ultimately becomes a psychological or mental process begins with a touch, sound, sight, taste, smell, or movement. The brain focuses, screens, sorts, and responds to this sensory information to organize feelings, thoughts, perceptions, and actions. This process is called *sensory integration*: the organization of sensations from out there as well as the sensations from your body that tell you who you are physically, where you are, and what is going on around you so that you can make sense of the world.[16] Sensory integration enables you to interact with the world accurately and efficiently and to learn and remember. It is the critical function of the brain that allows you to recoil at the sensation of an ant crawling on your arm but understand that the other sensation on your arm is your wristwatch and that is to be ignored. Sensory integration allows you to listen to the car radio and distinguish the violin from the other instruments in the orchestra, while tuning out conversation in the back seat of the car.

This organization relies on the modulation of sensation, on the brain's ability to calibrate sensory information, neither inhibiting relevant information and creating boredom nor flooding the system with irrelevant information and creating overload. When sensation is not modulated, perception gets distorted and disorganization ensues. This not only affects learning and memory but ultimately creates psychopathology—essentially the need to go to extremes to balance out the nervous system.

We can no more ignore sensory processing in studying behavior than we can ignore wind direction in studying weather. What sensations we selectively screen out and admit, and how we organize those sensations, determines how we make sense of our world. Sensory processing directly influences emotions, thoughts, the body, and, for some, the spirit and reflects the degree to which we lead a harmonious and meaningful existence: one of joy, engagement, exploration, intimacy, and optimism. If you are happy, calm, and positive—psychologically hardy—you have good nervous system organization, and what you see, hear, smell, and touch makes sense to you: you partake of the feast. If you are emotionally unbalanced, neurotic, or crazed—psychologically vulnerable—you have problems with nervous system organization and you feel easily overexcited or bored: you flee the feast or you focus on little else.

Lifting the cloud of defensiveness typically requires professional help from those trained in treating this condition, generally pediatric occupational therapists. The sufferer will follow a "sensory diet," a term coined by Patricia Wilbarger to indicate the optimum sensorimotor input a person needs to feel alert, exert effortless control, and perform at peak.[17] As the nervous system becomes less vulnerable to the onslaught of sensation, the defensive can evaluate sensation more accurately. If they are better able to make sense of the world, they are better able to manage their emotions and feel freer to be in the world.[18] As they are no longer just swimming against the tide, other treatments, like psychotherapy, can be more effective.

"So you're off to see the wizard," said a friend. Perhaps so. At the start of the new millenium, I left for a one-week intensive treatment in sensory integration at the Ayres Clinic in Torrance, California. Founded by A. Jean Ayres and maintained by her disciples after her death in 1989, the clinic is a teaching center for occupational therapists (OTs) and clients worldwide. At times, miraculous things do seem to happen there.

As I sat on cushions in a room darkened for my comfort and listened to nature sounds on a special CD, using earphones with bone conduction to stimulate balance and equilibrium, the OT sat behind me. She put her hands firmly on my back and, using craniosacral therapy, gently manipulated my spine to open my diaphragm and free my breathing, which she postulated to have been restricted since infancy by colic. This explained why, despite yoga classes, attempts at meditation, and breathing exercises, I continued to breathe in a hurried manner. To deepen my breathing, she gave me a breathing "whistle" and showed me how to invite three-dimensional movement of the diaphragm by placing my hand on my "power spot"—the upper abdomen just below the base of the sternum—or on the sides of my rib cage.

On the first night of treatment, I worked out at the athletic club, first on the weight machines and then walking and sprinting on the treadmill for 45 minutes. Amazing! I wasn't sprawled out on the couch. And I didn't feel noticeably bothered by the bright lights, the ongoing chatter, the close, sweaty bodies, or the clanking weights of the body builders.

This profound reduction in defensiveness in one short day was more than a result of treatment. I had spent a lifetime feeling overly excited, disorganized, different, and misunderstood. I felt like a lone violin playing out of tune. I assumed my crazy feelings resulted from anxiety, as did everyone else. At last I could speak openly about issues that went beyond the psyche—disorientation, confusion, the inability to make sense of what was in front of me. The therapist calmly listened and matter-of-factly explained my symptoms. Compounding my sensory defensiveness were other sensory issues that had never been incorporated in any diagnosis of my behavior: visual-spatial processing problems that explained why I didn't "see" and make sense of my world; problems with bilateral integration of the hemispheres of my brain that, together with the visual-spatial problems, greatly affected my spatial map. For instance, even after years of dance training, it always took enormous effort to translate the teacher's steps into my brain and out through my limbs, and I always lagged behind the class. For the first time, everything made sense.

What made me this way? My hunch is something untoward happened during a long birth. I emerged high-strung with a few crossed wires into a family of sensation seekers who, rather than calm me down, jazzed me up further, as they did what they could to satisfy their need for *excitement*. My overriding need for calm was rarely met. Head trauma at forty, from a fall down a flight of stairs, and changing hormones greatly exaggerated my defensiveness as I aged.

After a week of treatment, I was sent home with my "sensory diet." Daily, I brushed my skin at specific intervals. I listened to special CDs to reduce auditory and movement defensiveness and to better integrate sensory processing. I walked in water or danced freely to music to increase body awareness. I did breathing exercises and took yoga. Throughout the week, I jumped on a trampoline, bounced on an exercise ball, swung from a hanging hammock, and did exercises for bilateral integration and visual-spatial processing.

A week and a half later, I felt a calm that I had never known. I was breathing with ease, my whole diaphragm expanding. I walked to the supermarket and felt my body grounded, firm, and solid, my feet pushing off terra firma and my arms swinging freely. I saw the world anew. A few days later, I realized that I had spent the whole morning writing, largely unaware of the trees being cut down outside my window!

While teaching my class in child development, I noticed a different sense of being in the world. I no longer saw my students as a mass but as individuals. Rather than having to focus on reducing anxiety, I could concentrate on the material, choose my words, and hear and answer their questions. Teaching had long been drudgery and I counted the minutes until I could escape. For the first time, I knew its delights.

Of course, as stress increased, I still would go into meltdown. The nervous system does not transform itself overnight. With consistent treatment, it would take at least nine months to reorganize. But with a new perspective and my feelings validated, I felt less alone and strange. And now that I had the tools to ameliorate the defensiveness, which later on included more craniosacral work, neurocranial restructuring, and syntonic light therapy, I felt I could better take charge of the defensiveness.

Two years later, the cloud of defensiveness has lifted. My baseline arousal feels more in the normal range, and I don't go as easily into overload. My relationships with family and friends have greatly improved. The defensiveness is not gone but as long as I nourish my nervous system before it gets depleted, it's more manageable. When I start to feel scrambled, I tell myself "I'm not going there," and my mind generally obeys. If I do go over the edge, I know how to fix it. That's power! And I have written this book to empower you.

Part 1 describes the symptoms of sensory defensiveness, its origins, causes, levels of severity, and impact on daily functioning. Part 2 talks about how the stress and anxiety that result from sensory defensiveness unleashes and intensifies social, emotional, and physical problems. Part 3 outlines the different ingredients that go into a sensory diet, easing your nervous system out of a chronic stress mode and resetting it closer to a normal comfort zone. Part 4 discusses how to overcome potential treatment obstacles, such as poor nutrition, improper breathing, and incorrect posture, and the power of mind-body healing for relaxation and uprooting emotional trauma.

There is a disclaimer. Though this book will guide you in setting up a sensory diet, if you want to truly savor the taste of normality, an occupational therapist should evaluate you, figure out your specific needs, even if you are only mildly defensive, and carefully monitor your success. Evaluation and proper treatment require very sophisticated information about sensory integration theory and practice: for proper treatment, you must identify the cause of the defensiveness. As A. Jean Ayres pointed out, therapy is not just adding sensation: "The brain must be able to process the sensation so that the integrative mechanisms can develop and function."[19] If you only self-treat, your activity dosage or timing might be off, just as it would be if you took the wrong dose of a psychotropic drug like Prozac. Case in point. Without consulting my therapist, I decided to combine listening therapy with light therapy. Unknowingly, I chose a therapeutic nature CD that encourages one to close the eyes in order to reap its full benefits. Keeping my eyes open and staring at colored light caused stress, but I attributed this to special problems I have with my eyes from head trauma, and persevered, though I was not experiencing effects. It wasn't until I switched to a therapeutic Mozart CD, and my eyes more easily focused on the light, and afterward I felt a pronounced calm, that I realized my mistake. This book should be used as a backup.

Blessed are those who experience a rich sensory life and live within the comfort zone without effort. For the sensory defensive, it takes work. Fortunately, it's never too late to start. The rewards are beyond measure: You will feel safer in the world.

Begin your journey of self-discovery with hope.

Part One

Living Outside the Comfort Zone

To be thus is nothing;
But to be safely thus.

MACBETH V:3,
WILLIAM SHAKESPEARE

1

Senses on the Defense

I do not much like being touched and I have always to make a
slight effort not to draw away when someone links his arms in
mine.

—SOMERSET MAUGHAM, ENGLISH NOVELIST

Sleeping in a bed makes Emir feel lost in space. So he sleeps on his living
room couch, his back against the hard surface and his legs pushed up
against the raised end. He thrives on heat and eschews air-conditioning for
the breeze of the open window and a ceiling fan. Since most clothes make
him squirm, he wears as few as possible. His car radio blasts with hard
rock, but he cringes at the sound of someone chewing their food in a quiet
room. When he's outside, the sun blinds him, and he must wear sunglasses
or he gets a headache. Inside, lights must be dim. At night, he illuminates
his house mostly with eucalyptus- or jasmine-scented candles, scents that
relax him.

In the summer, Shannon sleeps with the air-conditioning set at 60
degrees and weighs herself down with three heavy blankets, which make
her feel held; otherwise she wriggles about and can't sleep. Rock music
puts her on edge, and she tunes to the classical station in her car. She likes

dim or bright light; anything in between seems dull and annoying. She delights and indulges in musky perfumes and light flower scents, which permeate her apartment. In the morning and before going to bed, she saturates her skin with fruity body lotions, like strawberry or peach. If not, her skin feels too rough, and she dislikes touching her own flesh.

Each sensory-defensive person has a unique set of sensory foes and comforts. People can show symptoms of tactile, oral, movement, visual, and auditory defensiveness or unusual sensitivities to taste or smell.[1] (For a detailed list of symptoms, see Appendix B.) One sense might be particularly involved, or hypersensitivity might reflect all the senses. In addition, a person may hyperreact to one sense, such as smell, but underreact to another, such as movement.

Touch: Too Close for Comfort

A wife, mother, and computer programmer, Madeline is a small woman with striking blue eyes, pale skin, and a nervousness that shows in rapid speech, tapping fingers, and a shaking leg. Introverted and intense, she keeps to herself but becomes friendly when others take the initiative. She seems perfectly normal—until someone gets too close.

Madeline doesn't like to be touched. When her sister greets her with a light kiss on the cheek, a shiver goes through Madeline, and she wipes the spot, much to her sister's dismay. When people touch her, Madeline feels like wiping, scratching, or squeezing the spot. In fact, sometimes when she touches *herself* lightly, she has to rub the spot. She can't help it—touch bothers her terribly.

Madeline is tactile-defensive, the hallmark of sensory defensiveness. Growing up, she often writhed when her father or mother hugged or kissed her, though both were caring and loving. Today when she hugs her 3-year-old daughter, it can feel like an obligation and she frequently draws back from her husband's unexpected love tap. When he crushes his powerful body into hers, she feels at once comforted and trapped. When she must hug friends or relatives, she squeezes hard enough so that she doesn't have to feel the other person touching her.

It pains her to be so touchy and makes her feel unable to satisfy her family's need for intimacy. She worries that her family might think that she doesn't love them, as her parents and sister used to feel when she denied their affection. Yet she loves them deeply and craves their hugs—but on her own terms.

About 18 square feet and weighing in at about 8 pounds, the skin is our boundary between self and world, and a constant source of information about our environment. It is studded with about 5 million tiny nerve endings, or touch receptors, generally larger than those associated with other senses and exquisitely sensitive: our brain registers touch at the slightest pressure.

The top layer, the epidermis, is tough and horny and replaces itself every 28 days, as dead skin cells flake off. The next two levels, the dermis, contain the nerves that set off the defensive reaction, along with blood vessels, glands, and the fibroplastic connective tissue that gives the skin its ability to spring back and retain its shape after a touch.

Touch receptors convey information about pressure, vibration, texture, heat or cold, and pain. Most people process these sensations normally and feel comfortable within their skin, largely unaware of clothes or another person touching their body and other skin sensations.[2] When touched lovingly, their body expands with pleasurable excitement, and they reach out to make contact with their world. They tolerate temperature changes and a normal amount of pain.

The brain of the tactile defensive registers some or all of these tactile sensations as unpleasant or threatening. Clothes feel coarse and pores start to itch; fashion choices are dictated by feel. "I base most of my fashion taste on what doesn't itch," the late comedian Gilda Radner quipped. The touch of others can prickle and elicit alarm even from the person they love the most, and especially when uninvited. The body shrinks away.

Unable to set their internal thermometer at a comfort zone, some feel hot all the time even in cold weather or cold all the time even when it is warm. Heaven is a hot towel out of the dryer. Quick temperature changes—for example, going from the warm bath into the cold air—throw them. As their nervous system is on high alert and blood leaves the extremities to deliver oxygen to internal organs and muscles, many suffer poor circulation and their hands and feet are always cold. Cold hands and feet might be one reason why the defensive have problems falling asleep. Research at the Psychiatric University Clinic in Basel, Switzerland, found that warm extremities, a sign of dilated blood vessels and healthy blood flow, were linked to falling asleep quickly. Booties, anyone?

Yet warm weather has its own perils as heat and humidity make the defensive feel sticky and clammy; tactile defensiveness increases along with the need for distance from others to cool off. (Moisture also increases sense of smell. When it rains, the low barometric pressure makes fluid spread even faster, and the defensive pick up odors that much more quickly.) Finding the right temperature balance is an endless struggle.

Pain can feel unusually intense. Some will get hysterical from a paper cut or faint from a needle drawing blood. Even the very thin needles used in acupuncture can be nerve-jangling. Certain parts of the body can be extremely sensitive—a minor injury on the foot may feel like a major blow.

Though each person describes unique areas of body sensitivity, different parts of the body are generally more sensitive than other parts and more likely to elicit a defensive response. The hands, dense with receptors for light touch, are more sensitive than the back; anything that feels gritty, sticky, slimy, slippery, gummy, greasy, prickly, or rough gives defensives the heebie-jeebies, and they wash their hands frequently. The fingertips, with 700 touch receptors for every 2 millimeters of skin, are more sensitive than the palm, but nothing like the face and especially the exquisitely sensitive lips. Skim your arm with the palm of your hand and then with your fingertips, and you will feel the difference in sensitivity. Do the same across your cheek and then your lips, and the sensitivity catapults. The area in the brain involved with the lips or the fingertips fills as much space as the area involved with the entire trunk of the body, far less sensitive to touch. Little wonder that many defensives find kissing to feel feathery and unpleasant.

Some parts of the body, like the bottoms of the feet, are ticklish, but they have fewer cold receptors than the tip of our nose or fingers. Other areas of the skin respond more when we itch, shiver, or get gooseflesh. Generally, the hairiest parts of the body are the most sensitive to pressure, as there are many sense receptors at the base of each hair follicle and a nerve ending senses movement. It only takes something pressing or tugging against one hair, or even the skin around it, for the hair to vibrate and spark a nerve. And the skin is thinnest where there's hair. In this way, displacing hair warns us of danger, like a piece of dirt alighting on our eyelash or a stranger breathing on our neck. It is primarily the light touch of hair displacement that causes the defensive response: If light and rough, the touch scratches; if light and feathery, it tickles. Deep pressure or firm touch reaches deeper levels of the derma, decreasing arousal and making us feel grounded and calm.

To understand the difference between light touch and deep pressure, squeeze the back of your hand. Now take your finger and very lightly catch a few hair cells. The light touch is more intense. If you are scratching, you have some degree of tactile defensiveness.

Timing, interval, tempo, duration, and quality of sensation also determine intensity of touch.[3] Slow touch as a rule soothes, while fast touch excites. Continuous and steady touch calms, while intermittent or vibratory touch arouses. (The skin is able to pick up a break of about ten-thousandths of a second in a steady mechanical pressure or tactile buzz, which is why the tiniest ant crawling along our arm bothers us.[4]) Touch of short duration excites, while prolonged touch calms. Rhythmic touch comforts, while arrhythmic touch stimulates. The quality of the sensation—silky or gritty, dry or wet—changes perception, as does the part of the body touched—e.g., the back or more sensitive neck.

Context matters. Relationship between the persons involved is crucial—

lovers, strangers—as is the situation in which the touch occurs—at home, in a crowd.[5] Control is another variable—is the touch a surprise or expected, is one touching or being touched? If a person initiates when, where, and how long the touch is, it's more easy to tolerate. One defensive woman would draw back if her baby touched her, but she could hug her baby all day. Also important is the person's current level of arousal—drowsy, in overload.

Imagine the ramifications of tactile defensiveness. Rather than being calmed by a cuddle or gentle stroke across the brow, a tactile-defensive infant may become more agitated. Rather than melting from a loved one's tender caress, a tactile-defensive spouse may tense up.

Body language speaks volumes. Somerset Maugham, the English novelist, hated to be touched and would greet his guests, "coming forward with arms outstretched in welcome, then dropping them to his sides to avoid contact."[6] These gestures represented his powerful need for human contact and also his terror of being touched. Even the anticipation of being touched can evoke a flight, fight, or freeze response, and the body begins to cave inward in self-protection.

To alleviate discomfort, some people rub and scratch at their skin until it reddens and even bleeds. For the severely tactile defensive, the skin feels like a pincushion. Touch can be perceived as pain and they may scream—recall Dustin Hoffman's autistic character in *Rain Man*. These people feel constantly vulnerable and imprisoned in their skin.

Touchy Mouth

For Manuel, eating a banana feels like eating mush and eating coconut or tuna is like eating hay. Gumbo soup feels slimy, like a raw egg. As for oysters, "God, if I even *watch* someone eat an oyster, I cringe with disgust." Manuel won't eat or drink anything too hot.

In some, tactile defensiveness extends to the mouth and certain food textures or temperatures irritate, as do some taste sensations, and the person gags easily. These picky eaters have long lists of food fetishes. Some seek crunchy food, like chips, or chewy food, like licorice, or squishy foods, like ripe bananas. Others feel repulsed by these textures. Some oral defensives need intense taste and pour on the salt, pepper, and chili sauce, while others find spicy foods irritating and need blander tastes.

Many dislike brushing or flossing their teeth or going to the dentist and will request novocaine, even when it's unnecessary. It's less the pain than the sensation of something in their mouth—the instruments, the dentist's finger, or the vibration of the drill.[7] One woman described it as feeling like her teeth had the "chills." Kissing may tickle unpleasantly.

Does any of this touchiness seem familiar to you? If so, chances are that you also feel out of balance: the senses of touch and movement form a close partnership.

LACKING TERRA FIRMA

Peggy remembers well her first roller coaster ride at age 13. It was a moment of sheer terror. Forty years later, she feels similar vertigo (dizziness, faintness, or lightheadedness that results from an impaired sense of balance and equilibrium) and anxiety going up and down escalators or walking down stairs. Yet she doesn't mind taking an elevator or traveling by air.

Her balance and equilibrium are off and she feels thrown when her head is tipped forward or backward. In an elevator her head stays level, so she feels fine. This sensation probably existed before her roller coaster ride and reflects less a learned fear than basic instability in her physical sense of space. Though she's probably unaware of its impact on her functioning, this primal fear creates insecurity in all aspects of her life.

We lose balance and orientation unless we know at every moment the relationship of our body to gravity and the physical world, our "place in space." A fog that created spatial disorganization and rendered John F. Kennedy Jr. unable to distinguish the black ocean from the black night sky is the hypothesized cause for his fatal air crash.

The vestibular system, the body's gyroscope, is located in the inner ear.

Inside three fluid-filled semicircular canals—one for side-to-side balance, one for up-and-down balance, and the third for back-and-forth balance—are minute calcium carbonate crystals ("rocks in your head") called otoliths. These otoliths press upon tiny hairlike filaments, called cilia, that line the inner membranes. Gravity acts on the otoliths so that they shift in response to head movements and the rocks "fall down." This bends the cilia, which, in turn, transmit signals to the brain. The brain then uses these signals to calculate the positioning of the head and, as we move it, to adjust our body to changes in gravity and body position. In this way, we know if we are moving or still, if we're going too fast and need to slow down, if we are moving forward, backward, or sideways, or if we're going to fall.

If the vestibular system functions poorly, people feel unsteady on their feet. Children will feel vulnerable when their feet leave the ground. If moved rapidly, spun, tossed in the air, or turned upside down, infants with gravitational insecurity will stiffen, arch back, and may start to cry. When they are picked up or put down, the sudden change from vertical to horizontal or vice versa can create terror. If the parent's movements are tentative or jerky, the infant may associate being handled and moved about with a feeling of dread, thus increasing tactile defensiveness.

These children grow up tending to dislike somersaults, slides, and monkey bars. Swings or roller coasters may create an unpleasant, frightening surge in the gut and such children scream in terror when riding the ferris wheel or become sick when riding in a car, because the inner ear connects to the gut through the vagus cranial nerve. They may feel unsteady and worry about falling on uneven terrain, such as stairs or curbs. Though no real peril exists, they grow up being afraid of heights, driving over bridges, and riding on elevators or escalators. Could movement defensiveness relate to nausea during pregnancy? In some cases, it may very well. During pregnancy sensory-defensive Teresita felt nauseated every time she moved. "I vomited the whole nine months."

Disordered or weak vestibular functioning can interfere with performing simple tasks that most of us take for granted. If moving back and forth or bending gets a person off balance and dizzy, caring for a young child can be disorienting. Housekeeping can be a challenge, as Sarah describes.

> I tend to avoid doing the kids' sheets and comforters. It's the stretching, getting off balance, leaning. I have a lot of vestibular issues, and I hate putting the sheets back on, because their beds are against the wall, and I have to lean way over.

Bending forward or backward over a sink to have their hair washed can create dizziness, and some defensives will avoid getting shampooed in a beauty shop. For Daphne, a shower is a shaky enterprise.

> I feel so out of sorts in the shower. I can't wash my face because I think I'll fall over if I do. And shaving my legs? Forget it!

Even sleep has its perils, says Susan.

> My husband and I used to have a soft bed that would bounce every time he rolled over or moved a leg. I couldn't stand it and would scream at him about an hour into the night. I would wake up every time he moved!

While those with an overactive vestibular system tend to avoid movement and dislike physical activity, those with an underactive vestibular system feel propelled to move. Some children rock and spin themselves, and train their caregivers to keep them in perpetual motion—to rock them, toss them in the air, swing them around. Many of these children look hyperactive, and some actually are. Sitting in a chair in school gives them the jitters. Bill Gates is well known for rocking back and forth while he works or talks to people, and he uses a home trampoline for extra up-and-down movement.

A person may seek one kind of vestibular sensation but avoid others. Batya adores the feeling of "flying" on a roller coaster and will happily go for fifteen rides in one day, but she gets disoriented and nauseated from spinning rides.

STOP THE NOISE

When the fire alarm went off in Tanya's kitchen, she didn't like the sound but tolerated it as she turned on the fan and opened the door to dissipate the smoke. Hands covering his ears, her husband ran outside until the alarm stopped.

All of us are surrounded by sound. At home, we might hear a fan, a ticking clock, the TV or stereo in another room, a door slamming, kids yelling, neighbors talking, outside traffic. Those with a modulated nervous system will tune out most of these sounds and remain only peripherally aware of them, or not at all. But the nervous system of the sensory defensive arouses easily to sound, especially if loud or sudden. And then the noise doesn't quit. "I neglect God and his angels for the noise of a fly, for the rattling of a coach, for the whining of a door," lamented English poet John Donne. Some react to routine noise with a whole-body startle rarely seen past infancy.

Located in the middle ear is the stapedius muscle. When sounds get too loud, it clamps down to dampen them and protects the ear. This is called the acoustic sound reflex.[8] As we speak, the stapedius clamps down to protect us from the sound of our own voice. But in flight, fight, or freeze, we need to take in all sound and the stapedius loses the ability to contract. Consequently, the constantly alarmed sensory defensives are alert to and get distracted by all sounds. Ambient repetitious sounds, like the humming from a fan or a tapping pen, catch their attention and they can't concentrate on anything but the noise. Normal noise levels can interfere with hearing conversation or concentrating; while on the phone, the defensive may snap at their spouses for the slightest movement. They may not eat certain foods, like celery, for the noise, or lose it upon hearing such sounds as running water or someone's footsteps on a carpet, for instance.

Low, deep sounds below middle C alert us to potential danger, like a thundering herd. For the auditory defensives, a low-pitched vacuum cleaner becomes a howling wind. Firecrackers on the Fourth of July become the thunder's whip. High-pitched sounds above middle C, like a siren or a fingernail scraping the blackboard, become an alarming scream. And though the human voice is more in the middle range of the scale, some auditory defensives find the human voice grating, especially if it rises in pitch and loudness. They might accuse their spouses of speaking harshly or yelling at them, when they're not.

The movement receptors are in the inner ear and responsive to vibration. As auditory defensives lay their heads down to sleep, they hear an internal "thump, thump" from the vibrations of motors of household appliances or passing trucks. Pummeling their ears with unbearable pressure, the pounding throbs against their bones and reverberates throughout their bodies, throwing off body rhythms and disturbing their sleep. They feel every quiver as an assault. Rebecca feels any electrical power on her body.

> Both my son and I can tell when the electricity goes off. I feel
> like a weight has been lifted. I can breathe again and perk up.
> This is why I like to be out in the middle of the woods. When
> the power comes back on, I feel it as a vibration. Some trans-
> formers on light poles leak energy, and I feel uncomfortable
> standing beneath them. I know when the TV is on, even if the
> sound is off because unless the TV is unplugged, there is still
> power surging.

After delivering a lecture at a hotel in Los Angeles next to the airport, Don Campbell, author of *The Mozart Effect*, felt exhausted and severe pain in his back. He knew he was stressed out from the jets taking off and from the "neon lights and air-conditioning noise, which contributed to mild, negatively charged energy." But he felt something else had to account for his pain. The next day he found "five industrial-size clothes dryers turning and humming. Although I could not 'hear' them, my body could feel their powerful vibrations."[9]

The human body consists of about 70 percent water and our bones are great conductors of vibration. The lower the sound, the more our joints and bones pick up the vibration. As sound is made up of air pressure waves that hit our bodies, we literally "feel" sound. Once a part of the body vibrates, the blood cells carry this resonance to the whole body very quickly. This is why the bass vibrations from a car radio can feel like giant fists pounding our chest and throw the body into turmoil. "It's like having a swarm of bees in my abdomen," described one sensory-defensive person. The experience sometimes evokes such a strong flight-or-fight response that normally cautious drivers will recklessly weave in and out of lanes to escape. Fortunately, some states, such as Delaware, have a noise code that prohibits drivers from blasting their bass. But the ticketing officer must speak loudly—many hard rock fans have lost some of their hearing!

Do You Hear What I Hear?

Sensory defensives often hear sounds before others, and even some sounds that others don't hear at all. As a child Barbra Streisand heard clicks and buzzing in her ears that evolved into a high-pitched, high-range noise, creating auditory defensiveness. She never heard silence. An ear exam revealed "supersonic hearing." As the fidelity was poor and as she concentrated on the defects, she seldom played the radio. She felt different, totally abnormal, and kept her hearing sensitivity a secret.

Not surprisingly, musicians have reacted defensively to unpleasant sound throughout history, most likely because of their extraordinary ability to discriminate sounds at high or low frequencies. Loud sounds made the infant Mozart sick. Handel refused to enter a concert hall until after the instruments had been tuned, and Bach would fly into a rage when he heard wrong notes.

Some sufferers hear the Taos hum, a low-pitched humming sound that people have reported around the world, from the marine base in El Toro, California, to Worlington in England. One person described it as sounding like the Goodyear blimp at a distance. Many who hear it also feel a certain rumble or vibration in their body. For some it stays the same loudness and pitch, while others complain of it increasing in pitch, sound level, or frequency.

People roam around their house, inside and out, to find its origin. Some of the suspects are electricity pylons, water mains, underground waterways and water pumps, generators, fans, transformers, microwaves and electromagnetic fields set up around radio or TV transmitters, though as yet no cause has been firmly identified.

Gathered in the same place, some hear the hum, some don't. Apparently certain people may have an extension of the normal spectrum of hearing that leans toward the lower frequencies, and they pick up noise that appears to go beyond the norm. Some hear it, get used to it, and tune it out, while the defensive find it incessant and maddening.

The hearing of certain autistic people is so acute it's almost impossible for them to live in modern society. Falling snow can sound as shattering as breaking glass! Occupational therapist Sheila Frick tells of how one autistic 2½-year-old, while riding in a car with his parents, started to scream when the road switched from asphalt to concrete.[10] The change in the friction grooves made the tires sound higher-pitched and intolerable to his ears.

CAUGHT IN THE GLARE

To most, the more light the better. The opposite is true for Shakir. Bright light makes him feel as if he can't breathe. At night he covers his car mirror with his hands so the light reflects less brightly, and he avoids lit-up places like gas stations or places where neon lights scream at his eyes. During the day he closes the blinds in his house to block the outside light and always wears a baseball cap outside to block the sun (the pressure of sunglasses sets off tactile defensiveness). Even when it rains, the outside light is too bright and he must have his visor down.

Like Shakir, many sensory defensives suffer from visual defensiveness, or photophobia, and find bright light painfully glaring. Shakir is brown-eyed, but blue-eyed people are probably more likely to be visually defensive, as blue eyes have less pigment than brown eyes and are more light-sensitive. Developmental psychologist Jerome Kagan of Harvard University found that more inhibited, fearful children had blue eyes, while more uninhibited, bold children had brown eyes.[11]

Bright light is not the only problem for the visually defensive. Any object moving close to the face can be distracting: the car visor, a baby's fingers, a dog's licking tongue, or overhanging branches. Flickering movements on the TV or some computer monitors can be maddening. Light-dark contrast between the bright picture screen and the dark all around can feel like being in a tunnel. Some defensives will avoid dark movie theaters and keep a light on while watching TV.

Busy visual fields, densely packed with images, high visual contrasts, shadows, or sudden movements can make shopping a nightmare. Scanning contents of the supermarket or a large department store feels confusing and disorienting. The visually defensive need mental blinders to tease out figure from background. In malls, crowds, fairs, or any place packed with activity and images, either static or moving, the world can seem like a haze and create acute discomfort. One art lover who visited small art galleries throughout the French countryside with great pleasure longed to get to Paris to tramp through the Louvre. But when she got there, she stood outside frozen. The thought of trekking through the mammoth block-long structure made her head spin. Visual clutter in the classroom and children in perpetual motion easily overstimulate defensive children who keep looking around, unable to focus their attention.

Some avoid the visual cliff, which is anything that goes down: stairways, escalators, balconies.[12] There are those who won't go to a theater or athletic performance if they can't sit on the first level. If they do go, they are unlikely to gaze easily into their companion's eyes. Eye contact easily overstimulates, and creates enormous social problems for the sensory defensive, who will look away to reduce the tension. This defensive reaction can be easily misconstrued as disinterest or rejection. In primates, prolonged staring might elicit aggression or fear. Few cultures find it socially acceptable to stare into another's eyes.

SNIFFING DANGER

At the dentist, Josephine would rather tolerate pain than the odor of anesthesia, and if a place reeks of cigarette smoke, she bolts. She can smell a dirty dishrag from the next room that her husband can't smell next to him. While taking the Métro in Paris one summer, she felt her head reel and began to feel nauseated from body odors. To her husband's annoyance, she demanded they get off at the next stop.

The nose can detect up to 10,000 different odors. Naturally, most people have odors that bother them, like cigarette smoke or a particular perfume. But being sensitive to an odor is different from responding defensively, as if it were a threat. Defensives react to more odors and with greater revulsion than others and detect faint, fleeting odors unnoticed by others. As Mandy describes:

> While visiting my mother, I kept asking if there was a candle
> lit because I smelled something burning. My husband, mother,
> and aunt smelled nothing unusual. I kept asking for about ten
> minutes and then finally had to search out the odor. I found a
> small fire in their laundry room, which we were able to extin-
> guish with a hose.

Even the subtle natural skin odors that mark a person and go unnoticed by most will disturb them and deter a friendship, a partnership, a love affair. Some sensory-defensives are sniffers and wrinkle up their noses at stale-dated milk or cheese or the sheets in the hotel room. Many are sensitive to chemicals, and their head will spin from the smell of detergents and cleaning fluids.

Such sensitivity cannot be tuned out. And though the defensive's sensitivity may be handicapping in today's world of chemical scents, smell remains a more important suvival sense than most realize: all are profoundly affected by the odors that surround us.

Each day, as we inhale and exhale nearly 20,000 breaths of life-sustaining air, we bathe our nostrils in a stream of scent-laden molecules that affect body and psyche. Guided by smell, a newborn placed on its mother's belly will crawl to her breast and begin to suckle.[13] If one nipple is washed with soap to mask the mother's natural odor, the newborn will crawl to the other breast.[14] An article of clothing imbued with the mother's natural body odor will help comfort a 1-month-old to sleep. Likewise, many of us have slumbered through the night wearing our absent lover's unwashed T-shirt.

Pheromones, biochemical molecules excreted in our sweat but undetectable to the nose, may play an essential role in sexual attraction. If you don't like the other's natural odor, no amount of perfume or aftershave will change that.

How can we begin to fathom why the sensory defensive so overreact to odors, touch, noise, lights, movement? Exploring how the normal brain integrates the sensations from the environment and from the body, and how that process gets distorted in the sensory defensive, provides insight.

2

Sensory Processing: The Touchy Nervous System

> We need above all to know about changes; no one wants or
> needs to be reminded 16 hours a day that his shoes are on.
>
> —DAVID HUBEL, NEUROSCIENTIST

David Hubel, meet the sensory defensive.

Why *would* a normal, healthy person pay attention to how the shoes on his feet feel? To find out, let's look at how the brain processes sensory information and how that processing differs in the sensory defensive. Traversing the brain can seem a bit complicated, but it will provide a road map for the rest of the journey.

SENSORY INTEGRATION

Inside our head lies a silent mystery: the human brain. Outside awaits an ocean of colors, shapes, sounds, scents, heat, cold, pressures, aches, and pains. Our bodies are constantly submerged in this ocean of sensation and our sensory antennas are extraordinarily sensitive. Standing on top of a mountain on a clear, black night you could see a candle flame atop another mountain 30 miles away. In a silent room, you can hear a watch ticking 20 feet away and smell a single drop of perfume three rooms away.[1] And on your arm, you feel the tiniest ant crawling.

How do these sensations get inside our head? Objects emit and reflect energy that our sense receptors pick up and our brains organize and try to make sense of.

The raw data (the input) is registered when the brain detects change: "I have been touched." Next, we orient our attention to the input: "Someone touched my shoulder." Our brain then integrates input across sensory modalities, and interprets it by scanning memory for prior sensory and motor experience, and by assigning emotions and meaning (the process). "This is a stranger whose intentions I don't know. The feel of his hand gives me the creeps and his aftershave is making me sick." Or, "The feel of his hands gives me a thrill, and I love the way he smells." We then organize our thoughts and emotions and ignore or act upon and execute the response (the output): We glare at him and step back to get away, or we inch closer with an impish smile. From that learning and memory, our brain initiates new actions, making our brain a self-organizing and self-perpetuating system.[2] In this way, sensory integration provides a crucial foundation for and greatly influences later, more complex learning and behavior.

As the brain attends, integrates, interprets, and organizes interesting sight, sound, smell, touch, taste, and movement sensations, neurons busily reach out to connect with one another and the brain bursts with activity. This steady stream of receiving and integrating sensation, especially from the body (from our movements; internal sensations) takes up 80 percent of the nervous system. Keeping us actively focused on the world, it gives us the means and energy to direct our body and mind adaptively and meaningfully and to work up to speed.[3]

That learning begins with sensory processing has not been the conventional view taken in psychology, which sees learning as a higher cognitive process in which hearing and vision are primary. But this view is changing, at least in the field of neuropsychology. Explaining how we process music,

Norman M. Weinberger, professor of neurobiology and behavior at the University of California at Irvine, notes:

> Neurons learn to prioritize some sounds. When a tone becomes important—because it signals food, for instance—the cells' response to that tone increases. This finding revolutionized thinking about brain organization by showing that learning is not a "higher" brain function but rather one that occurs in the sensory systems themselves.[4]

SENSES NEAR AND FAR

What is sensation? Most think of only the five senses: touch, vision, hearing, smell, and taste. These senses are sometimes called the "far," or distal, senses: they inform us of sensations coming from outside our bodies.

Yet they are bit players compared to the "near," or proximal, senses. Laid down before hearing and vision by evolution and by embryonic development, the tactile, vestibular, and proprioceptive senses inform us about what is happening inside our own bodies and allow us to examine the world up close: to interpret what our distance receptors perceive. For instance, if you see a person off in the distance, you know that it is not a tiny person. Your own experience of moving through space has taught you that people look small when they are farther away from you.

Tactile Sense

Including light touch, deep touch, vibration, pain, hot and cold, the tactile sense is both a far sense, as when we actively touch and reach out to the world, and a near sense, as when we are passively touched. To understand the difference, close your eyes and poke your finger into the palm of your hand. You feel touching, pressure, and some sharpness from your nail—the sensations of your own body—but can't describe your finger. Now grasp your finger and you can experience its shape, warmth, texture—you can discriminate what's "out there."

As the first sense to develop in the embryo, touch organizes other senses and is essential for the proper balance of the nervous system. A few weeks after conception, the human embryo consists of three layers of cells. The outer layer develops into the nervous system and skin, and by 6 weeks of age, the embryo experiences touch and vibrations. As both our nervous system and our skin come from the same origin, touch sensation flows throughout the entire nervous system and influences every neural process to some extent. If we feel "touchy," our whole nervous system is out of whack and affects other sensory systems as well: when you get a mosquito bite, chapped lips, or a hangnail, you feel on edge and the world gets louder and brighter. The discomfort occupies your thoughts, and it takes time and energy to cope and regroup. The defensive person may feel this way over seams in their socks, elastic around their waist, or the hem of their skirt touching the leg "all day long," sapping their energy and leaving them ill tempered and exhausted. "The skin should be thought of as our external nervous system," asserts Ashley Montagu in his landmark book *Touching: The Human Significance of the Skin*, "an organ system which from its earliest differentiation remains in intimate association with the central nervous system."[5]

How well we integrate other sensations relies on these first touch experiences and how our brain processes them: calming or upsetting, pleasant or unpleasant. The nature of these first touches has extreme importance for later development. Each touch nurtures psychological growth; stimulates physical and mental growth; impacts physiological functions like breathing, heart rate, and digestion; enhances self-concept, body awareness, and sexual identity; boosts the immune system; and enhances the grace and stability of movement.

In fact, touch is literally a baby's lifeline because touch releases growth hormone. Institutionalized infants at the turn of the century received little affection. As a result many died of marasmus, from a Greek word meaning "wasting away," without apparent medical cause. Today, in understaffed Romanian orphanages, some touch-deprived children achieve only half the normal height for their age.

The touching we encounter throughout life reinforces and continually affects how we perceive ourselves and the world. When warmly touching another, we feel in touch with ourselves. When uncomfortable with human contact, we feel a poor connection to self.

Vestibular Sense

Orchestrating balance, movement, and rhythm, the vestibular sense in the inner ear is intimately intertwined with the brain circuitry of the other senses, especially sight, hearing, and touch, and serves as a reference through which all stimuli get processed. Sensory neurons carry messages about sound, sight, touch, smell, or taste into our brain, and motor neurons deliver action: we squirm, sniff, turn our head, swallow our food. All this happens against the force of gravity.

The vestibular nuclei starts to develop nine weeks after conception and begin to function by the tenth or eleventh week; by the fifth month in utero they are well developed. As the mother walks, bends, twists, turns, she stimulates her fetus's vestibular system. When the mother's not moving, the fetus appears to seek out movement. During the day as mother moves around and the fetus gets jostled, it is relatively quiet. But at night when mother rests, the fetus gets more active, as if it needs to create its own movement and vestibular input.[6]

Movement becomes a language of the brain. Babies are quieted by rocking (as is the person rocking). On oscillating waterbeds that simulate gentle movement at an adult breathing rate, premature babies are less jumpy and more alert, and they sleep and breathe better.[7] To get children to direct their eyes toward a target and move in a coordinated manner, occupational therapists have them swing or twirl while doing an activity like throwing a beanbag into a hole. In one study of infants given supplemental vestibular motion, one 3-month old twin was part of the experimental group, while the other served as the control. Though both had started out with identical pretest scores, at 4 months of age the infant given the added stimulation had mastered head control and could sit independently, while the other twin was just starting to develop head control.[8]

If deprived of normal rocking and bouncing, infants may suffer effects as damaging as touch deprivation. In Harry Harlow's famous experiments with rhesus monkeys, baby monkeys were removed from their mothers and given a terrycloth mother for contact comfort and a wire mother with a bottle for feeding. As adults, the monkeys displayed abnormal behaviors, such as self-clasping and self-rocking. Another experiment compared a stationary terrycloth mother to one who rocked for 9 to 10 hours a day. None of the ten monkeys that were raised on the moving mother self-rocked, while all but one of the ten that were raised on the stationary mother did.[9]

Given the impact of vestibular processing on later learning, an increase in learning disabilities may relate to our more sedentary lifestyle: the developing fetus may not have had enough movement stimulation.[10]

Proprioceptive Sense

Close your eyes and extend both arms out to the side at shoulder height, then bring the tips of your index fingers together. You can do this because the proprioceptors in your joints tell you where you are in space. If you can't do this, something is amiss with your proprioception.

Giving us body awareness, the somatosensory system—skin, joint, and muscle sensation—tells us where our head, arms, legs, and trunk are; if our stomach is churning; if we are going to sneeze or need to urinate or defecate. It enables us to move muscles and limbs in a coordinated way so we can zip a zipper, get in and out of a chair, and sleep without falling out of bed.

When infants suck their thumb, they are engaging their facial muscles and jaw joints, which floods them with organizing and calming proprioception. In the womb, the tight, impenetrable space and uterine wall create steady pressure on the fetus's joints, as does the varying pressure created by the mother's breathing. When held, the infant's limbs naturally pull into a fetal tuck, containing and calming them. The never-ending need for deep pressure and joint and muscle sensation is why babies like being swaddled and tend to wedge themselves against their bumper pads in a corner of the crib.

When put down, babies will cry from the sudden loss of warmth and pressure. Similarly, we might feel a sudden loss of comfort when our spouse breaks from our embrace and rolls over to his side of the bed or when our fat cat jumps off our lap. And so we pull ourselves into a ball for comfort. During a particularly difficult period, one sensory-defensive woman spent hours in the "child pose," a yoga posture in which she lay prone on the floor curled up in the fetal tuck. Cracking our knuckles, grinding or clenching our teeth, or crunching away at the bag of potato chips are ways of getting pressure into our joints.

Unlike the tactile and vestibular senses, proprioception is not fully developed at birth but continually requires stimulation of the proprioceptors. Young children fall out of their bed but older ones don't.

As proprioception generally does its job automatically and unconsciously, it's hard to conceptualize. To sense proprioception at work and its importance in your bodily sense of self, try standing in a doorway and press as hard as you can against the door frame. Suddenly, your arms float up. Enjoy this sensation. Heavy resistance against your muscles—heavy work—invokes quick calm. As we'll learn later, figuring out ways to quickly get deep pressure into your joints is one of your magic bullets.

THE TRIPOD OF THE NERVOUS SYSTEM

The tactile, vestibular, and proprioceptive senses are the precursors to the development of the function of the far senses. Forming the "tripod of the nervous system," as neuropsychologist Steven Cool describes them, they are fundamental to accurately perceiving and processing sight and sound.

The ear is both the organ of sound and the organ of balance. In fact, hearing is movement speeded up. The hummingbird's wings move slowly and we see them but don't easily hear them. When wings move fast, like that of the bee, we hear a buzz. Feeling the music through their body as vibrations is what enables deaf persons to dance.

The ear evolved from the gill. Early fish had hairlike receptor cells on the sides of their heads to inform them of ripples in the water that might mean danger. Over time, membranes closed around these receptor cells and formed semicircular canals, gravity receptors to give the fish awareness of its own movements through the water. When the descendants of early fish flopped onto land, auditory receptors evolved out of the primitive gravity receptors. From fish to reptile, from birds to humans, progressive development of the organs in the inner ear evolved to enable us to move forward, backward, up, down, and side to side at will.

Though we hear from birth, it is initially a cacophony of sound. As an infant learns to integrate movement of the eyes, head, and body, he becomes able to locate sound in space. Gradually, infants learn to interpret what they hear, to pluck out their mother's voice from the surrounding sounds (auditory discrimination), and to learn verbal language.

Vision too depends upon the contribution of the vestibular, proprioceptive, and tactile systems. It is by seeing that you know where you are in space. If you close your eyes and try standing on one leg, you might wobble. Through movement, the vestibular system works together with the visual system to develop a visual map of the environment so we can place ourselves in space.[11] Picture how the vestibular system guides the movement of our eyes, enabling us to track moving cars. When learning to read, children will move a finger underneath the line of print, as following the moving finger is easier than focusing on the stationary letters. In fish and amphibians, the visual system is organized to respond only to movement. Every fisherman knows that bait must move for the fish to notice it. Bulls are attracted not to the red color of the bullfighter's cape but to its movement.

In a remarkable experiment, a subject wore special lenses that made the world appear upside down. After wearing the lenses for a while, the subject found that the inverted world appeared right side up. Presumably, the brain adjusts the visual field to be concordant with motion and the proprioceptive flow of information from joints and muscles. When people have a poor sense of balance, direction, or movement, they rely more on their vision to help balance and orient in space.

Treating the near senses influences the function of other sensory systems; activities like skin stimulation, swinging, and jumping and crashing down on a trampoline form the basis of sensory integration therapy. In her book *The Gift of Touch*, Helen Colton tells of Sterling, a brain-damaged infant, blind and having seizures.[12] The parents enrolled him in a touch-and-motion program. The child was moved in rapid, synchronized motions, spun in a revolving chair, rolled on the floor, massaged, squeezed, and tapped. One month after the program began, Sterling could see.

SENSORY TEAMWORK

Other than our aloof sense of smell, our senses massively intermingle in the nervous system, and input from each sensory system influences every other system and the integrity of the whole.[13] Hearing and touch inform vision, so we know where to look. Vision and touch inform balance, so we can maintain equilibrium (try closing your eyes as you walk down the stairs). Balance informs body awareness (sent by sensory nerves in the skin, muscles, and joints), so we know when we're on terra firma and when we're not. Body awareness informs movement, so we can direct our muscles to meet our goal. People look to their left to remember auditory information, like a favorite song, and to their right to construct auditory information, like to sing along to the radio. To access what a kitten's fur feels like, what newly mowed grass smells like, or a tart apple tastes like, people will usually look down and to their right.[14] The less integrated the senses, the more perception relies on utilizing two or more senses at once: a person must see *and* feel their keys for their brain to register "keys" accurately.

As one system is turned on or off—excited or inhibited—it works to turn on or off other sensory systems. To increase tactile sensitivity and better savor the rapturous sensation of a kiss, we dim the lights and close our eyes. If not, competing visual images, like our loved one's eyelashes, might distract us. To better hear Rachmaninoff's third piano concerto, we close our eyes to listen without visual distractions. This explains why churches are kept dark. Wrote D. H. Lawrence:

> I went into the church. It was very dark and impregnated with centuries of incense. It affected me like the lair of some enormous creature. My senses were roused, they sprang awake in the hot spiced darkness. My skin was expectant, as if it expected some contact, some embrace, as if it were aware of the contiguity of the physical world, the physical contact with the darkness and the heavy suggestive substance of the enclosure. It was a dark, fierce, darkness of the senses.[15]

When stimulation of one sense overloads the system, a person may need to shut out that sense not just for the pleasure of the music, for instance, but to make sense of the world. A defensive may wear earplugs while working at the computer to shut out distracting noise, or close her eyes to a busy scene to comprehend a phone conversation.

There are sensory cells that will not fire for hearing or vision unless preceded by touch or movement. Thus, when we meditate, we become quiet and still to tune the world out. When we are out of touch, we are off balance, literally, and tactile-defensive people often have problems with their place in space. In fact, if the sensory nerves to our hand were cut, in five minutes we would lose coordination.

In the movie *Awakenings*, based on neurologist Oliver Sacks' book of the same title, we see a dramatic demonstration of how the senses mutually influence each other. In one scene, encephalitic patients with symptoms similar to Parkinson's disease sit frozen holding forks in the air. Music they like begins to play. They take fork and knife, cut their food, and eat without missing a beat. Through the brain stem, the auditory nerve connects the inner ear with all muscles in the body, and the music apparently elicited coordinated movement.

Touch had the same magic on these patients—a gentle hand on the shoulder and they began to eat. So did vision; just watching another move somehow got them moving. This astounding ability for one sense to liberate another is sensory integration at work, the inner drive toward self-organization even when our nervous system betrays us. At the same time, the power of one sense to influence another can sabotage sensory integration, as when tactile defensiveness to clothing, a chair's surface, or the touch of another makes the person squirm and become overactive.

The senses integrate early in development in ways that scientists can't as yet explain. For instance, if you persistently stick out your tongue at a newborn infant, some will stick *their* tongue out—an integration of vision and movement. If given a regular nipple to suck or a nobbed one, a 3- to 4-week-old infant will look longer at the one he just sucked. Apparently, infants can identify what something looks like by what it feels like in their mouth—an integration of vision and touch.[16] This synergy of the senses is what makes sensory defensiveness a central nervous system problem.

In a rare condition called synesthesia, the customary boundaries between the senses appear to break down and people see a sound and hear a color. Many synesthetes suffer from sensory defensiveness. A well-known synesthete, Vladimir Nabokov found all music unbearable. Dr. Peter Grossenbacher, a senior staff fellow at the National Institute of Mental Health, suggests that neural pathways that normally act to suppress irrelevant sensory input and allow focused perception may be dysfunctional, causing one sense to bleed into the other.

BOTTOM-UP HIERARCHY

Sensory integration begins from the bottom up, as our brain has grown over the last 5 million years, with each higher layer representing an elaboration and improvement upon lower, more primitive parts.

As outlined by neuroanatomist Paul MacLean, a brain researcher at the National Institute of Mental Health, our "triune brain" consists of distinct, hierarchically organized levels that correspond to the evolution of the human species from lower animal form: the brain stem, the most primitive, communicates with motions; the limbic system, with emotions; and the cerebrum, with words.[17] How these brain parts commingle is a mystery. But somehow they function as an integrated whole and reciprocally influence each other.

The Primitive Brain: the Brain Stem

Starting at the top of our spinal cord and setting the conditions for self-regulation—for making our heart beat and our blood flow—sits the brain stem, our primitive, or "reptilian," brain and our first sensory register. Neither a thinking nor a learning brain, it is in charge of survival and drives the four F's necessary for self-preservation: feeding, fleeing, fighting, and . . . reproduction.

Comprising the brain stem's central core is the reticular formation (RF), the seat of the four A's—awake, asleep, arousal, and attention—and thus consciousness. Acting as a sensory antenna, the RF picks up sensory vibes from all sensory systems except olfaction and perks us up, quiets us down, or excites us. To go to sleep, we quiet the RF by toning down sensations and lie still in a warm, quiet, dark room. As we drift off into sleep, the RF ensures that we become less sensitive to the sensations around us. To wake the RF, we seek strong sensations—the light of the sun, the buzz of an alarm clock, a splash of cold water.

To prevent sensory bombardment, the reticular formation directs our focus by monitoring and filtering sensations, heightening relevant features, like the words you're reading, and dampening irrelevant ones, like the outside traffic. It also functions to set individual thresholds to stimuli: set at low, as in the sensory defensive, you take in too much stimuli; set at high, as in sensation seekers, you take in too little.

The reticular formation extends from the spinal cord to the thalamus, a joint pair of egg-shaped structures that is the sensory Grand Central Station of the brain. Excluding smell, which goes directly from the olfactory bulb in the cortex to the limbic system, sensory intake travels up the spinal cord to the thalamus. There, some information gets routed back to the reticular formation, which in turn routes the information to other areas of the brain, including the cerebrum, where it influences alert and sleep states. In turn, the higher brain returns some information back to the thalamus to route it to the medulla, which controls heartbeat and breathing, and to the cerebellum.

Wrapped around the back of the brain stem, the cerebellum is the puppeteer of the nervous system, responsible for coordinating muscle tone, balance, and all our body movements so we can move easily, smoothly, precisely, and with good timing. To plan and execute movement well, the cerebellum must receive clear vestibular and proprioceptive feedback. A ballet dancer doing ten consecutive pirouettes or a gravity-defying gymnast flipping backward through the air shows the cerebellum at peak performance. Poor coordination and stiff or flaccid (rag-doll) muscle tone convey faulty vestibular and proprioceptive messages that prevent the cerebellum from doing its job. They are a red flag for sensory-processing disorders.

Tactile impulses go just about everywhere in the brain. Touch receptors below the neck send impulses to the spinal cord and then get routed to the brain stem, where nuclei process tactile inputs to tell us that something is touching our leg and whether that "something" is pleasurable or painful, hot or cold, smooth or scratchy. Receptors in the skin of the head and face send impulses through cranial nerves directly to the brain stem—why our face is so sensitive.

The important components of sensorimotor interactions—the tactile, proprioceptive, vestibular, visual, auditory, and so on—must occcur in the cerebellum, the reticular activating system, and other parts of the brain stem for meaningful information transmission to take place and to enable the whole nervous system to organize for adaptive behavior. This total multimodal sensorimotor integration sets the stage for the cerebrum to function efficiently and effectively.

The Emotional Brain: the Limbic System

The next way station for sensations is the limbic system, our old mammalian brain and the seat of our feelings. It is here, thanks to neurotransmitters (like serotonin and opiates), and hormones (like oxytocin, the feel-good hormone), that we *feel* what has made our heart thump and our palms sweat: fun or fear, lust or disgust, titillation or ennui. And it is here, as noise annoys or as music evokes serenity, that our mood changes.

As all sensation, excluding smell, passes first through the gates of the primitive reptilian brain en route to the limbic system, our gut response to sensation and our feelings are forever married: arm in arm, the limbic system and reticular activating system modulate the nervous system. The emotional security of the embrace may emanate from a chemical buzz of oxytocin and other internal opiates, but it starts with sensation—warmth, deep pressure, and proprioceptive feedback from our muscles and joints. "*Hold* me!" we beseech when we are held too lightly.

To function we need a clear, calm sea of emotions. But that assumes modulated sensory receptivity. If one's senses feed ongoing negative information into the limbic channel, the person's emotional voyage is achingly intense and volatile. Easily provoked, the annoyance of sensory defensives can turn quickly to anger and then to rage. Easily alarmed, their apprehension can turn quickly to fear and then to panic. Readily hurt, their sadness can turn to melancholy and then to depression. When happy, defensives may quiver with excitement. When amused, they may laugh quickly, giddily, or even hysterically, tingeing their gaiety with confusing sadness. Such extreme emotions are stressful. Little wonder defensives desire solitude.

Could the strong emotions of the sensory defensive relate to their strong sense of smell? After all, the limbic system evolved from the sense of smell, which is why odors easily trigger strong memories and nostalgia. A person catches a whiff of orange blossoms and feels sudden sadness, her mind exploding with memories of a childhood friend who died young.

Fondly, she recalls snatching sprigs of orange blossoms together to place in their hair.

The Thinking Brain: The Neocortex

At the third level, we reach the neocortex, the seat of thought. Here lie the regions that interpret what the senses perceive—our conscious awareness. This part of the brain allows us to write, speak, scheme, decide what to eat for dinner, do a crossword puzzle, and, for a few, get into Harvard. All this gives us some control, or willpower, over the primal lower commands. But can it tell us not to startle from the motorcycle's roar? Can it tell us to ignore the grain of sand in our shoe?

THREE-WAY CHITCHAT

In humans, the cerebral cortex constitutes almost 70 percent of the weight of the brain system and has considerable plasticity—neurons have a remarkable ability to sprout new connections. This gives us clout to consciously modify our behavior.

Yet, even for those with a smoothly functioning nervous system, mind over matter is not easily achieved. The primitive brain stem sets up the integrity of the entire nervous system. To function well and permit more complex and specialized information, the cerebral CEO must rely on the maturation of adequate sensory organization and management at the lower, less complex levels.

When this happens, the connections between the three parts of the brain work in harmony and effective sensory integration occurs automatically. The person spontaneously adjusts his or her actions to signals from the environment, and the senses create curiosity and excitement. The brain responds by creating the necessary mental set for the activity at hand, and behavior is efficient, goal-directed, and purposeful. Good vestibular and somatosensory functioning produce a feeling of being centered and grounded—of having "a level head on your shoulders" and being able "to think on your feet."

But what if the neuronal connections between the three parts of the brain are not properly established and a person's brain cannot easily organize sensory messages from the skin, muscles and joints, inner ear, eyes, and the environment? A "traffic jam" occurs between sensory input and motor output: sensory neurons may send inefficient messages into the central nervous system, or motor neurons may send inefficient messages out to the body for correct action.[18] Without proper feedback the brain does not get the information that it needs to develop properly, especially the experience of support against gravity. The reptilian brain (defense) and the limbic brain (emotions) take over, short-circuiting thinking. The result is *sensory integration dysfunction* abbreviated as DSI, rather than SID, so as not to be confused with sudden infant death syndrome.

DSI can manifest as a problem with sensory discrimination, sensory modulation, or both.

Sensory discrimination enables a person to interpret sensory information, such as texture, shape, size, gravity, and body position, providing sensory feedback and enabling skillful actions. It enables her to know when someone is touching her back, rather than her shoulder, to unconsciously right her balance as she steps on and off an escalator, and to know the distance of her body from other passengers so that she doesn't collide with them.

If a snag occurs between sensory input and motor output, motor skills may not be smooth and efficient and the person may experience problems with balance, coordination, and body awareness. The muscles of these people may be weak or stiff and their body must fight harder to resist the force of gravity: uncoordinated, they bump into things, drop things easily, and tend to have poor handwriting. Poor handwriting is also related to poor eye-hand coordination. Activities that generally give pleasure, such as dancing or riding a bicycle, even writing one's name, may be effortful, demand attention, and cause frustration. The simplest activities create stress and anxiety and are likely to be misinterpreted. Until one woman discovered she had SI dysfunction, she assumed that she consistently lost her tennis matches because of poor motivation—she didn't try hard enough to keep her eye on the ball—or underlying psychological issues—fear of winning.

Some sufferers have diminished tactile discrimination and can't identify if someone is touching their knee or their leg or if the apple is heavy or light, smooth or rough. They can never be sure of what they're sensing. Other problems include poor bilateral integration, where people confuse right from left and hands and feet don't work well together. Speech or language delays and other auditory processing problems, visual-spatial processing problems, learning problems, or attention deficit disorder can be separate problems or tie into SI dysfunction.

Sensory modulation is the brain's ability to organize itself, inhibiting or suppressing irrelevant information and allowing one to focus on relevant information. Taking place in the primitive brain stem, it enables a person to recoil at the sensation of the bug crawling down her arm while ignoring the sensation of her bracelet gracing her wrist, to feel alarm at the smell of smoke while ignoring the smell of chlorine bleach. Those who have a problem calibrating sensory information are unable to maintain a normal level of arousal. The hyporeactive seek sensation; the hyperreactive or sensory defensive avoid it; and some vacillate between seeking and avoiding.

In a world bulging with confusion, those who suffer from SI dysfunction feel off center, out of focus, missing a beat, detached. Their spontaneous behavior is inefficient, excessive, or useless. They innocently say and do things at the wrong time, in the wrong place, in the wrong way; rejected, they chastise themselves for their stupidity. As such, it takes much effort and energy to reach their goal and they often fail: frustration, shame, and disappointment are ceaseless. Lacking self-confidence, they develop a negative, yet sadly realistic, belief system: "I can't do it." "I don't have fun like others." "I'm not normal." "People don't understand me." "People don't like me."

Health professionals who fail to realize or accept SI dysfunction as legitimate, misdiagnose and mistreat the behavior as anxiety. But just ana-

lyzing one's difficulty with succeeding in life or learning positive self-talk
will not bring about change. The nervous system must be fixed at the level
of the brain stem.

Some sensory defensives only have a problem with sensory modulation. Most, though, experience other sensory processing problems, compounding their dysfunction. But it is primarily the overarousal that throws
their nervous system into disarray.

AROUSAL CURVE

Everything we do requires a certain level of arousal to keep us alert,
focused, and emotionally stable: mental arousal to concentrate on reading
a book; emotional arousal to be up enough to converse with a 2-year old;
physical arousal to have the stamina to walk upstairs; sensory arousal to be
open enough to take in and explore life. Optimally aroused, we feel good
and alert and respond appropriately to our environment; underaroused,
we feel lethargic and not up to challenges, even if it is just brushing our
teeth; overaroused, we feel disorganized, anxious, and unhappy.

Upon awakening, our arousal is very low and our attention and concentration is limited. As arousal increases, we perk up and become alert
enough to do what we need to do. When we reach optimal arousal, we feel
at once relaxed and aroused, calm and alert, and carry out actions seemingly effortlessly. With eyes focused and body still, and without self-
consciousness or rumination, we direct our energy outward and freely
connect with what we're doing. The right and left hemispheres of the
brain chat back and forth easily.

But if arousal continues to escalate beyond the demands of the task at
hand—high arousal is fine during sex but not while eating dinner—we
start to feel anxious, disorganized, hyperalert, and unable to meet our
demands. If we cannot flee the situation, as when cramming for an exam or
running late, stress hormones do not dissipate and arousal continues to
rise: our heart pumps, our stomach churns, our breathing constricts.
Overarousal is so uncomfortable, even when feeling pleasure, that most

people will do anything to reduce it and relax. The burst of whole-body hugging often following athletic triumphs and other emotionally intense events neutralizes overexcitement. If arousal reaches very high levels, we get overly stressed and, in self-defense, begin to shut down information processing. At the end of a stressful day, our favorite TV program may seem like rapidly moving light and background noise, and we nod off.

Hans Selye, an endocrinologist and pioneer in recognizing stress as a cause of disease, discovered that stress itself is not necessarily bad.[19] The body responds with the same pounding heart and panting breath to a hot date as to a sudden temperature drop or viral infection.

Over limited time, mild stress enhances creativity and performance. The butterflies we experience before giving a speech psyche us up for peak performance. Selye called this state of high energy, low tension *eustress;* others call it an adrenaline rush. But if the stress is intense and prolonged, with too little time in between to recover, it creates high tension and high energy and evokes flight, fight, or freeze: eustress becomes distress, which diverts energy from performing to eliminating the source of the discomfort.

If the alarm system is constantly falsely triggered, distress piles up and the body stays in this heightened state for too long: over time distress becomes dis-ease. Dis-ease depletes the immune system, puts stress on the vital organs, and eventually turns to disease. It comes down to one's basic receptivity to sensation and arousability.

Nothing Stays the Same

Determined by our unique biochemistry, we each have a baseline level of arousal, set in the reticular activating system in the brain stem that, in partnership with limbic activity, sets our sensory threshold—the basic arousability, or excitability, of our autonomic nervous system. Receptivity to sensation ordains why some people are hotheaded and others stay cool.

From baseline, arousal moves up or down according to sensory input, which can be external (like bright or dim lights) or internal (like our heartbeat or thoughts), and which interacts with conditions such as time of day, health, state of mind, activity, fatigue, hunger, previous pain or pleasure experience, expectations, and motivation.

All these conditions vary according to our body rhythms, which orchestrate all of our behaviors. And these rhythms encompass far more than the notably rhythmic heartbeat. For instance, the blood pumped by our heart, along with the organs, muscles, and sinews nourished by our blood, moves in rhythm, whether we're conscious of it or not. The gastrointestinal tract contracts 3 to 12 times per minute. In REM sleep, our brain waves range between 8 and 13 hertz. When we dream, our body synchronizes with the earth, which vibrates at around 10 hertz.

Did you know that every 90 minutes or so we alternate which nostril we primarily breathe through? Research shows that when the left nostril is open, the right hemisphere of the brain, which processes spatial and visual material, dominates, activating the more creative, feeling side of the brain. When the right nostril is open, the left hemisphere, which processes verbal and analytic material, dominates, activating more rational, thinking activity.[20] In other words, brain dominance is constantly shifting: at one time of day we feel like doing a crossword puzzle, and at another listening to music. Yogis observed this shift thousands of years ago, and to balance their psychophysiology, they developed a breathing technique called alternate nostril breathing (ANB), in which they deliberately changed the flow of air through the nostrils. (ANB is discussed in Chapter 14.)

All these rhythms exist within a circadian, or 24-hour, sleep-wake cycle, an inner clock that synchronizes body rhythms by the ebb and flow of light and dark. Our body temperature, for instance, is higher by day and lower by night, while the right side of the body is warmer by day and the left side is warmer by night.

As these rhythms go up and down during the day, they change our biochemistry and sensory threshold, with resulting shifts in behavior and attention. If the phone rings at 2 o'clock in the afternoon, we unconsciously reach over and pick it up, barely breaking from activity. If the phone rings at 2 o'clock in the morning, our chemistry is in a different place and we fumble for the receiver. If we drink too many Cokes, we speed up our body rhythm—our heart rate, breathing, and brain waves—and reset the reticular formation to a faster speed and lower sensory threshold. If we play 2 hours of tennis, we slow our heart rate and breathing and reset the reticular formation to a slower speed and a higher sensory threshold.

In the sensorily nimble, rhythms hum in tune. But in the sensorily unstable, rhythms hum discordantly. Sensory defensives breathe too rapidly and their hearts beat too quickly. They don't feel like eating or can't stop. They urinate frequently and either eliminate irregularly or get the runs. They sleep too little or can't stay awake. They jitter and jerk or can't move. (In Chapter 4, I'll talk about the development of poor rhythmicity.) The challenge of treatment is to find what works to balance their system so that they can eat well, sleep well, love well.

It's not that the sensory defensive necessarily appear frenzied every moment. As varying rhythms change their biochemistry, so does how they code the world: okay or not okay.

APPROACH/AVOID

How does our brain maintain order? The answer lies in avoiding or approaching stimulation until we reach an optimal level of arousal, the midpoint between boredom and anxiety.[21]

At the slightest change—a light dims—the reticular formation in our brain stem perks up: "Something new!" All senses wake up to appraise the survival value of the stimulus. "Is it safe? Is it dangerous? Do we care?" If we care, the hippocampus, amygdala, and hypothalamus of the limbic system collaborate to evaluate the stimulus and, based on like or dislike (the emotional) and on pleasure versus pain or safety versus danger (the physical), make a decision: "Approach or avoid." The hippocampus, in charge of storing and laying down new explicit memories (numbers, dates, facts, names, colors, smells, touches) scans memory stores for past experience.

The amygdala, in charge of emotional evaluation, scans for trouble and adds emotional intensity: "I'm frightened. I'm intrigued."[22] If the verdict is danger, the amygdala signals the hypothalamus, the central control center of the brain, to convey the message back to the brain stem through the hormonal route and stir the sympathetic nervous system into action. The stress hormone cortisol is released into the bloodstream, which in turn stimulates adrenocortical glands to release adrenaline and spur autonomic activity: the heart pumps, breathing constricts, muscles tighten. Lastly, the limbic brain conveys outputs to the neocortical brain, which pulls together what the senses have perceived into conscious thought: "A ghost? Or a bulb gone out?" This entire cascade of events happens in milliseconds and integrates with multiple pieces of information coming in simultaneously—a nervous laugh, a whiff of brewing coffee, the dry heat from the overhead vent, a downcast look, a pain in the side. But the repercussions of this release of stress hormones can impact the entire body for hours or days afterward.

The brain craves novelty. If the brain evaluates a stimulus as too familiar, it becomes uninteresting—another sunset—and we quickly habituate and stop orienting toward it. In this way, our system remains open to take in the next new sensation. The quicker we habituate to the irrelevant, the more easily we adapt to our environment.

At the same time, the reticular formation continues to monitor the stimulus below the level of consciousness. This is why we can tune out bright fluorescent lights or a noisy air conditioner but still feel stressed by it. Often, we are not conscious of this stress until the lights dim or the air conditioner turns off and (sigh of relief) we suddenly feel a burden lifted. If there's a change and the light flickers, receptors will fire and we become aware. The more meaningful the stimulus—a nostalgic song—the longer it takes to tune it out.

But sensory receptors can be laid to rest simply by monotony. When most people pick up a baby, the feeling of silky soft skin and plump curves sends luscious warm waves through the body. But if the sleeping baby in your lap doesn't stir, the constant, consistent pressure becomes ho-hum and the brain says, "Ignore."

When our brain detects something meaningful, the *discriminatory sensory system* signals us to approach and take in the details. In this way we are at all times actively staking out what we need to stay alive, like fresh food, companionship, clothing, shelter, and financial resources, and what gives us pleasure. To focus our attention, activity stops, heart rate rises, the pupils dilate to take in more information, blood goes to the head and respiration stills: "Ah!"[23] A split second later we take in a deep breath, which lowers the heart rate so we can sustain our attention and observe the person's sparkling blue eyes, dimpled cheeks and dangling pink crystal earrings.

When we feel endangered, the older and nonspecific *protective sensory system* decides the relative safety or danger of a stimulus to ready us to initiate quick action: For instance, we snatch our finger away from the hot iron. Breathing and heart rate remain high, preventing sustained attention and we can't attend to and explore our world. If a person feels constantly threatened, this older more primitive system will rule and the person is in a constant state of flight, fight, or freeze. As the protective system decides whether we approach or avoid, occupational therapists Patricia and Julia Wilbarger propose that it is an imbalance in this system that biases the defensive to falsely evaluate harmless stimulation as a threat.[24]

In the cerebral cortex, the two sides of the brain function by similar guidelines. The rational, intelligent left brain will identify an odor. The emotional, hedonic, and less discriminating right brain decides if the odor is pleasurable or repulsive, without distinguishing the odor's source, value, or nature. The perfumer's ability to identify different scents in a fragrance indicates left-brain activity. The sensory defensive's quick, nondiscriminating emotional response indicates right-brain activity, affecting the ability to behave rationally and responsibly. How freely people move within the world and how wise their choices are relates less to free will than to the stability of their arousal level.

Staying Centered

When people have balanced biochemistry (not too much or too little adrenaline or serotonin, for instance), their nervous system is organized and they are better able to draw a curtain on irrelevant sensory information. Most irrelevant sensations wash over them like water off a duck's back. Even in the face of disruptive stimuli, their arousal remains steady. Going with the flow, they perk up to give a sales presentation, tone down to calm a crying baby, or wind down to sleep.

Those with a thinner stimulus barrier and greater sensitivity have a bias toward the avoid system and tend to be cautious and more introverted. Those with a thicker stimulus barrier—the "thick skinned"—have a bias toward the approach system and tend to be more bold and extroverted. Both are normal nervous system responses that had evolutionary advantages. Those with greater sensitivity could more quickly detect impending danger—like a snapping branch that might signal a predator—and help to protect the group. Those more fearless were the leaders of the pack—the first to hunt down danger in search of potential new food sources and stake out new territory.

When daily events send them out of the zone, they are generally able to quiet inner clamor with run-of-the-mill "self-stimming"—drinking hot coffee, stretching arms, sighing, bouncing a leg, humming or whistling, getting fresh air, chatting, joking, laughing. Experiencing a normal degree and range of emotions appropriate for a situation, they have the flexibility to modify emotion to suit circumstances, and their emotions neither run away with them nor stay hidden.

During unusual circumstances, the window of optimal arousal widens (on vacation) or narrows (when feverish and everything bothers us). In wartime, a sentry standing guard alone at night may notice, and spontaneously fire at, an almost imperceptible noise that he would barely flinch at under normal circumstances.

When threat is perceived, the brain's alarm signal matches the degree of danger and musters the appropriate amount of sympathetic activity needed for self-protection. If the person hears a jackhammer, he perks up, his brain assesses that it will not attack, and he ignores it. If he is walking alone down a dark alley at night, his brain assesses any change as a sign of potential peril. His arousal level elevates in preparation for flight, fight, or freeze, and he becomes vigilant to touch, sounds, smells, and unusual sights. When he reaches the safety of his car, his system works hard to tuck him back inside the comfort zone. He takes a deep breath and pulls himself together. The parasympathetic nervous system overrides the sympathetic, and he regains equanimity.

Quick recovery from danger and quick habituation to the irrelevant free normal curiosity and enjoyable engagement with the world, while the ability to take pleasure in sensation permits a bodily comfort that anchors him in the present: time seems full and expanded. It's not that he isn't monitoring his environment—we always are—but he can balance monitoring, or vigilant attention, and focus, or sustained attention.

As he processes information accurately, he has the ability to experience the depth and richness of sensations. The more fine-tuned the senses, the more information a person gleans. A perfumer distinguishes the orange scent from the tangerine; an artist discerns a face in a squiggle.

Going to Extremes

But what if a person's brain fails to accurately register sensation? The band of optimal arousal narrows and the person slips easily to either end—overaroused and threatened or underaroused and uninterested—or seesaws between the two extremes.[25,26] His emotions lack range and depth and, in relationships, may be inappropriately excessive or deficient.

The ordinary stimulation that succeeds in getting someone with a normal nervous system into a "just right" place does not have enough force for the starved nervous system, whether wired or sluggish. Possessing a runaway sensory appetite, this person requires extreme sensorimotor strategies to seek balance. To alleviate the deadline stress, he may chain-smoke, though his mother died of lung cancer, or loudly crack gum while coworkers try to concentrate—anything to momentarily drown out the internal chaos. Though irrational, impulsive, and seemingly destructive, this behavior is the best his nervous system can muster *in that moment* without disintegrating. The challenge is to live through the moment; the future cost is irrelevant.

Low Arousal

At the low end of arousal, the sensory valve is not open wide enough and sensations trickle in and take time to register. It takes a lot of input for these people to really feel something and someone might not notice an ant crawling on her arm. Those daredevils who swallow fire or lie on nails likely fall into this category.

Starved for sensation, the underaroused quickly become bored and need constant new, unpredictable, and intense stimulation to jazz them high enough to stay alert and function. At night, without movement, light, or noise to get their bodies going, they fall into a deep sleep in a wink, even in a strange environment.

Some underaroused may appear passive, lazy, quiet, or shy and shrug off responsibility that doesn't interest them. They are at risk for depression. Other underaroused are sensation seekers. Apparently both men and women have a high level of testosterone, and for life to sizzle they need constant uncertainty, challenge, or thrills. What is the difference between sensation seekers and extroverts with a normal nervous system? Like the overactive child who buzzes around the house past bedtime, the sensation seeker lacks the internal control to stop. Those with a normal nervous system can put on the brakes when caution is advised.

High Arousal

Now imagine life where the sensory valve is open too wide and sensations gush in without barriers of protection. One feels *too* much, *too* soon, and for *too* long. One is sensory defensive.

Presumably possessing a high baseline level of arousal, sensory defensives feel more aroused to begin with and their threshold for alarm is low. It takes only a small stimulus to charge their pulse; then they can't tune out the sensation. "There may be lower criteria for the sensory defensive that other people may never pay attention to," suggests Julia Wilbarger. "For instance, many sensory-defensive women complain that their bra hook bugs them all day long. They don't habituate to this sensation. It never goes away. They keep responding to the stimulus."[27] As their brain remains in the survival mode, all roads lead to danger and all sensations remain relevant: they startle to a minor sound, recoil from an insignificant touch, are alert to slight movement. Their window of comfort is pitifully narrow.

As sensations overwhelm the system, they attend to many sensations at once. Unable to screen out random noises, they will pick up ambient sounds. At a party, they feel thrown by the many conversations or the kids running around. As danger alerts them to high- and low-frequency sounds, they don't pay attention to speech and miss what people are saying to them. Peripheral vision rather than central vision dominates, so they can tell if someone is sneaking up behind them, and they pay attention to incidental movement, darting their unfocused eyes like a person dancing to strobe lights. Losing acuity, their world becomes a blur and they miss the big picture. Shown a picture of a baby wearing a pink dress and ribbon, they blurt, "Oh, how sweet. Girl or boy?" and then feel foolish. How do you explain a sensory defensive moment?

As mental fog descends, they become disoriented and slow to process information. Their minds go blank and pulling out a sentence feels like pulling taffy. Conversation becomes hard work. People describe them as "spacey," "in their own world," "out of touch." "I am always lost in a fog in public places and can barely understand what people say to me," says one woman. "Sometimes I have to sit down in the aisles and put my head between my knees for fear of fainting."

In many cases, other sensory processing problems make it hard to discern what primes the confusion. Inability to process language can result from feeling too overwhelmed to pay attention, from auditory processing problems that slow registration, or both. Inability to see what's in front of our nose can come from mental fog or from poor binocularity, where the eyes don't work together to focus and discern figure from background, or both.

As anything new elicits a strong response, defensives don't go far to seek excitement: it is jittering inside. Fearing new situations, they approach change cautiously, and on guard, greet the new with an "uh-oh." Bodily frenzy makes them want to escape the moment: time seems short and limited. Predictability, safety, moderation, and simplicity help minimize overstimulation.

To defend against overstimulation, defensives have primarily two strategies: fight or flight. The "fight" group shows an interest in new things, but poor sensory processing usually interferes, creating annoyance and frustration. They are easily angered—"Touch me and die!"— and appear stubborn, impatient, hostile, and explosive. Though alienating and seemingly self-destructive, this behavior imposes some internal organization, and the person can control his or her world enough to remain *in* it.

Others have a strong avoid and weak approach system. Feeling too overwhelmed to fight, they ignore the world by shutting down and retreating inside their quivering skin, imploding. They appear shy, inattentive, or self-absorbed. In fact, shyness is by definition a defense against overstimulation: averting eyes, standing outside the crowd, speaking quietly, letting the head and body posture droop—these all help tone down sensation.

Here, There, and Everywhere

If you can't quite decide where you fit in, this is not surprising. When does behavior ever quite fit into neat little theoretical boxes?

As conditions continually change and modify inborn disposition, or temperament, behavior is constantly changing. Though mostly hunting thrills, sensation seekers sometimes leave the party early. Though mostly withdrawn, the shy will explode and blast their stereos. At times, we feel at once bored and overaroused, as when listening to a dull lecture in a stuffy, crowded hall. At other times, sensations both bewitch and bother. The defensive might find crowds claustrophobic but exciting, rock music overpowering but exhilarating. Inconsistencies abound.

Nor can one necessarily discern inner state from a person's overt behavior. Someone may appear subdued because she is underaroused and lacks energy or because she is overaroused and withdrawing from stimulation. Seekers will get loud, giggly, and boisterous to self-stim, while the sensory defensive will do so to let off steam.

Some people are at once too low and too high. Zipping right through the safe middle zone of optimal arousal and barely stopping, they seesaw between seeking and avoiding. They can be simultaneously inquisitive and inhibited, gutsy yet anxious, easily bored yet easily hyped. Some of the later case studies on sensory defensiveness describe people so low that they need to down double espressos to get going, but they jump at the slightest touch.

That someone can be both unable to wake her body and to quiet it seems paradoxical, but in a state of overload, the body feels at once depleted (too low) and wired (too high). Sensations get processed at many levels; while organizing input to one sensation, a person is at once registering the input of others. As circumstance (home, away) and the body's rhythms (night, day) change, so does our receptivity to sensation. If our nervous system is unstable and our range of arousal narrow, sensory processing bounces all over. While we are avoiding some sensory input (light touch), we seek intensity (jiggling about) to maintain balance: to find a middle ground between not enough and too much is a constant battle. The trick in treatment is to find the sensorimotor recipe to broaden someone's band of arousal and increase their choices for self-organizing behavior.

OVERLOAD

Intuitively, the problem of sensory defensiveness seems one of immediate irritation and escalating arousal. In fact, the real problem is the failure to return to baseline once the defensive reaction occurs.[28] After the person gets home and rips off her bra or annoying piece of clothing, the conscious annoyance disappears, but the effect continues to resonate in the body like the aftershocks of an earthquake. Stress hormones linger for some 20 to 30 minutes in the bloodstream, and the person remains hyped and irritable. "I know it's normal to feel startled by firecrackers, gunshot, explosions and so on," says Hilary. "But I notice that it takes me much longer than most people to get calm after sounds like that. My body seems to go on feeling it long after everyone else's has forgotten it." In a Canadian experiment, highly anxious patients were compared to normal persons in their startle response to a sudden loud noise.[29] While the normal persons' muscles returned to their original state within half a second after the initial sound, the anxious persons' muscle tension remained high and continued to rise during the test.

As sensory and other disturbing events accumulate throughout the day, much energy goes into shutting out distracting sensation, and recovery to baseline becomes harder. If the person can't find his keys or if his boss wants the report yesterday, he begins to unravel. As defensiveness reaches intolerable proportions, the sufferer copes by isolating himself or lashing out. Stress chemistry spills over, and he goes into overload, where he feels too exhausted to move but jumpy on the inside. Even handwriting changes as the person heads toward meltdown and the tension in back and shoulders affects fine motor skills. Little things like errands can be rough, as Sandra attests. "The lights, everything distracts me—colors, balloons, signs hanging, announcements, so many people, different smells, especially the cars. Let alone trying to keep my attention on my children and what I have gone to do. By the time I am home, I am always exhausted and overwhelmed."

When things become too much, sufferers flip the switches off and go into shutdown, expending energy only for sheer survival. Sensation processing reduces to some or none at all. Sensations can't come in but neither can stress chemistry dissipate. To picture shutdown, imagine taking a deep whiff of ammonia. The odor would so overwhelm you that it would dull the nose; you could no longer smell anything and would feel momentarily traumatized. To shut out the world, people may retreat into their head or, like one woman, fall asleep. "On our trip back we had a lot of road noise. I slept almost the entire last day home. I was unable to keep my eyes open and deal with that constant noise. So my body escaped it through sleeping."

Going numb is the brain's response to trauma, whether from unbearable overstimulation, bodily injury, or an emotional blow. The brain releases endorphins, a hormone-like substance that is the brain's natural opiate: car accident victims or soldiers may not feel the pain of a broken leg or a gunshot wound right away. Children in shutdown, as the autistic, will fail to perceive noxious stimuli such as pinpricks, or dogs a lighted match to their nose. These children will bang their head and not feel pain. When victims start to come out of it, pain screams like a boom box in their ears.

If the shock is constant and intolerable, endorphins stream continuously and dull and anesthetize. When endorphin flooding is part of everyday life, the senses and emotions deaden and the person feels only intense emotions, such as anger, rage, sorrow, and fear. These trigger further endorphin release, which can lead to further emotional numbing and shutdown of sensory channels. While freezing or anesthetizing our bodies cuts off overstimulation, it cuts off pleasurable sensations as well: the sensory defensive rarely feel exulted.

Why can't sensory defensives talk themselves out of the defensive response? In life's drama, survival gets top billing. Sensations and emotions take precedent over thoughts—what Daniel Goleman, author of *Emotional Intelligence*, calls "emotional hijacking"—and intellect, or will, lacks the authority to override the automatic defensive response. Imagine if we had to *think* about fleeing the fire. Every night at work, for instance, Carolyn tries to prepare herself for the setting of the alarm system. "I continually try to condition my body by telling myself that sirenlike 'Beep! Beep' is coming, and to chill. But it makes no difference. I jump out of my skin. It's a knee-jerk reaction." Brain researcher Joseph LeDoux found far more connections from the amygdala to the cerebrum (from feeling to thinking) than the other way around.[30]

The cumulative effect of increasing irritation snowballs over the course of an hour, a day, weeks, months, and years. Each time someone smells that cologne he hates or anything similar, it burns new links into the brain, specifically in the amygdala, to strengthen the perception of certain harmless aspects of the world as threatening. Neurons that fire together once tend to do so again. As subtle changes accumulate, experience rewires the structure of the brain and the brain becomes "better and better at doing worse and worse." The more conditions overwhelm the system and elicit defense, the more this defensive pattern gets set as the person's truth and the more recoding needed to free a defensive mindset.

If extreme duress does not abate, physical illness and emotional collapse result. As we'll see in the next chapter, people at the severe level of defensiveness, whose system is constantly overwhelmed and needing to shut down, live in a state of perpetual post-traumatic stress. Fortunately, as we shall see in later chapters, activities that work directly on the reptilian brain can help tame the wild beast that pounces around inside.

Listed below are the various stages of sensory defensiveness, from mild irritation to shutdown.[31] They vary with each individual depending on the state of the person's nervous system. Some people experience all the stages; some vacillate from one to the other within minutes; others stay primarily in one or two stages for days, weeks, or years.

1. *I'm okay:* A person feels mild sensory irritation to things that don't seem to bother other people, but they are tolerable.

2. *Stressed:* A person feels tired, irritable, and short-tempered, and sensory irritation is more acute.

3. *Overloaded:* The person is in a disorganized frenzy—breathing is quick, body tense, balance unsteady and restlessness and anxiety constant.

Some connections are not being made, and verbal and physical responses are slow. Concentration requires effort, and it is hard to focus on others, on what they are doing, or on what's going on around them. Irritating sensations can appear life-threatening, and people may unwittingly strike out in anger, fear, or panic. They feel they must get away or snap.

4. *Out of Control:* The system has gone haywire. The body is exhausted, the mind is wired, and breathing is labored. It's hard to maintain balance, and even normal sensations, like people talking or sheets touching their bodies, become too much. Sufferers may feel crazy or severely depressed. Out-of-control crying or panic is likely.

5. *Shutdown/Depersonalization/Dissociation:* A cloud closes in and the world seems a haze. They feel unreal and can't see or hear clearly or feel the earth beneath their feet. It takes enormous effort to speak, move, or make sense of their surroundings. They escape into a twilight zone and do only that required for sheer survival. Dark depression and restless, nightmarish sleep is likely.

How many stages you go through depends on the level of severity, which runs on a continuum from sensation as annoying to sensation as excruciating. For some, just a few things annoy; for others, everything does. Let's now look at some examples of life experienced by those who are more or less sensory-defensive.

3

Levels of Defensiveness: From Mild to Maddening

> I discovered I scream the same way whether I'm about to be devoured by a Great White or if a piece of seaweed touches my foot.
>
> —KEVIN JAMES

If a person is mildly depressed or anxious—and who isn't at some point?—we assume that a dose of positive thinking and the passage of time will undo the situation and enable them to take control of their lives. And many do.

If a person is sensory-defensive, even mildly so, control is more elusive and the dysfunction has an insidious effect on a person's ability to control his or her fate and enjoy life day to day.

Though sensory defensiveness exists on a continuum of increasing severity, Patricia Wilbarger and Julia Wilbarger have delineated three distinct levels of defensiveness: mild, moderate and severe.[1] The mildly defensive do not relate to the moderate; the moderate do not relate to the severe.

GRIN AND BEAR IT

To an outsider, 36-year-old Hannah, a part-time lawyer, seems a typical suburban mom. She smiles and laughs easily and enjoys a warm and affectionate relationship with her husband and three children. But close inspection reveals exactness in her ways, a strong need for structure, predictability, and control, preference for solitude, and a carefully choreographed sensory environment.

Her clothing is cotton and loose and most of the labels and tags have been cut out (no surprise). Tastefully decorated in calming earth colors, her home is filled with windows that let in natural sunlight, minimizing the use of glaring indoor lighting. The house sits on an acre of land far from the madding crowd. Here she spends most of her time, away from "traffic, crowds, heat, and the sheer volume of noise from cars, planes, power machinery that works on my nerves and never seems to stop, even on Sunday." She used to take yoga to relax, but she quit. She felt the class was too crammed. Others didn't complain.

Her elevated shoulders and stiff posture reveal constant tension, and she feels a restlessness that increases in direct proportion to the noise and activity in her household. She loses patience easily with her children, and then feels guilty. Things must go as planned (rare) or she feels frustrated and gets steadily grumpier as the day progresses. By evening, she's wiped out and uses her last ounce of strength to get her kids to bed. She requires a half-hour scented bath to unwind for sleep, and if any of her kids yell "Mom" during her down time, she shrieks until they disappear. She considers her husband a saint to put up with her and works hard to pull herself together enough to have something left for the relationship.

Hannah is mildly sensory-defensive. Her normal state vacillates between feeling mild irritation to ordinary sensation—"I'm okay"—and stressed. Though more finicky than others, more easily irritated by her surroundings, by change and conflict, more difficult to console, and harder to please, she basically copes.

Most of us know someone like this. We call them touchy, emotional, high-strung, or neurotic. They may be withdrawn, set in their ways, and hard to get along with. Nevertheless, they can have good relationships and satisfying work, parent successfully and lead an otherwise normal life. Tension, though, sneaks out in rapid speech, nervous giggling, leg shaking, hair twisting, chewed-off nails, darting eyes.

Many crave hugs and love massages, unaware that they subtly withdraw if a stranger touches them. During infancy, they may have enjoyed being held, with slight tactile defensiveness apparent only with light touch, as during diapering and dressing.[2]

Even now, the defensiveness is barely detectable. Though choosy about fabrics and clothing preferences, most dress suitably. "If forced to, they will wear nylons but take them off as soon as humanly possible, and they may leave the party early," says Julia Wilbarger of the mildly defensive. These individuals may wear jewelry, though with distinct preferences as to how it feels against their skin, and they remove it as soon as they walk in the door. They may use lotions, deodorant, and makeup but only if a particular feel and fragrance.

They tend to prefer the comfort of home and avoid noisy, crowded places like malls, but they are willing to go almost anywhere. Yet, there's a cost. Grouchy and easily tired from the energy required to cope with sensory overload, at times they find it hard to get going. As small and large events add up, they are less able to hold it together. The effort required to succeed, as a spouse, a parent, or a worker becomes too much and they explode. Allergies and other stress-related health problems are common.

But they get by. At the next level of defensiveness, the person barely does.

BARELY BEARING IT

When Nicole feels most alone, she thinks back to the summer when she was 5 years old and on vacation in the mountains with her parents and grandparents. Her grandmother gave her an ultrasoft, shocking pink terrycloth jumpsuit. How different it was from her stiff school uniform, with its high collar that she wanted to rip off her neck. Having to wear it caused huge fights with her mother, who would say, "Everyone wears it. It's not scratchy. Why do you have to be different?"

Forty years later, this tall, soft-spoken nutritionist recalls the softness of the jumpsuit and her grandmother's soothing presence. That summer, the jitteriness, the intense, uncomfortable feelings, the feeling of being unsafe and unprotected lifted a bit, and the world took on a new meaning.

Nicole has always felt uncomfortably overexcited by people and victimized by a world too loud, too bright, and too close to her body. For years, she worked as a nutritional consultant in a hospital, and although she loved her job, her daily routine created enormous stress.

On winter mornings, she would stand shivering in the cold air waiting for the bus. "On the bus, the dry, hot air sucked the life out of me. My clothes felt horribly heavy, bulky, and sweaty. Those smells of strangers so close, sometimes squishing me—it revolted me. I felt claustrophobic. Sometimes I started to panic." At work, confinement in a windowless cubicle, surrounded by fluorescent lighting, stale air, and the inescapable smell of illness and antiseptics attacked her sensibilities.

Stressed before work, stressed during work, stressed on the bus, she would arrive home disintegrated. Too depleted to talk on the phone or make dinner, Nicole, the nutritionist, ordered out or ate leftovers. Then she collapsed into bed and listened to quiet music or half watched television. Tailed by exhaustion, she made constant excuses for not calling friends or family, sending birthday cards, socializing.

Those were the good nights. On other nights, she felt too stressed to tolerate the quietest sound or the dimmest light. She was barely able to crawl into bed. Her mind and heart would race, her hands would tremble, her legs would twitch, her gut would spasm, and her head and neck would throb. When she looked in the mirror, she saw a shocking image of lifeless, hollow eyes, dilated pupils, and a face drawn down like the mask of tragedy. Sleep seemed impossible. The feel of the sheets or a light blanket made her skin bristle, and she had to pile up blankets for weight on top of her, even in summer.

Today she works at home doing phone consultations with private clients. Better able to control the sounds, smells, and lights in her environment, her life is more manageable. But staying tolerably calm remains a full-time job. How could she fathom the responsibility of caring for a child or a husband, though she longs for both? Fortunately, Prozac helps contain a long-term depression, and weekly therapy sessions offer some relief from acute loneliness.

She tries to push herself to be with people but sags from the weight of these encounters. Animal odors, strong perfumes, or musty smells in someone's home distract her from enjoying conversation. The bright lights and overhead lighting that most people find necessary to stay alert seem like a blinding spotlight, disorienting her so she looks down, making people think she is uninterested.

Mostly she desires to be left alone—and people have complied with her wish. Throwing herself into her work helps her cope. Her supersensitivities and hard life have made her deeply compassionate to people in pain, and she has chosen to treat the seriously ill, people suffering from diabetes, cancer, and autoimmune illnesses. But extreme tension easily diverts her attention and makes it hard to listen to their woes. This makes her feel guilty, and she chastises herself for being insensitive and self-involved.

Even when she wishes to meet people, it is hard. Athletic clubs are a hotbed of sensation that can easily unnerve the moderately defensive, so Nicole boogies to an aerobics tape at home or takes a quiet yoga or tai chi class. Singles bars, where "an intimacy hound" might appear from nowhere, ready to menace her with an arm around her shoulder, are out.

As painful as loneliness is, love was worse.

When Nicole felt attracted to someone, thoughts that the man might fall in love with her, hold her protectively, and fill her profound emptiness would consume her and make her crazy. Perpetually anticipating his phone call, she would feel constantly excited, talk of little else, and fantasize obsessively about being in his arms. If he called, her neediness would destroy all equanimity, and she would be cool in defense. If they did get together, it was always the same: the more desire he showed, the tenser she became and the more she wanted to squirm out of his arms, at the same time desperately wanting to be held. Invariably men took her behavior as disinterest and stopped calling, leaving her devastated. For months, even years, she would obsess about the loss and not feel in possession of self.

On occasion, she would relax enough to enjoy an embrace—but not sex. She would feel easily aroused, but it didn't last. The more a man fondled her genitals, the more she felt unpleasantly overexcited. Sexual arousal and tension would increase in tandem and she would feel unsatisfied and frustrated. Her only enjoyment was when the man ejaculated and briefly stayed on top of her and inside. The weight of his body and of being "plugged" gave her a feeling of peace. But afterward, she would feel vulnerable and agitated by not having had orgasmic release and very anxious at having another person in her space. She couldn't sleep and constantly needed to urinate, which embarrassed her. Sex seemed hardly worth the effort, and for the last five years she has been celibate. Though her life lacks pleasure, excitement, and companionship, it's preferable to being a slave to uncontrollable feelings and in a state of perpetual mourning. No longer feeling consumed by a gnawing need for the other releases her energy and time for work and hobbies: a dull life is more easily tolerated than a constantly anxious one.

Nicole is considered moderately defensive. For people like her, a stressed state predominates. Feeling good means to feel only mild irritation to sensations other people tune out. Little stressors push them easily into overload, and then into out-of-control. Tactile defensiveness is ubiquitous and ruptures the thread that binds, alienating the defensive from the human connection and solace.

For those who are moderately defensive, anything they come into contact with—clothing, sheets, lotion, fragrance, soap, detergent or people—they scrutinize for comfort, warmth, and level of irritation.[3] Clothing must be made of soft, natural fabrics like cotton, which allows the skin to breathe by allowing air and light to enter. Synthetic fabrics like polyester don't breathe and therefore make their skin feel taut, sensitive, and sticky. Anything that puts pressure against the face, head, or neck—eyeglasses, face masks, hats, or chokers—is annoying, as is anything constricting, like elastic waistbands, cuffs, or turtlenecks, which feel like a noose on a tensed neck. "My extremely fashionable mother went nuts over my fiddling with tags, yanking at turtlenecks, refusing to wear certain styles. She'd just sigh and roll her eyes when I threw a fit," recalls one woman. At times, even air on the skin is annoying.

Most dislike anything snug on their bodies. Many will wear oversized well-washed cotton clothing and avoid belts, nylons, and gloves. If possible, women avoid wearing bras. The seams in socks irritate and socks are generally worn inside out. "The greatest invention in grade school was tube socks," remarks one man. "They didn't have those godawful seams." Shoes can make their feet feel squeezed. Jewelry irritates, and many defensives avoid wearing it. "I have never been able to wear my wedding band," laments one woman.

Because the head and face are exquisitely sensitive to touch, washing the face or using cosmetics and skin-care products can feel irritating. "To me, face makeup feels like a grease mask. I can't imagine how people walk around all day with it on their face," declares one woman. Lipstick must be a special brand; soaps and deodorants are chosen with great care.

Any pressure against the scalp can feel like a vice on their head and they struggle to find a hairstyle long enough for some weight and calming deep pressure, but not too long that the weight pulls uncomfortably on the scalp. And one that avoids little wisps of hair falling on the face, ears, and neck. Cutting or washing the hair can be unnerving, as can changing the way it is parted. For men, with more body hair, the problem is compounded. "At times my skin is so sensitive that my own hair plucks my skin," says one.

Any situation where people might violate their personal space, stand or sit too close, brush past them, or want to shake their hand feels like entering enemy territory, and they choreograph their movements accordingly. Exhausted at the thought of weaving through the sensory obstacle course encountered at supermarkets or malls, many will shop in small stores or on the Internet or through mail-order catalogs.

The litany of "can't go there, can't do that" can be endless. Uncomfortable with touching sand, mud, clay, grass, or snow, sufferers will avoid activities like going to the beach, playing golf, playing tennis on clay courts, or engaging in winter sports. Unable to tolerate being splashed or the sensation of dry to wet, swimming can be a trial and it takes a long time to get used to the water. Many experience some coordination and balance problems and will avoid activities that challenge equilibrium, which includes many sports. Many get carsick or seasick and fear heights, so vacations, which often involve flying and long car rides, induce anxiety and can become more ordeal than pleasure.

Beginning in childhood, fears are rampant and nightmares common. Sensitive and alert to nuances, these children more easily pick up noises, see shadows at night, and are terrified of most anything that might mean loud or scary noise, unwanted touch, or unexpected movement, like snakes, spiders, cats, dogs.

Because they experience the world as more dangerous than their capacity to protect themselves, anxiety is omnipresent. By adolescence, sufferers have likely been referred to as anxious, phobic, depressed, compulsive, hostile, aggressive, or controlling.[4] By adulthood, most moderately defensive people have been in therapy for anxiety, fears, or depression. They have taken tranquilizers, antidepressants, and beta blockers for panic, as well as alcohol and recreational drugs to help them calm down—but often to no avail. And they experience a slew of stress-related complaints.

How do they cope?

They minimize helplessness and loss of control over events that throw them by seeking to control what they can, especially when it comes to touch, thus their avoidant behavior. They increase predictability by compulsively adhering to strict schedules and rigid routines for eating, waking, going to sleep, and so on. But the cost of such behavior is huge. A rigid structure allows a modicum of control over their environment but it makes the defensives' behavior inflexible and places severe restrictions on all life choices: where to live, work, dine, play, vacation, socialize. Living with them is a challenge—if they even find a mate.

Tactile defensiveness makes sexual relationships traumatic. The defensive obsessively yearns for the enveloping hug, but it comes as part of a sensual package that includes kissing, petting, and intercourse, all of which may cause chills of terror. "I thought I was looking for a partner with a libido to match mine when all I really wanted was the deep touch," says Maggie. "I found the partner and ran from his touch."

The lips, tongue, and genitals all have similar neural receptors and are highly charged. If your skin is ultrasensitive, it's not surprising that tactile defensives' sexual touch receptors are easily driven to overstimulation, creating uncomfortable overexcitement that triggers alarm and the need to reduce intensity. The body electric surges less with desire than with shock, and as arousal escalates, so does tension; the body stiffens, the back arches and breathing becomes shallow and forced. Intercourse feels overwhelming, even painful. "Very frequently, before orgasm, I break contact," admits one woman. Some never reach orgasm.

Great sex is a spontaneous loss of self in a mutual sea of rapture, thrilling all the senses. But a body can't flow with sensuality if touching the erogenous zone causes a rush of panic. Or if the slightest sound, body odor, or the light seeping through the blinds distracts you. Or if your partner must watch his every move so as not to irritate you. "I have a problem maintaining arousal," says one woman. "If my husband makes one wrong move, I react defensively to his touch and it can ruin the whole night!"

Because sexual encounters evoke anxiety, it might take a long time to relax enough to feel sexual. When feelings start to open, the defensive become quickly overwhelmed with need and overexcitement, feelings that they can't easily turn off. This powerful need for and fear of sex can make sufferers feel crazy and out of control. To compensate, they may deny their sexual feelings or inhibit their expression. Some may unconsciously make themselves unappealing to the opposite sex.

For others, the thrusting of intercourse creates intense pressure that relieves tension. Although they may dislike foreplay, which involves light touch, intercourse relaxes and distracts them. Interestingly, sex therapists generally recommend that a couple with sexual problems cease intercourse and spend long periods just tenderly touching, which may be the tactile defensive's worst nightmare. Because of constant tension, some masturbate excessively. But as you can't self-stimulate heavy pressure, masturbation may create the same defensive reaction as foreplay and rather than orgasmic release, some experience increased tension.

There's another impediment in the sex life of the sensory defensive: boredom. Many need routine to control what happens, so they may avoid variety.

When a partner doesn't feel free to explore a loved one's body, intimacy issues inevitably emerge and create much misunderstanding. If a husband rolls over in bed to stroke his wife's hair and she recoils, he can't help but feel that she doesn't love him. She might find it hard to convince him otherwise and wonder what's wrong with her. The nondefensive spouse may attribute the rejection to something undesirable about him- or herself. This happened to Bonnie. "I've been married sixteen years and long thought I was unattractive because my husband isn't that interested in things physical. It always has to be on his terms. Now I finally understand that it's his hypersensitivity."

Imagine what intimacy issues do to parenting. Feeling uncomfortable about physical intimacy, a mother may not feel maternal, especially if she was not securely attached to her own mother. Handling an infant might feel uncomfortable, as little fingers and hands offer lots of feathery, wispy strokes. Unwittingly, a tactile-defensive parent may appear to reject her infant's need for physical closeness. In studying mothers with intimacy issues, presumably emotional rather than sensory, attachment researcher Mary Main found they would position themselves indirectly to avoid physical intimacy.[5] The mother would stiffen up and hold her baby away from her body or bring her baby toward her body but with the baby facing out. When her baby's arms would fly open to be picked up, the mother would leave her arms at her side. When her baby would crawl toward her, she would cross her arms and legs to make her body a barricade. These mothers were less likely to breast-feed and if they did, it was often perceived as a chore and quickly given up. Some defensive mothers have described breast-feeding as feeling overwhelming and overstimulating.

As if there wasn't already enough to handle, sensory defensives commonly have a sensory-defensive child or two. Talking about working overtime, the parents must keep not only themselves but their children calm. If the defensiveness alone hasn't made them sleepless, stressed, and exhausted, caring for defensive children will.

Few moderate defensives live happy lives. Nevertheless, there are times when life can feel pleasurable. This is rare for severe defensives, who can hardly stand being inside their own skin.

UNBEARABLE

To Joshua, a pale, blue-eyed, burly, and reticent 24-year-old, the less the world notices him the better. His work as a security guard stands as a metaphor for a life spent sniffing out danger in his environment, and it allows him to observe rather than participate.

His appearance is unremarkable, but for one peculiarity. Even when it is 95 degrees outside, he wears a long-sleeved buttoned shirt with a high collar. In this way, *nothing and no one can touch his skin.* Even leaving one button undone makes him feel bare and vulnerable to attack. His stiff raised shoulders ready him to ward off any intrusion.

From waking to sleeping, Joshua screens the world for what might invade his bubble of space. His entire body is ticklish to soft or intense touches, especially his toes, feet, sides, and neck. Most textures feel prickly against his skin and his clothes must feel like butter. Even if his skin does not directly touch a rough material, like a berber rug or a tweed-covered chair, he will squirm upon contact. His clothes must be of heavyweight material or they sit too lightly on his body; he will not wear a cotton T-shirt even though it is soft. But if his clothes are too stiff, like jeans, he feels like he's wearing a suit of armor.

He wriggles from dirt anywhere on his body and washes his hands constantly. When he touches anything greasy, gooey, or sticky, his teeth feel "strange." Grass feels like "sticks poking my feet," and the pavement is always too hot or cold. He won't let anyone touch his hair; cutting his toenails or fingernails is agony. He can't stand anything inside his mouth, hates to brush his teeth or go to the dentist, and hasn't gone to one in over fifteen years. Nor has he gone to a doctor, as the probing is torment, though he has suffered from allergies, upset stomach, and temporomandibular joint dysfunction (TMJ) his whole life.

Rules provide Joshua the only control he feels in his life. Before going to sleep he checks every room to ensure that nothing is out of place. The dishes must be done, and the bed ready for sleeping. To minimize the light touch of the bedding against his body as he moves, and especially against his ultrasensitive neck, he sleeps without a cover sheet and with cotton pajamas up past his neck. Two thick, heavy comforters create warmth and heavy pressure against his skin. Still, he can't find a place in his bed and will fidget and wiggle for hours before falling asleep. Once he's asleep, any minor noise or smell will awaken him, as will his own movements, and sleep is not restful. Most mornings he awakens with his hands clenched, teeth gritted, chest tight, and breathing hard. If it's too bright, hot, or noisy or if the blanket doesn't feel right, he can't get out of bed.

Disgusted by bodies, smells, and textures, Joshua feels extreme distress when he is physically close to others, even an acquaintance. In public, he is stiff and on guard, especially when confronting strangers such as store clerks. If someone unexpectedly puts an arm around his shoulder, he jumps a foot and angrily removes it; though nonaggressive, he has even punched someone for this intrusion. When Joshua knows he will touch someone, he prepares himself mentally and makes the first move to shake a hand or hug someone with a quick A-frame hug and then backs off.

As a child, Joshua hung out in a concrete barrel used for water drainage often seen on children's playgrounds. Cool and dark, it was a place where he could be alone and safe from others' touch and where he didn't have to move his flabby, clumsy body or listen to the children taunt him. They laughed when he fell off the monkey bars and called him scaredy-cat for refusing to ride on swings or the merry-go-round. He wanted to do these activities, but they made him dizzy and frightened. His balance was so unsteady, even a tap would make him feel as if he would totter and fall.

Desperate to be like other children, he tried to play baseball but consistently dropped the ball. He attempted to play basketball but constantly missed the hoop. When he was 11, he tried to brave a helicopter ride, but as he approached the door he burst into tears. He has never flown in an airplane, fearing that he will faint or fall out.

Noise has always been a calamity. If a dog barked or a truck roared by, he startled and angrily covered his ears and closed his eyes. A hearing exam in second grade diagnosed hyperacuity ("sensitive hearing"). A thud sounds like a grenade and ordinary background conversation like bellowing tumult. If his fiancée, whose voice is pleasant and modulated, speaks animatedly, he snaps at her to stop "yelling," as she is hurting his ears. Even normal voices sound like megaphones and create "static" in his ear. He feels nervous from vibrations, and his "teeth" feel irritated when he hears someone biting or picking her nails. Nor does he like total silence, as he hears a slight ringing in his ear. To sleep at night, he requires the white noise of the air conditioner or fan to distract him from the ringing and from the reverberating sound of his pulse pounding in his neck.

In school, fluorescent lights made him want to close his eyes and go to sleep. Outside, he has always had to wear sunglasses to block out the light, even when the day is overcast. When he has to chase a felon through a store, he experiences tunnel vision and doesn't see anything around him. At this point, his arousal has reached a dangerous level and he has to flip off sensory channels not directly related to sheer survival and shut down.

Too shackled by his sensitivities to enjoy the company of others, he grew up horrifically lonely, with only wooden soldiers to occupy his time. In his early twenties, he met Amelia. Easygoing, warm, and a born caregiver, she made his creature comforts her priority. Initially, he kept her at bay, physically and emotionally, and didn't initiate kissing or even handholding. When she did, he would often draw back. When he finally opened up, he latched on, dependent on her solicitation, encouragement, and reassurance.

Plain and obese, Amelia worried that he found her unattractive. In fact, her size attracted him, as her embrace was enveloping and her heavy movement engendered less light touch. He permitted intimacy—up to a point. When she took his hand or gave him a love tap, he screamed silently inside. When her lips approached his, he would turn his head to the side, and he would roll away from her immediately after sex. If her foot grazed his, he would bridle and retreat tightly into his corner.

The predominant state of the severely defensive vacillates between overload and out-of-control, and relatively little challenge sends them into shutdown. Life can feel an unbearable burden. Generally, the severely defensive are given other diagnoses, like autism, Asperger syndrome (normal and even bright but emotionally deficient and unable to pick up normal social cues), severe developmental delay, schizophrenia, agoraphobia, or borderline personality.[6] Some, though, will be diagnosed only with sensory integration dysfunction and live presumably ordinary lives.

Kayla is married, works, and is going to have a baby. Yet her skin is so sensitive that even taking a shower is agony. The water against her skin, especially her face, feels like daggers and she has to ease in slowly to adjust. "I can't wash my face in the shower. When I shower with my husband, I actually have to turn around and not watch him wash his face because it upsets me so much."

She only has to take a shower once a day. But she has to deal with her hair twenty-four hours a day and this is maddening. No matter how she wears it, every nerve on her scalp feels raw. When anyone or anything touches her hair, she feels as if she's losing her mind. She doesn't share her misery. As far back as she can remember, she has been told that "hair shouldn't bother you." One day, in a fit of rage, she cut it off. "Weightless" and without a mane of protection from the world, she felt perpetually agitated and traumatized. "I was so out of sorts, I couldn't get out of bed, I couldn't sleep, I couldn't get dressed, or take showers. I didn't have the ability to force myself to do what was always so hard for me." She quit her job, and she and her husband moved in with her parents.

She got pregnant and hoped that it would help ease her supersensitivity. But the added weight increased her tactile defensiveness. "I can't stop feeling the extra skin, my thighs rubbing, my breasts touching, my tummy, my hips. It's terrible. It's just like the problem I have with my hair. I just can't stop feeling it." When she felt the fluttering of life, it created an internal tactile defensiveness and she became terrified. Every time it happened, she wanted to cry. She hated not being able to control what was happening inside her own body.

Alice Gerard, a writer, could commiserate. To escape overwhelming sensations, she retreated into a fantasy world. As a child, her mirror image became a friend she could talk to.

> I looked at my mirror image and she looked at me. I talked to
> her. . . . I wondered what her world was like. . . . Did teachers
> honk like geese in her world? Did the screams in the gym class
> bounce off the walls and into her ears? Did snapping gum
> explode like little bombs? Did flying baseballs look like mis-
> siles? How did she feel when her clothing scratched or when
> people brushed up against her little body?[7]

She tried to force herself out in the real world. One night she went on a date to a fund-raiser. But the sound of the speaker's voice over a microphone and people clapping and whistling made her ears feel as if "someone were jabbing at my eardrums with seam rippers" and voices around her became distorted. And the smell of perfumes, aftershave lotions, and stale cigarette smoke started to turn her stomach. She wanted to run out but stood frozen—many people milled around the door and she couldn't get by without someone touching her. Arriving home extremely distressed, she gave in to an urge to flap her hands "as ferociously as possible," which relieved a little tension, a behavior that might seem strange to some, but it was what *her* nervous system demanded. When she awoke the next morning, her ears still hurt, her eyes felt puffy, and she felt too exhausted to get out of bed.

How irritating could another's innocent touch possibly be? Maddeningly so, beyond imagination. Patricia Wilbarger's first adult case was an attractive 21-year-old man who would get into "knock-down fights" any time he was inadvertently touched.[8] One night, he was in a restaurant with his girlfriend. She reached over to tenderly touch his arm. It hit like a lightning bolt. He flew out of his chair, ran into the bathroom, and smashed his fist into the mirror. He was taken to the emergency room and required twenty-six stitches. "What could I say to her?" he thought. "That I was just nuts, that I was crazy? What could I say to myself, that I was psychotic?" For the first time in his life, he felt suicidal.

When someone is this severely tactile-defensive, the need to avoid light touch but seek deep pressure can lead to unusual sexual behavior, such as sexual fetishes and sadomasochism.[9] As tender touch creates agony, and heavy pressure and even pain create ecstasy, some will select abusive mates who will punch them, bite them, pull their hair, and pin them down.

As tactile defensiveness is not widely known or treated, people can make it to old age with severe touchiness. James Hardison, in his book *Let's Touch*, writes about an elderly lady in Chicago, who carried a cane to keep people at bay.

> One of her daughters spoke of occasions when her mother used
> the cane as a shield to keep her two grandchildren from coming
> into contact with her. On no occasion would she allow anyone
> to touch her, even for services like having her hair cut (she did
> it herself) or for medical services; she explained to the doctor
> where the pains were and how they felt in her body, but he was
> never allowed to touch her in an examination.[10]

Perhaps no one is more victimized by sensory defensiveness than the autistic. And though few can communicate well enough to put their experiences into words, Temple Grandin, a remarkable autistic savant who holds a Ph.D. in animal science and teaches at Colorado State University, has broken the autistic barrier to reveal this strange world.

At 6 months, Temple started to stiffen when her mother gathered her into her arms and, a few months later, to claw her "like a trapped animal."[11] At age 2 or 3, her ears felt like "helpless microphones," transmitting everything, regardless of relevance, at full overwhelming volume: a foghorn on a ferry caused excruciating pain; the ringing of the school bell felt like "a dentist drilling down my ear."

Her world was one of heightened, sometimes excruciating, sensations. To escape, she focused her attention on something no one could break into.

> I enjoyed twirling myself around or spinning coins or lids round and round and round. Intensely preoccupied with the movements of the spinning or lid, I saw nothing or heard nothing. People around me were transparent. And no sound intruded on my fixation. It was as if I were deaf. But when I was in a world of people, I was extremely sensitive to noises.[12]

As a little girl, she ached to be loved and cried out for human contact, but she was terrified of engulfment and withdrew from it "in pain and confusion." She dreamed of a magic machine that would embrace her with a gentle but powerful hug but be under her control and command. Later, she invented a squeeze machine, a device that she could crawl into that exerted firm but comfortable pressure on her body, from the shoulders to the knees. "I could satisfy my craving for contact comfort without flooding my senses with massive amounts of input my nervous system couldn't tolerate."[13]

The mildly defensive experience somewhat unstable arousability, get more quickly on edge and, as the day progresses, find it harder to recover until they feel exhausted. The moderately defensive experience more unstable arousability and more quickly ratchet up into overload and exhaustion. The severely defensive experience extreme arousability that precludes comfort and live in a state of overload and shutdown. As arousability becomes increasingly unstable, various forms of psychopathology and disease become increasingly more inevitable. In the next part we look at developmental dynamics that lead to this point.

Part Two

Secondary Effects:
From Dis-ease to Disease

I'm like a cat on a hot tin roof, jumping as soon as my skin
touches a surface. I have felt anxious every moment of my life.

—JOHN

4

Weaving a Web of Fear: Sensory Defensiveness Across the Lifespan

When my body becomes a safer place to live, I will interact with
you differently.

—ROSIE SPIEGEL

How do we know ourselves? There are many ways—by feelings, body sensations, thoughts, relationships.

At the core of psychological health lies a sense of self as complete and viable. Appraising sensations accurately, the normal person maintains a comfortable steady state and regular body rhythms for sleep, rising, eating, eliminating, loving. The ground feels steady beneath his feet, and he moves as a compact presence in the world, freely connecting to the community of others and loving and receiving love. He feels competent to do what he needs to do and in control of his destiny.

At the core of psychopathology lies a sense of the self as incomplete and deficient in any or all of these areas. Sensory defensives experience overarousal, irregular body rhythms, atypical attachments, and a distorted body sense. As the sensations coming from her body overwhelm her ability to cope, she encounters internal chaos when stress threatens. Efforts to connect to the world engender frustration and confusion and render her emotionally and socially powerless. Overwhelming feelings and poor connection to her body and to the world at large create a fragmented self. Her true self is entangled in a defensive cobweb.

From the beginning of life, the infant attempts to ward off the world more than embrace it. By adulthood, this psychological warfare is well entrenched in a highly protective lifestyle that greatly limits normal participation in life.

Inborn Style

Each baby is born with her own style based on how well she organizes sensation. A baby whose nervous system can ingest a wide range of sensation is cheerful, alert, and easy to please: a delight. Resilient, she adapts easily to change, calms herself easily, and recovers quickly from stress. Often these babies love to snuggle, and she will mold her body into yours but not fret when she's put down. Able to maintain optimal arousal, she can fall asleep peacefully in the middle of a thunderstorm. Blessed is she *and* her parents.

A baby whose nervous system cannot easily digest sensation is edgy (most babies fall somewhere in the middle), prone to howling, and slow to calm. He seems content only when held, though he may not be cuddly. He exudes an aura of dissonant tones—hypersensitivity, colic, fussy eating, poor sleeping, poor adaptability, moodiness, and distractibility. Around two-thirds of these infants are shy and inhibited; the other third are crabby but feisty.

Differences in sensory reactivity and recovery from disturbing stimuli are obvious from the start. One of the many behaviors rated on the Brazelton Neonatal Behavioral Assessment Scale (NBAS), an assessment employed in infant development research, is how quickly the newborn habituates to sensation.[1] An examiner will repeatedly shine a flashlight into the newborn's closed eyelids or jingle a bell near his ear until he tunes out the sensation. Some newborns stop responding in two to three trials, some in five or six, while some remain red and squirmy even after nine. The "consolability" part of the examination measures the steps it takes for a crying newborn to quiet. Some remarkably organized newborns will curl up, find their fist, and self-calm. Some need to be swaddled, held, and rocked. Some only become consoled when they are swaddled and left alone, as any stimulus from the environment seems to disturb them. On the "cuddling" test, most infants nestle into your neck as you hold them upright. A tactile-defensive newborn will resist snuggling and stiffen, push away and thrash about. In some, this overreactivity is a temporary response to maternal medication or birth trauma. But if it's still present by two weeks of age, sensory defensiveness can be diagnosed.

For over twenty-five years, Harvard developmental psychologist Jerome Kagan has been studying the highly reactive inhibited child. These cautious, sensitive infants become more easily aroused and distressed by novel stimuli—a stranger coming into the room, a noxious smell—as if any new person or situation were a potential threat.[2] Especially noted is a difference in heart rate. Ordinarily, our heart rate rises and falls slightly as we breathe and speeds up under stress: the faster the heart rate, the less the beat-to-beat variability. From infancy, these inhibited children show a high and invariant heart rate when stressed and even when asleep. In fact, Kagan discovered a correlation between inhibition and fetal heart rate, which was consistently over 140 beats a minute, faster than the heartbeats of other fetuses, and suggests a higher baseline arousal even before birth. These hypersensitive infants don't need to be traumatized to feel afraid. Born with the physiology of an animal under stress, the slightest pressure pushes their fear button. Throughout their lives, they become easily anxious when faced with challenge, depressed from chronic stress, and compulsive to cope. And they are more vulnerable to stress-related disease; for instance, many exhibit allergic reactions starting in infancy (see Chapter 6).

These infants' biochemical reactions show similar vulnerability. Following exposure to stress, inhibited infants show high levels of norepinephrine (the brain's version of adrenaline) in their body fluids and stress hormones like cortisol that activate the amygdala, heightening the senses and putting them on edge. Psychologist Nathan Fox of the University of Maryland has further filled in neurological details to explain this trait. He found that these fearful infants had greater activity on the right side of the brain, where more negative emotions reside. Bold children showed more activity on the left side of the brain, which plays more of a role in positive emotions and an upbeat disposition. These patterns held true not only under stress but even when the children were resting, and continued into adulthood.

Kagan has not investigated tactile defensiveness per se in these inhibited infants. But Steven Suomi of the National Institute of Child Health and Human Development has discovered a correlation between "uptight" monkeys and tactile defensiveness. Suomi bred monkeys to be reactive. By age 2½ years, those who at 1 month showed an accelerated heart rate in anticipation of irritating noise reacted defensively to human handling.[3] The two most tactile-defensive monkeys shared the same father, as did the three least defensive, suggesting a strong genetic link for sensory defensiveness.

Not all infants fuss because they are hypersensitive. Some are excitable and impulsive but underreactive to sensation. However, occupational therapist Georgia DeGangi and colleagues found 87 percent of difficult infants to be hypersensitive to sensory stimuli and show some degree of tactile defensiveness.[4]

The difficulty of the child's behavior increases in proportion to the severity of the defensiveness. The mildly sensory-defensive infant is fussy and moody and has some feeding or sleeping issues but, when comfortable, can be cheerful. As crying is an intense respiratory effort that helps these infants balance their overloaded systems and shut out overwhelming sensory input, colic is common. The moderately defensive infant is highly irritable, cries a great deal, is hard to calm, clings, sleeps poorly, seems often unhappy, and may have more serious feeding problems, like projectile vomiting. The severely defensive infant cries all the time, seems inconsolable, doesn't eat or sleep well, makes poor eye contact, and doesn't thrive. Often these babies look autistic, and some actually are.

If the infant constantly fusses, he will be unable to concentrate on taking in and enjoying his world. "The learning that then takes place," explains occupational therapist Patricia Oetter, "is related to personal comfort and safety, defense, control, survive, demand."[5] Their play might lack joie de vivre, their interactions mutual delight.

Experiencing their world as very stressful, these infants stress their parents. And though colic usually ends at 3 months, symptoms shift over into other systems. The oral-defensive infant will reject solid food and resist weaning. Arousal problems will generate sleep disturbances, fears, and inconsolability. Kagan found that about half of the 4-month-old infants who had overreacted to sensation were still highly fearful at age 2. As adolescents, their heart rate stayed elevated longer when exposed to a harsh smell than that of their more outgoing peers, and they were prone to panic attacks from normal events, like a first date. In moving from sitting to standing, they had larger rises in blood pressure—a sympathetic nervous system response mediated by the vestibular (balance) system.

As these children develop, they become increasingly more sophisticated as escape artists. As infants, self-protection is limited to squirming, arching their backs, stiffening, averting their eyes and turning their heads, or crying. Once the infant can crawl and then toddle, he adds movement to his armament and will move away from people who might come too close or from normal activities that might be messy or loud. This gives him greater control but restricts exploration. These children tend to look for hiding places where they can play alone. The mobile child, however, can also more easily initiate when and where he wants touch, making it more tolerable and even pleasurable.

By the second year, the word "No!" becomes a power tool and the sensory-defensive child may express excessive negativity, explosive behavior, or temper tantrums. Over time, these defensive patterns gel into a template for interacting with the world. By preschool, these often unhappy children may whine, cling, have tantrums, or become aggressive.

Some become more withdrawn as increasingly more sophisticated thinking allows for a larger repertoire of ways to keep people at arm's length. As one women describes her experience, "I tried to become invisible when I was a child. If no one saw me, no one would come up and hug me and I could feel safe. I tried to act like a grown-up so people would feel less of an urge to 'coochie-coo' me. I would situate myself at a distance, like a corner, so people couldn't rub up against me."

A double-edged sword, the child's increasingly more complex strategies for escaping unpleasant sensation enlarge his means of self-protection while at the same time creating ever more defensive armor. Take language. By preschool, language enables the child to effectively convey information to his parents. "I don't want to go to the birthday party. The balloons will burst and hurt my ears." But language also creates anticipatory anxiety, or rumination. The day of the party, the child gets a tummy ache.

The more severe the defensiveness, the better the child becomes at letting the world know how not okay things are, and the shakier his developmental course. How parents interact with the child can increase risk and further destabilize or serve as protection to guide the child down a more stable developmental path.

THE MOTHER-BABY DANCE

Mothering (and fathering) is about touch. As the normal infant reaches out to his world, the parent's tender and reliable cuddle or kiss comforts and encourages the infant to explore the world, confident that should he get in harm's way, loving arms will scoop him up. Trusting that others will care for him when he is in peril lays the foundation for forming healthy human connections and building a viable self.

Also furthering healthy relationships is clear communication between mother and infant. If a baby's nervous system permits engagement with the world, most of the time he will generally convey his needs well enough for his mother to read his cues and satisfy his needs. Thus, the infant receives accurate information about the effects of his behavior: he learns that when he signals a need, he can *expect* a prompt and soothing response. This permits self-efficacy—the feeling that one's actions result in needs being met. As his feelings are accurately responded to, he learns to recognize when he feels angry, sad, or fearful, and to comfortably communicate these feelings. Aware of his own feelings, he responds more empathically to other people, enhancing his relationships. Life is inviting.

The Out-of-Step Baby

With the sensory-defensive infant, the rules change. Rather than do his best to keep his parents close, the infant may inadvertently drive them away.

A loving mother will affectionately rub her infant's head, trace her finger along his brow, and gently kiss his nose, but rather than coo or cuddle, a tactile-defensive infant may fret. Confused, the mother may feel she has to be gentler and inadvertently offer a more light touch, thus exacerbating defensiveness. During diapering and dressing, which often involve light touch, the infant might squirm away and fuss. During bathing, which involves splashing and water that may be too hot or too cold, the infant might scream and flail about.

Oral-defensive infants will fuss during feeding and may reject the mother's breast.[6] Explains Patricia Wilbarger, "They will suck long enough for their blood sugar to rise and to fill their immediate hunger and then they spit out the nipple or breast. An hour later, they're screaming to eat and they seem hungry all the time."[7] Consequently, rather than a time of quiet lingering gazes that fill the heart, feeding becomes a struggle and the mother feels incompetent. At the same time, these infants often dislike rubber bottles or pacifiers and want only the breast—and often. Mothers lose sleep because they need to comfort and feed these infants frequently, and they end up exhausted and at risk for depression.

During ordinary play, which involves light strokes and little pokes, especially from Daddy, defensive infants can get easily overloaded, fussing and looking away, twirling their hair, sucking their thumb, or staring at their feet to reduce sensory input. Or they may look at the parent with a hypervigilant wide-eye stare, which the parent may misinterpret as alertness and desire for more play. Even when content, the facial expressions of sensory-defensive infants are often hard to read. Constantly feeling threatened, their face muscles tend to be tight and they find it harder to smile or convey facial expression.

In an experiment called the "still-faced paradigm," mothers are asked to play normally with their babies for 3 minutes and then change their expression to a flat, impassive look—a "still face"—with no talking or touching. A normal, securely attached baby looks happy and in sync with the mother during the play segment and then looks upset after the mother freezes, as this violates the infant's expectation of the mother's usual warm responsiveness.

But occupational therapist Marie Anzalone found the opposite to be true with a 3-month-old moderately sensory-defensive infant.[8] As the mother chatted and gently touched the baby's face, the infant became disorganized and bounced around jerkily, looking at anything but the mother, and vacillated from crying (overload) to drowsiness (shutting down). When the mother went into a still face and withdrew almost all stimulation, the infant pulled herself together: her body quieted and she smiled and glued her eyes to her mother. Without moving or touching the infant, the mother joyfully smiled back and suddenly this out-of-sync dyad was briefly in a lovely rhythmic dance. "Mother wasn't doing anything wrong," explains Anzalone. "Everything about her was loving, caring, nurturing. But there was no goodness-of-fit that this infant could manage."

To further confuse the mother, the defensive infant's receptivity to sensation varies unpredictably depending on where her biochemistry is. At one time of day, the infant may smile and gurgle during a diaper change; at another, flail and fuss. After a feeding, she might accept the hug, but squirm later when she is tired. How can a mother decipher her baby's needs? How can she know how to make her baby happy? What happens to bonding when frustration rather than enjoyment dominate the mother-and-baby interaction?

When a mother can't discern her baby's cues, she can easily misinterpret his needs and respond inappropriately: feeding a tired infant; putting a hungry one to sleep. She may ignore his cries. As she sometimes soothes her infant and sometimes not, the infant is unable to predict comfort. Confused, he feels a desire for closeness to the good, loving mother but anger toward the mother who misunderstands his needs. An infant may toddle to his mother to be picked up, but then he will angrily arch away from her body, demanding to be put down and seemingly inconsolable. Unable to derive comfort from Mother, the child cries angrily for long periods, sometimes hitting and kicking in frustration. Both the infant's expectation of comfort and the mother's need to provide that comfort get violated.

To those who study attachment, the child's ambivalence and fussiness are viewed primarily as a response to a moody and erratic mother. But tactile defensiveness can invoke the same pulling back and inconsolability; maternal inconsistency can be the result, not the cause, of the infant's behavior.

Caring for defensive children stresses the parent in other ways that can create inconsistency. As the infant's range of optimal arousal is narrow, parents must work hard to provide the right sensory input for play, feeding, diapering, and sleep. To reduce threat, the parent might take the long route to the supermarket rather than the noisy highway or wash the new jeans twenty times before the child tries them on. Since change will throw these children, these parents must provide constant predictability or spend their days putting out fires. Says one, "If the bagel is toasted too much or not enough, my daughter has a fit." As parents are not always in the mood to meet these demands, especially if they are under stress, lacking sufficient supports, or inexperienced, they can feel victimized by their child's whims and become resentful.[9]

The constant fussiness of these infants also puts them at risk for rejection. If a mother can't stop her baby from crying, she will feel her baby doesn't like her and she will hold the baby less and with less warmth and affection. The oversensitive infant picks up on this and becomes distressed by cues of anger and disapproval, like a mother's frowning face. Perceiving the mother as rejecting, the infant begins to withdraw, which further increases the mother's feelings of rejection and ineptness; the cycle continues. In the face of a consistently emotionally unavailable mother, the infant is in a constant state of despair. To cope, she learns to inhibit her need for comfort and becomes emotionally detached. She grows up seemingly independent, but inside feels empty and starved for human connection.

Fortunately, insecure attachment is not irreversible. If a mother can understand and empathize with the infant, she will eventually catch on to the signals. She will hug a child when he wants to be hugged and back off if a child signals "don't touch," though it breaks her heart. She will learn to refrain from touching the child with light, tickling touch; not wash or cut her hair often; buy soft fabrics and cut out labels; turn socks inside out; and allow the child to saunter about without shoes and hats.

As children get older, when attachment relies less on the embrace than on a warm smile or kind word, even the moderate to severely defensive child will look securely attached to an emotionally available mother. They may not want to be touched, but if they can feel confident of their mother as protector, they will turn to her unhesitantly when life becomes too much. Deborah, an occupational therapist, and her two children, ages 4 and 7, are all sensory-defensive. Yet Deborah is a loving mother with apparently normal, though overactive, happy children. Having given herself a proper sensory diet, Deborah has her defensiveness under control most of the time and is patient and warm with her children. The children's defensiveness, in turn, is helped by a strict home sensory diet and occupational therapy three times a week. There's lots of laughing, smiling, sharing, *and* loving touch, though the uninitiated can't detect that even the love pats are deliberately firm.

Because of Deborah's constant hard work in managing her own and her children's defensiveness, these children can more easily know the solace of their mother's body. As such, they will feel better about being inside their *own* bodies.

Mother's Rhythms

All feeling starts with body sensations: feeling happy is directly proportionate to how good it feels to be inside one's body. This begins with the mother's body, inside her womb and outside in her arms.

The human infant is born the least mature of all mammals. The mother's body provides sensory qualities to continually balance her infant's physiology. What seems like a simple caregiving function, like rocking the infant, provides touch, warmth, movement, smells, sounds, and the sight of the mother's face—all helping to organize the infant's rhythms, its regular heartbeat and breathing, smooth, quiet body movements, body temperature control, ease of digestion. If the newborn is cold, the mother's body temperature rises to provide warmth. If the infant is hot, the mother's body temperature cools. When the infant's body reaches thermoregularity, the mother's temperature returns to baseline.[10] Apart, the young infant loses this primary source of stability and must struggle alone to maintain physiological harmony. The longer the separation, the quicker the infant plunges into body disarray.

The less regulated the infant's body rhythms, the more the child depends on the mother's body to calibrate his physiology. Ironically, the more a sensory-defensive infant squirms away from his mother, the more anxious he feels and the more he depends on his mother's organizing touch for self-regulation. When separated, the child feels boundless, as if nothing holds him, and becomes alarmed and often inconsolable. Thus, the sensory-defensive infant may protest even more when put down than when cuddled.

Does the mother calmly quiet the child? Or does his distress make her too jumpy to do so? The answer to how she reacts can be the sensory-defensive infant's saving grace or spiraling downfall.

The Calm Mother

A mother who remains calm in the face of the storm will pick up the wailing infant and hold him firmly to her chest, where the infant will feel the mother's slow, steady heartbeat. She sways the infant slowly and rhythmically at a beat that unknowingly matches her resting heart rate. "Entraining," or getting in sync with the mother's rhythmic movement and her slower heartbeat, the infant becomes programmed to these regular rhythms and eventually calms. Researcher Tiffany Field found that even when a mother and her infant or toddler are not in physical contact, they often have synchronized heart rates.[11]

When a nervous system matures in a low-key, protective environment, the mother offers an external order, or scaffolding, that teaches the defensive child how to independently manage some physiologic rhythms to buffer his overreactivity. Research shows that if you place a "breathing bear" set at a normal neonatal rate inside the incubator of a premature infant, it will scoot over to the bear and soon start to entrain to the bear's rhythms.[12] Before long it is breathing at a more normal rate, developing better respiration and sleeping more quietly.

After countless occasions of maternal comfort, the infant learns to self-calm, reducing internal emotional pressure and presumably building more little branches in the brain for handling adversity. Better able to regroup in the face of stress, the defensive child becomes more resilient to its degenerative influence. When uncertain or insecure, he moves in close to his trusted attachment figure, retreats into safety, or cautiously observes until the unfamiliar is deemed safe. Sensory defensiveness becomes more manageable.

In a compelling experiment conducted by Steven Suomi, nervous monkeys reared by a bold, easygoing, exceptionally nurturant foster mother took on her easygoing ways and even her low-norepinephrine (one of the chemicals released during stress) chemistry.[13]

Jerome Kagan found that in a group of highly reactive inhibited children, a third to half of them had lost their basic shyness by age 7. The ones who learned how to cope with mild anxiety and frustration tended to have mothers who scaffolded their children's environment but at the same time gently prodded their children to explore new people and situations. Apparently, these mothers did not overreact to their children's fears, thereby broadening the child's safety net and permitting them a greater range of exploration. This greater exploration in turn fed their nervous system with organizing proprioceptive and vestibular stimulation, emhancing sensory integration and healthier development. But parental influence was not enough to change the inhibition of those with the highest heart rates in infancy, suggesting more severe sensory defensiveness. These children remained in a constant state of high arousal, with high levels of stress hormones and a high and invariant heart rate.

Having internalized the benefits of good mothering, many sensory-defensives later marry patient, understanding people who learn to modify their behavior accordingly. As authors Thomas Lewis, Fari Amini, and Richard Lannon sum up in *A General Theory of Love*, "Stability means finding people who regulate you well and staying near them."[14]

The Nervous Mother

But what happens when the mother's body does not offer this stability? Like a lifeguard who can't swim, the unstable mother's efforts to save her sensory-defensive child from chaos often backfires. When her infant cries, the body of the anxious mother tenses up. Frantic, she shakes, pats, and rocks her infant in a rhythmic reflection of the baby's distress, matched by a verbal torrent: "Sh! Sh! Sh! Sh!" Entraining to these faster, discordant rhythms, the infant's system speeds up and the infant cries harder, making mother and infant feel increasingly more anxious. Calming the infant can take forever until both get exhausted from the effort.

The more the mother's ministrations create intolerable overarousal and unrelieved tension, the more the infant feels helpless—in effect, punished for asking for help. The infant comes to associate closeness with discomfort rather than solace, intensifying or even creating socially mediated tactile defensiveness. The more unrelieved his tension, the more he grows up feeling unworthy of help and comfort, and the more his core experience becomes one of depression, unmanageable anxiety, frustration, and anger.

How does the infant protect against unremitting distress? He behaves to reduce contact by dampening the display of discomfort; over the first year, he expresses anxiety less and less. By the second year, this pattern is well entrenched. Except under extreme circumstances he exhibits only muted distress and anger.[15] If overloaded during play, the infant may squirm, look away, and kick the chair but not cry or flail. If the mother misses these cues and, feeling snubbed by her infant, intensifies stimulation to engage him, she further overstimulates the baby, who may now openly fuss.

A nervous mother interferes with development in other ways. Falsely perceiving the environment as threatening, she will overreact protectively: "No! You'll hurt yourself!" A bold child may disregard her hysteria, but a vulnerable child becomes more frightened. This can limit normal activity that helps organize the nervous system, like climbing out of the crib or up and down stairs. The mother's excitability further hypes up her child, intensifying defensiveness and a perception of the world as dangerous. Overprotected, misunderstood, and feeling constantly vulnerable, the child might react with helpless dependence, defiant misbehavior, or both.[16]

If the infant's distress does not get buffered, the stress hormone cortisol pours through the bloodstream regularly. Brain researchers in child development have discovered this constant infusion to eat away at pathways for handling stress. It increases especially in the area in the brain involved in vigilance and arousal, and so sensory-defensive and abused children are on continual alert. As the system is so revved up, it no longer responds to ordinary forms of regulation, and the slightest stress can trigger an out-pouring of stress hormones. Such reactivity persists into adulthood. A minor stressor sets the system fluttering with anxiety, while a larger or longer one plunges the person into depression—psychological shutdown.

As stress activates the attachment system and as these unstable children depend on something external to steady them, they will look to the attachment figure for protection, even if severely defensive or severely abused. They cope by staying close enough for protection but far enough away to avoid intimacy.[17] Lost in a sea of chaos, they experience life as an ongoing, often fruitless quest for an external anchor.

THE MELODY LINGERS

What happens during infancy leaves an indelible mark that gets stored in the crevices of our psyche and plays out repeatedly in profound and unsuspected ways. Memory is not just cognitive and emotional. Sensitivity, or the memory of the body, is more primitive and, unlike incidents that we "remember," always true.

In his book *Touching*, Ashley Montagu relates the story of a 2½-year-old child who had been referred to psychiatrist Philip Seitz for pathological hair pulling that appeared with the onset of a punitive toilet-training program. While drinking from her bottle, the child would pull out some hairs from her head and roll them up against her lip and nose.

Perhaps, thought Dr. Seitz, the child had once been nursed and the mother's nipple was surrounded by hair. This behavior would then be an attempt to re-create this early experience.

Indeed the child was nursed—but only the first two weeks of her life! How could she have "remembered" the experience two and a half years later? What was remembered was not the actual episode—early memories are not stored in a verbal filing system so they cannot be verbally retrieved. The memory is implicit—sensory impressions like the taste, feel, shape, contour of the breast and the nipple, and the tactile sensation of the mother's coarse hair against the baby's face. Later, to re-create the comfort, the child tried to re-create these sensations. When she matured, she may have found herself attracted to men with beards and hairy chests. Why, she couldn't have said.

Memory gets stored as a few prototypes in our brain: mother/loving; father/adoring; brothers/fun; teachers/bossy. As experiences repeat, the brain unconsciously extracts the rules that underlie them. When a baby cries and a mother's arms generally quell, the archetype imprinted in the brain is one of a mother who brings sensations of warmth and calming envelopment, happiness and solicitude. Similar situations jiggle this perception, and later we perceive loved ones as protective, concerned, and relaxed and look for those who match our expectations.

When a baby cries and the mother's presence brings increased distress, for whatever reason, the child unwittingly memorizes a different script: those who love you get uncomfortably close, make you angry, tense, anxious, and uncomfortably dependent, or any number of crippling scenarios. If our mind did not create similar scenic structures for our stories, changed here and there by adding or removing props and dialogue, we would live in chaos, as we would be continually constructing reality anew. As subtle changes accumulate, experience rewires the structure of the brain: the more meaningful the experience, the more indelible the imprint and the less amenable to change. Trauma gets burned deep into the brain.

Each part of the body has its own memories—the infant's cheek against the mother's warm breast; the schoolchild's cheek slapped. These memories are recorded not just in our minds but in the cells of our body and can remain locked in for years: unknowingly, memory's ghosts trample us.

Brain researchers such as Candace Pert at Georgetown University School of Medicine have discovered receptor sites for neuropeptides (brain chemicals) that reveal the "brain" and its functions, including our emotions, to be actually located all over the body. Functioning as messengers between cells and various organs and other mechanisms in the body such as the immune, endocrine, and gastrointestinal systems, these neuropeptides, or "molecules of emotion" create a transit system to and from the brain to systems throughout the body and form a dynamic information network.[18] "The body is the unconscious mind!" asserts Pert. High concentrations of almost every neuropeptide receptor exist in locations such as the dorsal horn, or back side of the spinal cord, the first synapse within the nervous system to process all somatosensory information. In the sensory defensive, even innocent memories get stored throughout the body as trauma—like your grandmother lovingly combing your hair into banana curls or your father running his fingernail down your back.[19] Later, dating and sexual experiences can get lodged in the cells as trauma.

Anything that reminds you of the traumatic memory trips the alarm system in the brain and anxiety, fear, or terror floods the body. Subjected to painful medical procedures like heel sticks and insertion of feeding tubes, premature infants are at risk for tactile defensiveness and some will grow up with various parts of the body extremely tactile-defensive.[20] One man born prematurely could never stand his feet to touch any surface. He stands on a terrycloth towel while taking a shower and always wears socks. Nor could he stand his chest being touched, where he had a chest tube inserted during newborn hospitalization. He overreacts to noise as well, possibly as a result of his days in the loud newborn intensive care unit.

Memory gets laid down even before birth, as the fetus entrains to maternal rhythms. If the fetus has a reactive nervous system and a higher heart rate, the fetus will become agitated every time the mother's heart spikes. If you have a nervous mother, you have a nervous, traumatized fetus. Even the environment inside the mother's protective belly can be too stimulating, as Sonya discovered.

Swinging back and forth on a glider swing during an occupational therapy session, she listened to *Chakra Chants* by Jonathan Goldman. Chakras are what some believe to be auras or whirling vortices of colored light in the electromagnetic field around your body that converge at seven major points: sacrum, belly, solar plexus, heart, throat, brow, and crown of the head. When the music got to the heart chakra, Sonya complained that the "drums" were pounding her head like hammers, suggesting a primitive experience of the heartbeat as stressful.

Her sensory defensiveness began in the womb, either created or exacerbated by her mother's erratic physiology. All her life she recoiled from her mother's nervous screaming and could not tolerate to be near her, repelled by the touch of her body. Love begins with sensory compatibility.

DISCONNECTED FROM ONE'S BODY

Our "sense" of self starts with body awareness—what the body does, how it feels, and the knowledge that it belongs to us.[21] Through the felt presence of another, the infant becomes aware of her body's boundaries: she learns that her fingers feel differently in her mouth than in Daddy's mouth. This enables her to differentiate "me" from "not me" and to know where she begins and ends in space, encouraging a greater awareness of her body—proprioception.

The more time spent in her mother's arms, the more the infant experiences another human being and receives sensory stimulation to develop her body map. In *The Natural History of the Senses*, poet Diane Ackerman writes, "Touch teaches us that life has depth and contour; it makes our sense of the world and ourselves three-dimensional."[22] The more solid the child's body sense, the more solid her sense of self, and she grows up to feel attractive, close to others, and endowed with a healthy sexual identity.

But what if normal touch sensation feels uncomfortable and the infant rejects certain tactile experiences, even subtly? She fails to receive adequate tactile and proprioceptive information to feel connected with, and get a sense of, her body and lacks a well-developed body map. Thus, she "loses touch" with her body and grows up not feeling grounded, or "inside" her body. When tension rises, she feels easily "out of it," as if in orbit, and loses her sense of time and space. (Think how foreign your body feels when you get a shot of novacaine or your foot starts to fall asleep.) As one woman describes, "I feel completely unconnected to my body, like I'm floating. Some times are worse than others, but its always there and always has been. I used to stare at myself in the mirror when I was little and try to get all the way out of me."

What does feeling grounded mean? To find out, try this exercise offered by Alexander Lowen, the creator of bioenergetics. Stand with your feet about 8 inches apart, knees slightly bent, and reach out as if to shake someone's hand. Now press the corresponding foot into the ground and lean forward slightly as you extend your arm. You will feel the movement extending from the ground up through your arm and a lifting and elongating through your central axis. This whole body connection gives you a sense of self as whole and present.

To feel more whole and solidly in touch with her body, a tactile-defensive person needs constant weight against her body and seeks the other to define her edges: as a child she clings; as an adult, she looks for the perfect lap to curl into.

To get pressure, children may use rough-and-tumble play: the loving hug becomes an aggressive bear hug, the embrace a wrestling match. The tactile-defensive adolescent may engage in contact sports, such as wrestling and football, or even in self-injury, such as cutting or burning the skin, or become sexually promiscuous. At the same time, poor body awareness inhibits them from moving comfortably in a sexual way or expressing sexual signals in a relaxed manner. They may be unaware of their sexual appeal. "When I was young and thin, with my large bust," says one woman, "I had no idea that I turned men on. I didn't even think about sex. I couldn't 'see' what I really looked like." Nor will the oversized clothes many tactile defensives wear impart evidence of desire.

When they don't have weight against their skin, defensives feel constant skin hunger—an "unbearable lightness of being." Lamented poet Rod McKuen, "The need to touch someone can be so great at times that it's as close to madness as I ever hope to come."[23] For Marla, skin hunger becomes actual pain.

> I feel constant sensations on my skin like tingling or like there's something crawling under my skin, though I can't say that it literally feels this way. If I go too long without being held, I physically feel pain. Often, I feel like tearing off my own skin. Sometimes I think that this is just all in my head, because others may feel the same things that I do, but I just handle it worse. But I've been told that it is indeed not normal to feel like something is crawling in your skin.

Yet, defensives feel compelled to erect a mental suit of armor to protect people from violating their tenuous space. Life is constant irony.

The drive to establish boundaries may even motivate repeated pregnancies. The fetus filling the empty belly with deep pressure and extra weight offers proprioceptive input to the hips, knees, and ankles, and many sensory-defensive women report feeling more in touch with their body during pregnancy. Some don't want the pregnancy to end.

DISCONNECTED FROM ONE'S FEELINGS

To feel belonging—to a partner, a family, friends, a community, and a higher being, whether the divine or nature—is a basic and essential need. To feel different creates alienation. "I've never been able to speak to anyone about my hypersensitivity," said one woman. "I thought I was the only one to feel this way."

The young egocentric child assumes that everyone is like him. If the tactile-defensive child hates to wear woolen mittens, he assumes that is so for all other children. The more he interacts with peers, the more he realizes that few share his feelings about the world and the odder he feels. He doesn't know how to process why he is different or explain his idiosyncratic behaviors, like having to sleep wrapped like a mummy in a sleeping bag. By the time he is school age, he starts to think, "I'm weird." Language reflects defensiveness: "I don't want to," "I can't," "I shouldn't."

If a parent understands and accepts the child's feelings, the child feels affirmed and better able to cope with being an outsider. To the teachers and professionals in her school, the behavior of severely sensory-defensive Alice Gerard seemed strange; at one point, a psychiatrist diagnosed her as psychotic.[24] But to her parents, Alice's fantasies and odd behavior were a sign of being bright, inventive, and unique. In spite of not fitting in, she prevailed and went on to use her enormously imaginative mind to become a writer.

Not all parents empathize as did Alice's. Research has found that mothers tend to underestimate their children's tactile defensiveness.[25] Some will even ridicule the child for refusing to eat the "mushy" pudding or wear the "itchy" new dress. Clicking their tongue or rolling their eyes, they make comments like, "Stop being so finicky," "You're too sensitive," "Why do you have to be so difficult?" They will tell their child to "Just ignore it" or assume the child is being lazy or stubborn or dramatic. They may punish the child. Consequently, the child too may assume her feelings are not real and deny them. "So many people got mad at me for so many things," says one woman. "They thought my sensitivities were in my imagination. So I did too. Thank God it's not only me."

In school, children might feel similarly misunderstood. For instance, a child may tell his teacher that he can't concentrate on his work because the ceiling fan is too noisy and be accused to trying to get out of work. "None of the other children are complaining," says the teacher. Such misunderstanding increases their sense of being strange and an outcast. They learn that their feelings, fierce and inarticulate, are an oddity that should be hidden, lest others see how crazy they are. They cope by learning to deny and ignore uncomfortable sadness, distress, anxiety, and hurt and to falsify display of feelings to please others. Hiding feelings helps them to fit into the crowd better, but further reduces another person's ability to read and know them. As they may also be too overwhelmed to pick up facial expressions, they may not easily read others' cues, further interfering with their ability to relate to others. Unlikely to find many kindred spirits, they grow up feeling inauthentic, crazy, and painfully alone. "I feel I must be wrong to feel this way," says Daria. "Or maybe everyone feels like this and doesn't talk about it! I think, 'Be quiet, you're so annoying to everyone. Stop saying ouch when someone bumps you, stop saying you don't feel well. You're fine. You're exaggerating.' And then I feel really alone."

This flawed perception of self peaks in adolescence, when fitting in with the crowd takes priority and kids are supposed to enjoy dating, parties, football games, and going to the mall and they wonder why *they* don't—why everything makes them feel uncomfortable, overwhelmed, overexcited, overloaded. How do they explain to friends that dating means discomforting eye contact, distasteful odors, uncomfortable touching, and emotions crazily out of control? That going to the disco means loud music, crammed dance floors, and the uncomfortable closeness of slow dancing? That going to the pizza parlor means being squished in a car or a restaurant booth? Even worse, how do they tell *themselves* why they are different from other adolescents? Interactions often feel like a lesson in managing anxiety.

To feel more like others, the teen might go to the party. But as he enters the door, his body says, "Beware," and he focuses his mind on the emergency exit. Overloaded and horrifically uncomfortable, he converses with a pasted smile, hunched body, and uncomfortable stare. His laughter is frantic, his movements jerky. Rushes of heat or cold or goose bumps unrelated to the outside temperature and waves of tingling or buzzing may permeate his body. Slowly he gravitates to a corner and glues his back to the wall, where he safely observes with despair "normal" people laughing, touching, and flirting. The contrast between his discomfort and the enjoyment of other people intensifies his feeling of being an outsider. Here's how Holly describes it: "Being and doing things out in the world reminds me of how different I am. Checking out the personal ads—'normal' people—who they are, what they're looking for, things they like to do—nothing like me. Meeting new people, going on dates, trying to be normal, do normal things; it doesn't work—just reminds me how different I really am."

Unable to sort out intense and confusing feelings and exhausted at the effort of trying to fit in, many defensive teens become reclusive and look for hiding places. Some will fall into books like Alice falling down the rabbit hole, which shuts out the peripheral world in a socially accepted way. Few date. If they get involved, it tends to be with a sympathetic person that they've first gotten to know casually.

By adulthood, denying their feelings, while feeling acutely uncomfortable and crazy, is deeply ingrained, and defensives learn to pretend that all is okay long enough for social acceptance.

They put great energy into developing strategies to not give themselves away. To defend against inadequacy, they may shift blame to others. To avoid socializing, they may throw themselves into work or a project. To get other people to accept their idiosyncrasies, they may become self-effacing and be the first to laugh at their finicky ways or spacey behavior. To compensate for feeling inherently flawed and to hide their terror, they may put on a cloak of perfection, arrogance, or super strength. "When I think of doing something where I have to endure unwanted sensory invasion, I get a sinking in my stomach bordering on nausea and anxiety, and then I get angry," says Mandy. "I walk around afraid all the time. But I hide it and show overconfidence, perfectionism, and strength, when that is the last thing I am really feeling. Even antidepressants and anti-anxiety medications cannot relieve the feelings entirely. I have spent half my life waiting for the men in the white jackets to come to take me away." Some become overly apologetic for their complaining or refusals. Others let their annoyances slide and hesitate to complain to the dentist about getting zapped simultaneously by the drill and Led Zeppelin. Such effort at pretense is exhausting.

Years of ongoing bodily upheaval have taken their toll, and recuperating from stress becomes increasingly harder; these sufferers get quickly saturated and run out of steam. As most have children, spouses, and jobs, they push beyond their limit and further deplete their system. Or they become spoilsports, leaving the party early, and feel like a disappointment to loved ones. Says Millie, "Getting together with my family is hard because they all think I'm antisocial, or a snob because it's exhausting just to talk. Lots of people think I am unfriendly, or angry or a party pooper when I want to leave early because it's hard for me to communicate with new people or in crowds. I just get too overwhelmed."

As they are productive at times, family and friends find it hard to understand why they can't work, clean the house, go shopping, or go to the movies. Life is filled with false accusations of thoughtlessness and laziness that few perceive as symptoms of defensiveness.

Defensives too don't know why they can't meet their responsibilities. They may perceive their impatience with their children as bad parenting rather than an intolerance for noise and mess. They may perceive their dislike of housework as a basic character flaw rather than a dislike of the feel of dirt or grease. "Do I dislike doing the dishes because it's boring," wonders Pamona, "or because I don't like the feeling of getting my hands wet and the irritating smell of the dishwashing soap? Do I not vacuum often because I'm lazy or because I can't stand the sound of the vacuum cleaner? Is my house messy because I won't take the time to clean or because I'm too tired, having used up all my energy and resources just to make it through the day?"

Because their feelings have not been affirmed, they mistake their own intentions. They assume they can't get close to others because they are uncaring. They think that they don't want to take their children to the amusement park because they are selfish. They believe they are always late because they are inconsiderate.

This estrangement from self is further intensified by constantly changing moods and a varying level of comfort with each person that makes them feel different in each interaction—fragmented. To get people to finally understand and validate their feelings, giving them a desperately needed connection to others, and to strengthen their identity, they may spend much time explaining themselves, which other people find tedious and narcissistic.

Sensory defensiveness often begins at birth. Throughout development, it steadily robs the individual of a sense of self, disrupts personal relationships, distorts body image, and makes one feel powerless and out of control. The result is social and emotional dysfunction.

5

From Anxiety to Addictions

> It is a pity that just the excellent personalities suffer most from
> the adverse effects of the atmosphere.
>
> —GOETHE

The latest edition of *The Diagnostic and Statistical Manual of Mental Disorders* (DSM-IV-TR, 2000) of the American Psychiatric Association lists over a dozen major disorders relating to anxiety. Sensory defensiveness is not one of them. It is neither recognized as a condition that leads to excessive stress and anxiety nor as a cause of psychopathology. Yet problems with sensory modulation, from sensory defensiveness to sensory seeking, might underlie much of what appears to be psychological at root.[1] Perhaps one day in some future edition, *sensory affective disorder* will be added to the list.

Sensory defensiveness creates *anxiety*, intensifies unpleasant emotions, exacerbates stress, and leads to extreme and often uncontrollable behavior.[2,3] If you're constantly anxious, you cope poorly with stress and with life transitions, such as marriage, divorce, childbirth, changing jobs, and so on, and suffer an *adjustment disorder*.

Poor vestibular functioning causes many sensory defensives to experience some degree of vertigo and disorientation and mild anxiety can erupt into intense fear, or total *panic*. If sensory defensiveness becomes severe, touch, loud noises, or bright lights will trigger panic

Some sufferers will experience panic on an ongoing basis and bury themselves in their homes. They have become *agoraphobic*, a serious disorder in which the person fears harm in open space, away from the security of the home and a safe person. Sensory defensives can also become reclusive because the home is the only place where they can reasonably control sensory input, and as a result they appear agoraphobic when they are not. In fact, the two disorders share many behaviors in common. For instance, to insure a quick escape in case of panic and to prevent loss of control, agoraphobics sit in aisle seats in theaters or churches; the sensory defensive do so to avoid closeness and other unpleasant sensations. Both drive down deserted streets at odd hours to avoid traffic and seek out all-night stores to avoid standing in line; the agoraphobic do so to flee faster, and the sensory defensive to control noise, traffic, or a stranger's touch.

As glaring light, overstimulating eye contact, sudden touch, and other people's odors overwhelm the sensory defensive, they disengage from social contact and appear to be *socially phobic*. Expressing a desire for affection, acceptance, and friendship, while having few friends and sharing little intimacy, many might be labeled *avoidant personalities*.

As the sensory defensive feel victimized by sensations they cannot control, they go overboard trying to control what they can. Their rigid behavior, along with compulsive eating, shopping, sex, and so on, predispose them to an *obsessive-compulsive personality* style. Acutely bothered by certain sensations, some will wash their hands constantly, wear gloves when preparing meals, and obsess over getting dirty, suggesting *obsessive-compulsive disorder* (OCD), a serious and debilitating condition. Other behavior can mimic OCD. For instance, the sensory defensive might engage in rituals, like repetitive rocking or counting, as a distraction. The repetitive, rhythmic behavior might lower their arousal enough that whatever else is going on doesn't come in with such intensity; repetition also boosts levels of serotonin in the brain, regulating their mood and balancing their neurochemistry. Rocking four hours a day but unable to convince her parents to take her for an occupational therapy evaluation, one teenager made the rounds from psychiatrists to neurologists, all convinced that she had OCD and insisting she be put on medication. She reluctantly agreed but the rocking continued unabated.

To create a steady flow of pleasurable vibes and to blunt feelings of tension, anxiety, and frustration, some develop *addictions* to controlled substances, like alcohol or tranquilizers.

Loneliness, anxiety, extreme fatigue, sleep problems, and lack of human affection set up *depression*, as does learned helplessness, the passive resignation that what you go for you don't get, so why bother. And the extreme stress associated with sensory defensiveness depletes serotonin. Marked shifts in mood, impulsive and unpredictable behavior, and great difficulty in personal relationships, which are often transitory, have earned many sensory-defensives the diagnosis of *borderline personality*.

Refusing to get dressed or unintentionally punching someone who bumps into him, the tactile-defensive child will demonstrate wild mood swings and unpredictable *aggression*, and might get diagnosed with *oppositional defiant disorder.* Tactile defensiveness resulting from physical or sexual abuse contributes to the tendency of some victims to become *violent.* Prison inmates with histories of violent crimes accuse others of being "in their faces," and "crowding" them at distances most people consider acceptable and unthreatening.

When life inside one's body becomes unbearable, sensory defensives shut out the world and *depersonalize*. Some even *dissociate*, which entails loss of memory, as in amnesia or multiple personality disorder.

When anxiety, panic, depression, isolation, and bodily upheaval reach intolerable proportions and feel beyond control, some sufferers contemplate and commit *suicide*.

Let's look more closely at how sensory defensiveness might underlie some of these psychological disorders.

GENERAL ANXIETY DISORDER

A successful model since adolescence, tall, blond, and lanky, 38-year-old Jackie is warm and friendly. She seems to have it all. But when you talk to her, you notice a wariness: a body hugged tight into a ball, a cautious smile, averted eyes.

Moody and on edge, she worries about seemingly silly things. When taking an escalator, "I obsess over falling or tripping. I imagine the escalator opening up and chewing up my leg." When sitting in night class, she worries that her mind will blank out when she takes a test, even though she studies hard and usually gets A's.

As a small child, she couldn't sleep and would often awaken from a nightmare that a million coins covered her body, weighing it down. Only her head was free. Lately she's been having panic attacks out of nowhere in which her heart pounds and she feels unable to breathe, though they are brief and relatively mild.

From morning to night, anxiety, stress, and worry rule Jackie's life. According to DSM-IV, her symptoms indicate generalized anxiety disorder (GAD), which is characterized by muscle tension, fidgeting and restlessness, irritability and perhaps angry outbursts, sleep difficulties, concentration difficulties, and fatigue. People with GAD experience some combination of sweating, dizziness, pounding or racing heart, hot or cold spells, cold and clammy hands, upset stomach, lightheadedness, frequent urination or defecation, lump in the throat, high pulse, and fast breathing. They worry about the future, people close to them, and even their valued possessions. Hyperaroused, they constantly scan the environment for danger, get easily distracted, and have problems falling asleep.

Sounds a lot like sensory defensiveness. In fact, a sensory intake might reveal that sensory processing is the trigger for GAD in some cases. Jackie is one example.

The weight in her dreams was the unbearable pressure of the sheets and blankets against her body—tactile defensiveness. Her fear of taking an escalator comes from feeling off balance—movement defensiveness—which likely triggers her panic attacks as well. Her worry about blanking out while taking a test appears triggered by the glare of the overhead, fluorescent lights—visual defensiveness. Bright light "shoots" into her light blue eyes, especially when she feels stressed. Momentarily unable to see clearly, she can't make sense of things and "freaks" out.

Yet, most clinicians would not consider sensory processing when assessing Jackie. The recommended treatment would be cognitive-behavioral therapy to work on her negative thought patterns, along with an anti-anxiety drug like BuSpar to calm her. This therapy might desensitize her fears, and she could learn to not let panic get out of control, but it would do little to stop her from startling each time she hears a loud noise or squirming from unexpected touch. Nor would it enlighten her as to *why* she overreacts.

Is Jackie's case unique or could sensory defensiveness underlie an untold number of cases of ongoing anxiety and worry? As sensory defensiveness has not been well researched, we can only speculate. But if someone does not respond well to drugs, or talk or cognitive therapy, the problem could be sensory based and should be dealt with for any lasting improvement.

Anxiety is defined as a state of unpleasant emotions, physiological stress, and thoughts of apprehension, guilt, and impending doom. It covers a broad range of symptoms that look a lot like sensory defensiveness. Yet there are clear distinctions between the two.

Thought or socially mediated anxiety is cortex-based, meaning it refers to highly evolved, complex, human thinking, and starts from a thought (conscious or unconscious) that elicits dread and psychic terror. The brain negatively appraises an event. This produces overarousal and leads to flight, fight, or freeze symptoms that encompass bodily distress, anxious thoughts, and feelings of dread: you are in a crowd; you worry that someone might grab your wallet or push you off the curb; you get hyped and, body and mind running wild, take flight. As the defensive response notches up sensitivity, everyone under stress experiences increased tactile sensitivity. But the sensitivity is a *result* of anxious thoughts, not the *cause*, and psychotropic medication or therapy alleviates the symptoms.

Sensory defensiveness, which is brainstem-based, meaning it refers to reflexes and instinctive reactions, starts from bodily sensation, triggered from external or internal stimuli. Overaroused, you feel your body tense up as the person in the crowd swipes past you. This leads to flight, fight, or freeze behaviors and ends with an appraisal of the threat: "Crowds make me jumpy." As thoughts of dread don't necessarily accompany the experience, your body can be jumpy from overwhelming stimulation, but your mood may be upbeat if you are at a concert of your favorite band, for example. Occupational therapy and sensorimotor activities such as skin brushing or jumping on a trampoline reduce the defensiveness, while anti-anxiety medication may make barely a dent. "The nerve attacks, complete with pounding heart, dry mouth, sweaty palms, and twitching legs, had the symptoms of 'stage fright,' but were actually more like hypersensitivity than anxiety," writes Temple Grandin. "Perhaps this accounts for the fact that Librium and Valium did not provide relief to my trembling body."[4]

Both sensory defensiveness and mental anxiety can look, and in some ways feel, the same because both are a stress response that create sympathetic nervous system arousal, edginess, difficulty concentrating, hypervigilance, avoidance, and lack of control.[5] And both have vulnerability at the core.

When a situation both overstimulates and elicits dread, sensory defensiveness and mental anxiety interact and become indistinguishable. For instance, your boss, wishing to speak to you about your tardiness, beckons you into her cluttered, smoky office. Or you panic when someone touches your highly sensitive neck.

Sometimes the feeling of overstimulation includes genital overexcitement in nonsexual situations, as with a parent, a sibling, or a friend, and this elicits terror. Sufferers describe themselves as not feeling sexual desire but more like prepubertal genital arousal, perhaps initially set off by a seductively overstimulating parent. Later situations in which the person feels close to but overpowered by a loved one evoke similar feelings, a bizarre experience that makes one feel crazed and few share.

Once anxiety is set off, whether triggered mentally or by sensory defensiveness, it perpetuates itself and spawns anticipatory anxiety. After numerous occasions of tensing up in a crowd, the thought of trekking through the mall drives the sufferer's system up and throws it into a negative feedback loop. Anxious thoughts fuel sensory defensiveness and sensory defensiveness fuels anxious thoughts. Because avoiding overstimulating situations reduces anxiety, the person may duck the very experiences that can balance the nervous system, like sex, camaraderie, or a workout at the gym, thereby increasing defensiveness and avoidance.

As sensory defensiveness and mental anxiety require different treatments, it's important to know the underlying mechanisms, especially since anxiety can erupt into panic.

PANIC AND PHOBIAS

At 15 while driving in a car with her parents, Estella suffered her first panic attack. Going through a long, dark underpass, Estella felt that she couldn't breathe. She felt that if she didn't get out of there that second she would explode. She screamed. Her father slapped her and she stopped.

In her twenties, she went with her father to the immigration department in New York. It was dark and crowded and the room seemed terrifyingly huge. As they stood in line, people seemed horrifically close. She felt very shaky and couldn't catch her breath. She told her father she was suffocating. He ignored her. She screamed. Again he slapped her to calm her down.

At 56, space-related fears continue to permeate Estella's life. Terrified of heights and claustrophobic in enclosed spaces, she still won't drive in tunnels, take subways, or ride elevators. She refused to take magnetic resonance imaging (MRI), as she was afraid to go into that tomblike box.

Before flying, she takes the anti-anxiety drug Xanax but nevertheless has panic attacks. Once, she was unable to breathe and passed out.

Estella is tactile defensive, light defensive, and movement defensive. At times, she feels so unsteady on her feet that walking down a street feels like walking along a precipice. Jumpy, impatient, and at times hysterical, she has not found either tranquilizers or talk therapy to reduce her fear of flying (aviophobia), fear of heights (acrophobia), or fear of enclosed spaces (claustrophobia). Could her phobias be triggered by her sensory defensiveness?

Indeed.

Phobias, an inordinate fear of a situation or a thing, afflict one of nine adults in the United States to the point of seeking psychiatric help. They represent a conscious fear of physical harm and draw their energy from the primal need for self-protection buried deep in the primitive brain.

Some phobias are realistic and occur after a traumatic event in response to a real danger: for example, after a serious car accident, you panic when you need to drive a car. Some come from learning. If your mother pulled your hand away as you masturbated as a child and warned that God would punish you, self-stimulation may elicit panic. Others come from unresolved childhood fears, like being left alone. While others come from imitating a fearful role model, like a nervous mother who would worry that a sneeze meant pneumonia.

But these kinds of phobias are in the minority. Most pop out of nowhere; one day you get on an airplane and become terrified that you will fall out. Or they are held in check and then suddenly intensify, or randomly come and go. What accounts for their haphazardness? Psychologists aren't sure.

Dr. Harold Levinson, clinical associate professor of psychiatry at New York University Medical Center and author of *Phobia Free*, spent years grappling with the origin of phobias.[6] As a practicing psychoanalyst, he mostly treated private patients. But starting in the 1960s, he quite fortuitously began treating dyslexic children. The conventional wisdom was that dyslexia was due to a disturbance in the cerebrum, or thinking brain.

But after examining 1,000 sufferers, Levinson found only 1 percent showed evidence of cerebral dysfunction, but 750 of the children exhibited problems with balance and coordination. He concluded that dyslexia correlated with problems related to inner-ear, or vestibular, dysfunction. This was at the same time that A. Jean Ayres discovered most learning disabilities and hyperactivity to be a by-product of sensory integration dysfunction, characterized by tactile and vestibular processing problems.

Faced with this startling discovery, Levinson decided to treat dyslexia with anti–motion sickness medications, antihistamines, and other drugs useful in treating inner-ear problems. To his delight, a whole series of sensory and motor symptoms improved—including visual, auditory, and tactile functioning, exactly what sensory integration theory would predict.

But he found something else. The dyslexic patients reported that their phobias—motion-related, direction-related, balance-related, and coordination-related—disappeared or were substantially alleviated by these medications.

The next logical step was to see if the same correlation between inner-ear dysfunction and phobias existed in his psychiatric patients. This is precisely what he found in *90 percent of his cases*, with similar treatment success using the same medications. It now became clear why many phobias seem to behave randomly. They are primarily physical, not psychic, in origin. The notion that phobias and panic are primarily psychological was turned on its head.

Shaky Place in Space

Clinical evidence indicates that an integral part of the anxiety-control network is mediated in the vestibular system in the inner ear. "If the inner-ear system is impaired, the entire anxiety-control network may be affected," explains Levinson.[7] Under ordinary stress—physical, emotional, hormonal, sensory—your system may be unable to dampen or regulate anxiety properly. You quickly reach your sensory threshold and mild to moderate anxiety erupts into panic.

This makes good sense. As the vestibular system controls our sense of balance, direction, and the coordination and sequencing of movement in time and space, inadequate feedback from this system will, in certain circumstances, make the person feel dizzy, disoriented, light-headed, floating, faint, or nauseated—the symptoms that sufferers of panic attacks report.

If balance and coordination are off, heights, bridges, stairs, escalators, and wide-open spaces can destabilize. If a person doesn't feel confident of landing on his feet if he falls, he will fear heights. Even looking out at the horizon can evoke panic:

> I . . . liked standing at the edge of the water and having the waves roll up over my feet . . . But then I'd look out at the horizon and I'd feel dizzy. I was afraid that I'd sort of go out there.[8]

If a person has a problem with orientation in space, then tunnels, shopping malls, or other disorienting situations aggravate their problems with sense of direction:

> I had what would be called a panic attack of some kind in the fun house with those mirrors, and I just fell apart. . . . They were everywhere you looked and you're supposed to remember what direction is straight ahead to get out and everything was spinning. People came in and tried to get me out and no one could make me move. I just sat down and cried.[9]

If a person is movement-defensive and hypersensitive to change in direction, speed of movement, or sudden movement, riding in a vehicle, elevator, escalator, or even a rocking chair can provoke panic, as it does for this woman. "It seems like cars are closer than they really are," says Katia, "seems like we're going faster than we really are, feels like we're 'falling' going around corners. Riding with my daughter going over the Chesapeake Bay Bridge it sometimes looks and feels like she's going to drive into and over the edge."

Dependency on visual input to orient you in space complicates the problem. One woman becomes dizzy and anxious watching someone rock in a rocking chair. Disorientation and dizziness intensify in the dark. Afraid of losing their footing, some defensives will not take a shower in a dimly lit bathroom. One woman sleeps with the lights on and wears her glasses or wakes up dizzy and in a panic.

Many childhood fears emanate from fear of the dark. Tamika was so afraid of the dark as a child that her parents sent her to a child psychologist, who asked her to draw pictures of what she feared. "I drew monsters and gnomes because I thought that might be something normal people are afraid of. But there really was nothing. I would just wake up terrified!"

As she grew up, the terror continued. Feeling she was about to be murdered, she would sleep with one eye open and the lights on. She couldn't leave the house or breathe normally and felt dizzy all the time.

> Every time I have to go up and down stairs I feel anxious. I feel
> like I might fall or miss a step—like I'm being pulled down. I
> end up running or walking fast up or down to get it over with.
> If I go slowly the bottom seems really far away and I feel
> pushed from the top like something is chasing me, and I feel
> dizzy. I don't clean my house upstairs very well, and my laundry,
> which I do in the basement, is always piled up.

Anti-anxiety medication didn't alleviate the problem. Fortunately, an occupational therapist identified her as being gravitationally insecure, and gave her daily exercises for vertigo. Within a week, she was amazed to wake up in the middle of the night and not feel frozen in fear. "I can actually get up, go to the bathroom, or get a drink of water—things I could never do before."

Auditory defensiveness can contribute to panic as well. All auditory information is filtered, sequenced, and fine-tuned by the inner ear. When this processing is off, certain noises or vibrations can trigger panic, as Sandra describes.

> When I was young, my imagination would go wild at night, try-
> ing to see what was making the sounds, trying to figure out the
> sounds of the wind in the trees, bushes, etc. I would see ghosts,

goblins, demons, outside from my imagination. I always felt like
I was halfway crazy to go through such weird pathways trying
to explain the sounds I heard. Even today I feel paranoid at
night, not being able to see what is causing sounds.

If specific stimuli trigger panic, as taking an elevator, the person has a
phobia. If panic occurs without a cue, the person has panic disorder. One
woman describes her experience, "I was sitting and waiting for the train.
Though the tracks were over twenty feet away, they suddenly seemed dangerously close. I felt as if a magnet could pull me onto them. I feared that
if I got any closer I would fall onto them or someone would push me."

Panic originates from Pan, the Greek god of woods and fields, who was
blamed for the inexplicable dread sometimes felt by travelers in lonely
places. Different from anxiety, which has an external trigger—a first date,
performing in front of an audience—panic is triggered from internal stimuli, from a biochemical imbalance. People with *panic disorder* may not be
anxious all the time, but have unanticipated anxiety attacks that psychologists can't explain. In many cases, inner-ear dysfunction may be the missing link. It could certainly explain why, after an especially stressful day, one
person may feel anxious sitting in a vast, dark subway station with a pre-
cipitous drop, and many people milling about, while another becomes disoriented and panics. This condition is so disabling that 20 percent of those
suffering panic disorder have attempted suicide.

Space-related phobias are not the only ones implicated in faulty
vestibular processing. So is agoraphobia. The poorer the vestibular functioning, the greater the likelihood of having a panic attack in situations
that challenge balance, orientation, and movement. When panic attacks
occur often, sufferers begin to associate these attacks with situations where
they might feel trapped and where escape would be difficult and embarrassing—sitting in the middle row of a dark movie theater, driving over a
bridge or through a tunnel. To protect against overwhelming panic, they
begin to avoid these "unsafe" places and to live their lives by how quickly
they can reach safety. In wide-open space especially, the visual perception
of space as vast creates anxiety and a desire for escape.

Even social phobia can have roots in movement defensiveness. Social phobics are painfully shy people that tend to show a persistent fear of social contact, worrying that they will blush, their voice will tremble, their hands will shake, and they will embarrass themselves. Fear of public speaking is common, as is fear of using a public bathroom. But they also fear situations like writing or signing their name in front of others or eating and drinking in public. In some, this self-consciousness may emanate from problems with coordinating fine motor movement—from either flaccid or stiff muscle tone—which reflects problems with vestibular processing. If a person has poor coordination, anything that involves movement can create anxiety and feel humiliating if other people are watching.

CRAVING RELIEF

If you put a rat in a maze with food at the end and throw in a cat, all priority changes and the rat will claw, eat through, or kill to get out of that maze. If you put people in danger, they think only of what they can do to escape to safety.

Sensory defensiveness creates ongoing threat. Pleasure releases endorphins that block the distress. People will continue to avoid or seek stimulation until they reach an optimum level of arousal, and so the sensory defensive will compulsively eat, take drugs, and do whatever it takes to lower his or her arousal and feel safe. Their addictions are self-soothing gone amok.

Eating for Modulation

What does "hungry" mean? It can be physical hunger. Or it can represent a need for self-regulation—for comfort, stimulation, pleasure, diversion, love.

Doing something with our mouth is our first way of getting into the comfort zone—think of the crying infant's pacifier. When we are frustrated or tense, we chomp on potato chips, chew licorice, suck on candy. A cold drink perks us up, while a warm cup of tea calms. Intense taste, like very salty potato chips or spicy nachos, boosts arousal.[10] The lower our arousal level, the more we go for cold or spicy foods and the more we tend to abuse coffee, soda, and chocolate. The higher our arousal level, the more we go for hot and blander foods. In a nervous system that vacillates up and down, food choice may reflect a need at once to calm and arouse. A compulsive eater, Ruth has to eat three foods together, usually one chewy and salty, one sour and crunchy, one sweet and creamy. If she finishes one food before chewing all three, she feels compelled to take more of the missing food to maintain equal amounts of all three choices in her mouth at the same time. If you compulsively need oral tranquilizers, you not only overeat, but chew on your pens, or smoke, anything to stimulate the mouth.

Overeating serves another purpose: it helps balance our biochemistry. Eating has a biochemical effect. The stress response uses up sugar, or glucose, the very substance that provides the energy to sustain life, and depletes serotonin, the brain chemical that controls both emotions and eating. To restore balance, we crave sugar naturally in the form of sweet or starchy carbohydrates: devouring candy or cake, pasta or potato chips, is self-medication to help raise the serotonin level in our brain.[11] The more prolonged the stress, the greater our need to restore serotonin. Chocolate, especially, has a euphoric effect.

Compulsive overeating is also about chronically elevated cortisol, the stress hormone. When you feel stressed, cortisol rises. Normally, it rises briefly while you adapt to the stress and then returns to baseline levels. But when stress is chronic, as it is with the sensory defensive, cortisol stays at a constant high and you feel jittery, irritable, and hungry. Cortisol stimulates appetite because it is responsible for refueling you with carbohydrates and fat after you have completed the flight-or-fight response. If you never complete it, and remain stressed, your appetite is insatiable for sweets, and you feel a false sense of stress relief—and an expanding waistline.

If you are oral-defensive, different food textures feel unpleasant in your mouth. Eating to satisfy hunger and eating to satisfy oral motor input can produce unusual cravings and eating patterns, as we saw with Ruth. If the problem is extreme, stress will exacerbate the defensiveness and in some cases lead to starvation.

Anorexia as Response to Sensory Defensiveness

At age 8, Serena stopped growing. In seventh grade a doctor put her on growth hormones, but by her freshman year of high school, she was only 4 feet 9 inches and 55 pounds, so the doctor continued with the hormones until her junior year of high school.

At age 16, she became anorexic. "I hated my parents, hated myself. I was depressed and suicidal. I worried about everything and took everything to heart. I thought, why eat?" So she starved herself. For weeks, she ate a bag of chips for the day or nothing.

Anorexia is intentional starving—a compulsive drive to not eat driven by an unrealistic fear of obesity and a faulty perception of the self as fat. A serious and complicated disorder, it includes biochemical imbalance, a low self-concept, distorted body image that suggests depersonalization (the anorexic looks in the mirror and sees not emaciation but fat), faulty thought patterns, and often enmeshed family dynamics.   •

Typically, a middle-class female adolescent goes on a diet and can't stop. As a child, she is well behaved, overcompliant, and a bright, high-achieving perfectionist who seeks to please her parents. As adolescence hits, with its hormonal changes, maturing body and mind, and new expectations and responsibilities, she can no longer hold in feelings of fear, sadness, anger, and profound inadequacy. Nor can she face becoming a mature, sexual woman. Eating for these girls becomes one of the few things she feels she can control; controlling food intake becomes an addiction, as well as a way to avoid budding sexuality, as starvation and lowered body fat inhibit menstruation and body maturation.

On the surface, Serena might fit this description. She was a depressed middle-class female adolescent who used not eating to feel some control in her life and, like many anorexics, had a childlike body and barely budding breasts. But Serena didn't feel too fat or worry about getting fat, as anorexics do. "I didn't want to be skinny. I just hated food."

If desire to be thin didn't motivate her starvation, what did?

Serena is oral-defensive. Always a finicky eater, she finds certain foods in her mouth irritating and she gags easily, preventing her from eating many foods, which compromises nutrition. She won't eat anything mushy, like pudding, mashed potatoes, or thick soup, or anything creamy, like chocolate or soups or yogurt. Nor will she eat meat or fish, as she hates their smell and texture.

Contrary to the anorexic's avoidance of sweets and fats, which put on calories, she craves ice cream for the fat, sugar, and cold but, disliking the texture, she can only take a few licks and then can't eat anymore. She especially hates it when the ice cream melts but will suck on Popsicles for the intense cold as they have more texture. Compounding her eating preferences is low blood sugar and she keeps candy in her car.

Primarily, she seeks crunch, as in chips, granola, crackers, croutons, and salad, though the only vegetables she'll eat are lettuce, carrots, and broccoli stalks. These food textures cause her to bite hard, creating heavy work for her jaw that helps her to regulate her aroused level. Looking for things hard to chew, she will bite gum, pencils, pens. "If I can put it in my mouth, I will."

Too anxious to sit down to eat, she grabs a small amount of food at a time and will munch on crunchy food until she no longer feels starved, a snacking pattern started in infancy. A half hour later, she's hungry again. Allergies to pollen, cat hair, and dust leave her nose constantly stuffed, affecting her taste buds, and this adds to her difficulty in finding food satisfying.

With intense oral defensiveness, tactile defensiveness will likely be equally debilitating and, predictably, Serena can't stand to be touched. "I squirm when I touch myself," she says. Though her skin is smooth, it feels coarse and porous. If tickled, she gets the goose bumps and has to "shake it off." When her mother wants to hug and kiss her, Serena pushes her away and this turns into a fight. "I just want to tell you how much I love you," her mother says, calling Serena "standoffish." If her cat brushes against her, she shudders and rubs her body. She hates cutting her nails or washing her hair and will not go barefoot in grass or sand.

Before she goes to teach her preschoolers, she must prepare for light touch. "Okay, I can do this, I can handle it," she tells herself. If possible, she initiates contact by giving the child a bear hug and then pulling away quickly. At 6 feet 5 inches tall her boyfriend allows her to feel enveloped and safe. She has taught him to avoid touching that irks her and especially never to tickle her.

Getting dressed is a nightmare. The less clothing that touches her body, the better. The clothing she does wear cannot be too stiff, too tight, or too loose but must fit so it flows with her movement and not move around on her body. To avoid any material touching her arms, she wears tank tops. To avoid any material hitting her legs, she wears shorts or long pants. "I should join a nudist colony," she says. She can only sleep on cotton jersey sheets and on her stomach, a position that provides the most pressure. In the morning, she can stand in her closet for sometimes up to two hours, trying to decide what is comfortable enough to wear.

Serena fits the classic hyperactive tactile-defensive, first described by A. Jean Ayres. Tactile defensiveness, noted Ayres, leads to overalertness, distractibility, and hyperactivity.[12] In fact, many ADHD sufferers are sensory defensive. With hands animated and body constantly changing position, Serena chatters cheerfully in a childlike manner and hops from one subject to another in a nonstop flow of words, as if on speed; at times, her voice gets inappropriately loud. To stay interested in the world, she must do many things at once and will play solitaire and watch TV while glancing at the newspaper.

As a baby, Serena was happy but fussy, couldn't sit still, and would fidget all night in bed. In school, she was called a "chatterbox" and "social butterfly." Feeling unsteady but in perpetual motion, she was out of her seat at every opportunity—running to chat with a friend, throw something in the wastebasket, go to the bathroom, deliver a message for the teacher.

Starting out low and then going like a whirlwind, which further burns precious calories, Serena quickly overshoots and then can't unwind. She tosses and turns when trying to go to sleep, but once she's asleep, she sleeps soundly and then can't wake up. In the morning, she feels drowsy and keeps falling back to sleep. To stay alert enough to care for the children at the day-care center, she drinks three cans of Coke. She regularly smokes half a pack of cigarettes a day and drinks one or two cups of strong Cuban coffee.

Upon graduating from high school, she tried going away to college but couldn't focus. Her parents sent her to a psychiatrist, who diagnosed her as suffering anxiety and depression and prescribed Prozac. But she became a "zombie" with the first pill and didn't take another.

Luckily, Serena's starvation abated by college and she was not diagnosed as anorexic. But she could have been. And not just because of her starvation. The profile of the anorexic and the sensory defensive is strikingly similar. Both are hypersensitive and emotionally unstable; have low self-esteem, intimacy and sexual issues; have a poor body image; and compulsive personality tendencies. Both are described as having been unregulated, fussy infants who cry for long periods, and, seemingly insatiable, confuse frustrated parents who may feed them when they are actually tired or put them to sleep when they're hungry. Poor body schema prevents these infants from learning to rely on their own body signals, and they grow up confusing bodily tension and emotional states: "Am I eating because I'm hungry or because I'm frustrated?"

Could sensory defensiveness underlie some anorexic behavior? Without systematic research, the answer is unknown. But evidence suggests a link in some cases. If eating has been a lifelong issue, it makes sense to choose an eating disorder to broadcast that life has become more than you can stomach. And issues with intimacy and sexuality, poor body schema, and withdrawn behavior suggest tactile defensiveness. Often, for instance, anorexics describe eating as "messy." They are also infamous compulsive runners, presumably to run off calories but perhaps in some cases to also get needed heavy pressure.

Anorexia is poorly understood and extremely difficult to treat. It can create such conditions as retarded bone growth and osteoporosis, anemia, dry skin, low body temperature, and cessation of menstruation. In some 15 percent of cases, anorexia leads to death. Identifying when sensory defensiveness might be a contributing factor to anorexic behavior could save lives. Two days after Serena started doing a simple intervention to combat oral defensiveness, devised by Patricia Wilbarger, she was eating and enjoying soft, mushy foods, such as ice cream and bananas for the first time in her life.

Drugs to the Rescue

Food addiction is one way to relieve the sufferings of the flesh. Alcohol and drug addiction are another. Some sensory defensives become addicted to anti-anxiety medication, as did Estella, who relied on Xanax to make her feel calm enough to get out the door. Others turn to a warm glass of wine to relax enough to do something they know will make them anxious, like having sex, or to ease into sleep.

For Joe, a 51-year-old medical courier, alcohol has been a steady companion his entire adult life. When he finishes his shift at 8 P.M., he generally goes bar hopping and will down fifteen scotches, spending $50 to $100 a night on drinks. If he goes straight home, he drinks a glass of vodka before going to bed.

The alcohol drowns out intolerable tactile defensiveness: everything that touches his skin bothers him. Constantly tugging and yanking at his cotton T-shirt and adjusting his clothing, he wiggles, jiggles, and stirs as if he has ants in his pants, which is how his skin makes him feel. If touched suddenly, he goes "ballistic." He wears a ring on his finger for "status" but takes it on and off "a thousand times a day." His nose hair tickles him and he trims it every morning. He wears no socks and, at work, keeps taking off his uniform hat, as it creates unbearable pressure against his scalp. His mother is also touchy, and he thinks he inherited her sensitive skin.

Joe is friendly and outgoing, but he talks constantly, perhaps as a need to rev up his system enough to function or to release tension. Consumed with his unease, he can't stop to listen and tries to dominate the conversation. He will ask a question and before it is answered, ask another or bolt up and pace. By ruling the exchange, he circumvents the confusion and embarrassment he feels when questions and comments derail him.

Unable to tune out or organize sensations, he could not concentrate in school or sit still long enough to learn and though he scored highest in his grade on the scholastic aptitude test, he had the lowest grades. Reading has been torture, as he can't read fast enough to comprehend the material and his mind wanders. For this reason, he didn't go to college.

Sensory issues have cost him heavily in every aspect of his life. He never married and lives alone. Most nights he comes home drunk and collapses on the couch in front of the TV, which he keeps on all night as a distraction. He never sleeps in his bed unless he's "dead drunk," as he needs the feeling of something rigid against his back. Sometimes he sleeps on the hard floor. Movement defensiveness compounds his instability. Though he loves to party, he won't dance. "I can hardly stand up straight without wavering," he says. Alcohol further destabilizes his equilibrium. To compensate for lack of control over his world, he is a neat freak, and before he leaves his apartment, he will check everything five or six times.

He has no idea what it means to relax. His shoulders are tensed up to his ears, as if pulled by marionette strings. "I'm like a wild animal, surviving minute by minute, like a predator." When frustrated, he often mutters that he will feel better if he could "just kill someone," though he doesn't behave violently.

Living in an unsteady, itchy world, for which he has no explanation or control, he feels like a "loser," a "psycho." "Are they going to lock me up?" he asks half in jest. Alcohol is his way to numb the pain. And though emotionally addicted to alcohol, he is not physically dependent on it: when he can't afford to drink, he has stopped for as long as ten months at a time and he rarely drinks during his 9-hour work shift.

Occasionally, Joe walks to the ocean from his home and swims for an hour or so. On these days, he feels more together and can manage a normal conversation. But in flight, fight, or freeze, people need an immediate fix. Vodka fills the bill.

Watching the World Reel By: Depersonalization

Major depression, post-traumatic stress disorder, borderline personality, panic disorder with agoraphobia, depersonalization, dissociation—these were some of the diagnoses given to Trish, a bright 43-year-old cook and twice-divorced mother and grandmother. Yet at times she seemed so strong and competent that people told her nothing was wrong—she was just a spoiled, lazy snob.

From an early age, she was aware that things that were hard for her didn't seem to bother other people. She wanted to participate in doing fun things like going to the beach or amusement park or just getting together with friends, but everything was "too much! too much!"—the smells, sounds, lights, touches, crowds, and hectic activity—and she got overloaded every time she tried. At the same time, she felt too lethargic to get going without several Pepsis and cigarettes—and then she couldn't slow down. If she didn't stop and regroup, she crashed. There seemed no quiet middle ground. "I was always trying to rev up or calm down." Any change in routine set her off. She felt like a cork bouncing on a raging surf.

Her mother hated to take her shopping because she was so "picky." If Trish complained, she struggled with two blows: overstimulation and misunderstanding:

> I would say, "That hurts" and my parents would say, "No, that doesn't hurt, I'm only touching your hair." Or, "It's just a scratch and nothing to whine about, you are being too picky, sensitive, nuts, a baby, crybaby, cranky, and just not normal." Or, I would hear "Stop crying or I'll give you something to cry about."

The more people tried to make her respond, the more she learned to restrain her feelings. Nevertheless, she coped.

Then, in seventh grade, she got her first pair of glasses. From that moment on, her life changed irrevocably.

Most people put on their glasses and tune out the sensation of the frame resting on their nose, face, and ears. But Trish's face and head were severely tactile defensive, and touching her hair or head caused extreme discomfort. Though not consciously aware of it after a while, she continued to respond at a subconscious level to the unbearable pressure of the glasses against her face and ears. This irritation evoked a defensive response. But as she could neither escape from nor fight wearing her glasses, she was constantly on guard from unknown threats that no one could explain.

When threatened, you need to see everything around you. But Trish felt the frame of the eyeglasses obstructed her peripheral vision, an area of potential visual processing weakness, and shut out some light, making the world appear dark. Blocked vision increased her sense of danger, compounded by a poor sense of balance that left her more dependent on vision to navigate her world.

To escape escalating tension, her sensory systems started to shut down. She felt in a daze, out of touch with her body, and only perceived bits and pieces of the world, as if in a dream. She would sit in the local park aimlessly watching the cars and people go by. "It was like looking through a long, dark tunnel—the world so very far away. I sat there for hours, for days, for weeks at a time."

Depersonalization is a defense mechanism to escape from extreme tension, anxiety, and stimulation. A surreal experience, it makes sufferers feel estranged from their body and experience body distortions: their body seems far away or inordinately small or large. Says Trish:

> I remember passing by mirrors and wondering whose reflection that was. It certainly didn't feel (or look) like *me*—floating and unconnected. I had problems trying to describe or remember what other people looked like or how I looked to others. I could only see myself through others' eyes.

Actions or speech feel labored and objectified rather than spontaneous, and hearing seems distorted, as if you are in an echo chamber. Says Trish:

> What I hear is very hard to describe—just distorted, not right, kind of muffled, yet at the same time, more distinct . . . sometimes a hollow feeling. Like being in a big empty cavern, yet hearing and feeling every little sound. A very frightening and lonely feeling.

At times, sufferers doubt their own reality and feel as if they are losing their mind. If the shock is especially traumatic, they may dissociate and lose time and memory, as in amnesia or multiple personality disorder. To cope, Trish put her feelings into separate categories that became separate personalities, so she would only have to deal with one at a time. Different personalities emerged. She felt possessed and spoke with a priest. Integrating her alter egos into a cohesive self took years of therapy.

In most cases, dissociation is a defense mechanism to escape from severe childhood physical or sexual abuse. To stop the horror, the child disappears into the crevices of her mind. Trish experienced neither. Dissociation came from extreme muscular tightening that shut off some felt body frenzy. While offering some relief, withdrawing from sensation eventually resulted in her oscillating from numbness to free-floating anxiety or panic. Her bodily states were cut off from the awareness of feelings or thoughts that could give them meaning.

To feel real, Trish needed a body against hers. By 18, she was married, and by 22, she had four children. Pregnancy, with its added weight and pressure, and the healing sensations involved in holding, carrying, and rocking infants, unbeknownst to her provided a terrific sensory diet to balance out her system. She felt less crazed and at times even happy.

When the last infant toddled away, she had less modulating sensation and broke down. She divorced her first husband and married a man with the "right touch," who made her feel more grounded. But they divorced as well, and afterward she felt an almost constant state of overload—"misfiring."

She was put on the antidepressant Zoloft for depression and spent three weeks in a psychiatric hospital for evaluation.

Alone again, Trish turned to an old love. But she found the sexual encounter excruciatingly overstimulating. Traumatized, humiliated, and deranged, she fled in panic. For the next six years, she walked around crying and terrified, moaning and rocking herself to sleep. Agoraphobic, she panicked when she left the house unless someone was with her.

Through therapy and dogged determination, she slowly began to allow the world to seep in and to feel the full extent of her pain. She found outlets of expression in reading and writing poetry. Yet her emotions remained unstable: one minute she was laughing wildly, the next sobbing convulsively. And she didn't know why her senses were on red alert.

One day her granddaughter came home from school with information on sensory integration dysfunction. There it was at last—the missing piece to explain her hypersensitivity, her erratic behavior, her extreme and uncontrollable emotions, inability to cope, and her omnipresent exhaustion. She was sensory-defensive, and had other sensorimotor processing problems, like low muscle tone and poor postural control, that interfered with her normal functioning. "The more information I found, the more I knew I had found my answer."

Yet her safety net still remained relatively small. Sensations still felt overwhelming. The world was chaotic and confusing. She barely knew what people said to her, and figuring out how to respond was exhausting. She generally held it together enough to function minimally, but her behavior remained unpredictable and often emotionally inappropriate.

Then, one day, at age 43, she decided to buy contact lenses. She put the new lenses in her eyes and looked out at the world. *The wall disappeared.* "I could feel my body in space and the world didn't seem at a distance. I could see *people*, not just a swarm of cloudy, faceless bodies." Free from tactile irritation and hearing and visual distortions, she didn't need to shut down sensation and dissociate.

She barely noticed when her daughter left the radio on loud and hardly heard her neighbor's barking dogs. Her balance and orientation seemed better, and she felt less vertigo. She was able to read books out loud to her grandson, whereas before it was an effort to speak the words. "I feel normal in ways I never imagined."

She wrote this poem in celebration.

To go up and down steps and know where my feet are;
To be able to breathe;
To be able to move.
Such an amazing thing—Just to BE
In the mall, and not alone.

Children at the carnival—My grandson
Going round and round on a swirling swing, his face alight
With wonder "I'm flying like an airplane!!!"
No longer disoriented, I share his wonder—
At the lights, the sounds, the movement
At the laughter and the life.
Such an amazing thing—Just to BE
At the fair, without running away.

A bedtime story, a tuck goodnight,
To reach out and touch; to share the smile of a child—
To respond with a smile of my own;
Answering questions—to hear and be heard.
Such an amazing thing—Just to BE
With my grandchildren, feeling the bond between us.

A busy day at work, listening, watching
Others as they work, as they talk, as they play—
Sometimes even joining in—sometimes even smiling.
Such an amazing thing—Just to BE
At work, seeing and being seen.

One night, after taking her contacts out, she put her glasses on. Though she saw the same as with the contacts, she felt instant agitation and the urge to smash them into pieces.

As Trish emerged from her frozen state, she started to feel some sensations more intensely than before. She felt more touchy and noticed more clothing irritations. It was harder to tolerate another's mess or smell. It took her about a month to reprocess everything. As she was not used to hearing and seeing the world, she found it distracting at first. Yet, despite whatever else she needed to work on, she felt *in* the world, a sense of self and personal control.

Six months later, her tactile defensiveness had abated enough for her to cut her hair, which she had always worn long for the needed weight. "It felt like I cut off my past," she said.

In this chapter, we've seen how the repercussions of sensory defensiveness attack the psyche to create *dis-ease*. Now let's look at how they attack the physical body to create *disease*.

6

The Body Erupts: The Psychosomatic Side of Sensory Defensiveness

> I feel like my '76 Chevy pickup truck: irregular electrical problems that create little sparks of ignition that die out a few times before it gets going (I get energized enough to do some little thing, but it doesn't last and I'm back trying to get that starter to kick in again); often misdiagnosed; affected by poor-quality fuel (sensory stim); bad tires (feet); rusted (chemically sensitive); very slow to get warmed up and moving (low arousal); bad brakes (crash and screech rather than gradual slow down—high arousal); worn-out battery that didn't seem to hold a charge (once I've done something, no more energy); caught on fire three times (meltdowns!); totally "falling apart," but just kept on going.
>
> —PATSY

At 38, Sandra suffers from severe sensory defensiveness and a slew of unenviable psychosomatic complaints: chronic fatigue syndrome (CFS); fibromyalgia, a condition that causes weak and aching muscles and sleep disruption; constant headaches; allergies; and asthma.

Sandra always had a weak immune system and a sensitive constitution, possibly as a result of trauma before and during birth. During pregnancy, a doctor put her mother on diet pills, causing her to weigh less at delivery than when she got pregnant, which may have starved her baby's developing nervous system. Sandra was born with the umbilical cord wrapped three times around her neck and remained in an incubator for close to two weeks.

As a child Sandra remembers having allergies and hypersensitivities, but after a car accident in her twenties, she developed asthma, severe allergies, and severe sensory defensiveness. Two more auto accidents caused soft-tissue damage to her neck, back, shoulders, wrist, and knees, as well as a broken hand, further exacerbating these conditions. Today, every part of her body feels "ultrasensitive in a most unpleasant way." Constantly irritable and moody, she is on antidepressant and anti-anxiety medication.

Nevertheless, most noise makes her feel like she is "having a heart attack" and sends her running for her inhaler. At work, the overhead fluorescent lights and every ring of the phone increase her headache. Living in Norman, Oklahoma, her hearing sensitivity is compounded by the Taos hum—"a low-pitched, dull hum with almost an oscillating quality"—that she hears just before dawn or at any quiet time.

Midway through her day, she begins shaking from the noise, lights, and odors. By the time she leaves work, she usually feels nauseated and teary-eyed and arrives home "practically crawling." Her keyed-up state worsens her fibromyalgia, and sleep feels impossible.

From Stressed to Sick

The stress response was designed to enable us to survive an immediate threat. The bear in the cave, the sudden crack of a branch overhead, or the shadow of an intruder signaled life-threatening danger and required an immediate response: energy-producing chemicals released in the body to prepare for fleeing or fighting danger. If that wasn't possible, the animal played dead long enough to escape the predator's attention and to run for its life. The flight, fight, freeze response was not designed to be experienced chronically and keep our bodies flooded with toxic stress hormones. *It was not designed to be itself damaging.*[1]

The nervous, endocrine, and immune systems are interconnected. To maintain systemic harmony all three must work in concert or the body cannot resist disease—the blood, lymph, and other fluids don't circulate efficiently, and the liver, spleen, and kidneys lose integrity. Symptoms in one trickle eventually into the other and inhibit progress in any one system: sensory defensiveness throws off your hormone levels and immune system, and vice versa. Anyone who's ever had a fever and the flu knows how light hurts your eyes, noise jars you, and touch irritates your skin.

How does this happen? The immune system exchanges information with the brain and the hormone-secreting endocrine system. In response to overstimulation, the brain secretes stress hormones, which in turn suppress disease-fighting lymphocytes, the white blood cells that hunt and destroy foreign bodies. If overreactivity is chronic, stress wears down the body. Eventually the immune system is depleted and the body succumbs and breaks down. This process happens in three stages, as outlined by Hans Selye: alarm, resistance, exhaustion.[2]

Alarm

When the sensory defensive first encounter overwhelming sensation, it sets off an alarm reaction in the amygdala of the limbic system. The adrenals hyperfunction and secrete high amounts of the hormone adrenaline (epinephrine) and noradrenaline (norepinephrine) to energize the body massively for flight or fight, as well as steroid hormones such as cortisol. Noradrenaline raises blood pressure, helps transmit messages in the nervous system, and acts on the immune system and emotional reactions. Mechanisms needed for immediate high-energy action take priority, shutting down bodily activities directed toward growth, reproduction, and even resistance to existing infection.

Resistance

If the stressor remains and the sensory defensive do not recover back to baseline, as they generally don't, the body continues to cope by sympathetic nervous system activation and hormonal release, though not as high as in the alarm reaction. The body draws on available nutrients and energy reserves to repair damage and increase resistance to noxious stimuli.

To prepare for a long battle, the pituitary secretes hormones:

- Vasopressin, which raises blood pressure by causing arteries to constrict.
- Thyrotropic hormone, which stimulates the thyroid gland to increase production of the hormone thyroxine, accelerating metabolism.
- Adrenocorticotrophic hormone (ACTH), which acts upon the outer part of the adrenal glands to release a number of hormones referred to as corticosteroids, which help the body respond to stress by fighting inflammation and allergic reactions (such as difficulty breathing). Cortisol is an important corticosteroid which, among its effects, raises blood sugar level to increase energy, alters the immune system, and increases blood platelets (blood-clotting elements), which can adhere to artery walls, narrowing them.

Under prolonged stress, the adrenal glands become overtaxed and go into a state of temporary underfunctioning. If you are relatively healthy, the glands will try to compensate, actually rebuilding themselves to the point of hypertrophy (growing larger).

Prolonged stress will also cause the body to form free radicals. These undesirable chemicals cause damage to cells, impairing the immune system and leading to infections and degenerative diseases and hastening the aging process. The immune system can err by overresponding and attacking the body's own tissues, causing arthritis or an allergic reaction, or by underreacting and, for instance, allowing cancer cells to multiply.

Exhaustion

Over time, constant stress uses up the defensive's energy reserves and they eventually reach the last stage of exhaustion. The body becomes overworked and depleted of its normal energy reserves. Fatigue becomes chronic, and the sufferer tends to have a difficult time handling any stressful situation without overreacting or becoming unglued.

Without sufficient rest to restore and rejuvenate, the body is in a state of disequilibrium and the basic sleep-wake rhythms are disrupted. While awake, the defensive feel agitated and exhausted and get increasingly more overloaded and depleted as the day goes on. While asleep, they feel restless, startle easily from noise, arouse from temperature changes and their own movements, and awaken fatigued. While dreaming, they may have nightmares. A tight, hard, drawn face and body and wan eyes make them look old.

At this stage, the adrenal glands remain in a chronic state of underfunctioning. They overproduce adrenaline some of the time, causing panic or mood swings, and underproduce adrenaline the rest of the time. Autopsies of adult suicides often show the adrenal gland enlarged.[3] The body is so revved up, it fails to respond to ordinary forms of regulation, and the stress hormone cortisol will remain high even if the sufferer is given a substance to decrease the body's output. Even if someone was not sensory defensive previously, she will feel increased irritation to light, noise, and touch. Depression, lack of attention to personal care, and addiction to coffee, cigarettes, stimulants, alcohol, or drugs are likely.

Because of exhaustion, resistance to disease decreases and chronic conditions emerge, including:

- Tense muscles, with increased headaches, back pain, or stiffness and tight jaw, which affects chewing and inhibits breathing
- Suppressed immune system, reducing the white blood cells critically important to fighting a cold, flu, or even cancer and shrinking the thymus, spleen, and lymph nodes
- Retention of excess sodium and fluid, which elevates blood pressure with slow, steady damage to the heart, kidneys, and entire cardiovascular system
- Increased abdominal fat
- Increased "bad" low-density lipoproteins (LDD), elevating total cholesterol levels
- Depletion of calcium from the bones, leading to osteoporosis
- Spasms of the gastrointestinal tract, which can cause irritable bowel or spastic colon
- Excess secretion of digestive acids that eat away parts of the lining of the stomach or small intestine, creating ulcers
- Tearing of arterial walls and elevation of clotting elements in the blood, both of which increase plaque formation and clog the arteries
- Rapid heart rate and electrical conduction problems, which can cause cardiac arrhythmias
- Decline in sex hormones
- Killing of brain cells, premature aging of the brain, and interference with neurotransmitter function
- Decreased learning ability, memory, concentration, and even IQ

Long-standing addictions to caffeine, sugar, nicotine, or alcohol worsen adrenal insufficiency and exhaustion. Continuing stress, inadequate sleep, sudden trauma, severe physical illness, prolonged exposure to heat or cold, exposure to toxins, pollutants, and substances to which you are allergic, as well as prolonged medication with cortisone, all aggravate adrenal exhaustion.

DISEASES OF ADAPTATION

As the body ages, it becomes less flexible and able to recuperate. By adulthood, the body of the sensory defensive is torn apart from stress-related health problems, what Selye called "diseases of adaptation." Allergies, asthma, fibromyalgia, CFS, arthritis, cystitis, irritable bowel syndrome, headaches, high blood pressure, and coronary heart disease are just some diseases that sufferers get depending on what is the weakest point in their system. If it is their cardiovascular system, they may develop high blood pressure or migraine headaches. If it is their digestive system, they may develop irritable bowel syndrome, hiatus hernia, colitis, or ulcers.

By middle age, functioning becomes seriously compromised. Exhaustion, weakness, and frequent illness affect the ability of the sensory defensive to assume normal responsibilities of home and work. Type, place, and the number of hours of gainful employment a sufferer may assume, already severely limited by the challenge to find a work environment that doesn't overstimulate, become so restrictive that supporting oneself and one's family may be difficult.

In addition to the impact of ongoing stress on the immune system, the symptoms associated with sensory defensiveness increase vulnerability to disease in other ways.

- Sleep deprivation, a common symptom, is known to affect immune system functioning.
- Premenstrual sensitivity is exaggerated, PMS is inevitable, and menopausal symptoms are pronounced.
- Heightened smell triggers allergies.
- Skin sensitivity triggers skin disorders. As the skin is both the visible physical boundary of the self and an immunological organ, with every type of immune cell presented in its grooves, it is a choice medium for psychosomatic expression. Psoriasis, eczema, warts, and chronic acne all are exacerbated by stress.[4]

- Constant physical tension can produce myofascial pain syndrome, TMJ, and fibromyalgia.

Though the sensory defensive will display a multitude of symptoms, most, if not all, suffer gastrointestinal problems, allergies, and extreme hormonal fluctuation in women.

Allergies

Allergies are a defense against some kind of danger that triggers the immunoglobulin E (IgE) system. They are provoked by pollens, fungal spores, animal danders, and mite feces; by skin contact with many different substances; by eating certain food, like peanuts or shrimp; by drugs, like alcohol; by injections of drugs, like penicillin; or toxins, such as bee venom.

As infants, the sensory defensive have more allergies than the average child. How might sensory defensiveness contribute to allergies? Allergies *are* hypersensitivity. If you are highly vigilant around smell, it's as if the chemicals in the air convey to your immune system the need to be highly alert to the danger of this odor and trigger an allergic reaction to rid your body of the offending toxins. The sensory defensive often react to chemicals, like chlorine bleach, that others tolerate without discomfort, and many become physically ill from chemical exposure.

If the system becomes overwhelmed, you shut down to smell. Ella is allergic to dust, mold, pollen, feathers, and tobacco smoke, which make her nose itch. Though she had an exceptionally strong sense of smell as a child—"too deep, too intense"—and bad odors often made her nauseated, she lost her sense of smell twenty years ago. Now her sinuses are constantly stuffed and she can't even smell smoke. Dave too was strongly allergic as a child and had a strong sense of smell—his earliest memory is of feeling sick at the smell of dead fish. He too has constantly stuffed sinuses and has lost much of his sense of smell.

As sensory defensive infants often have allergies, it's unclear what came first: the chicken feathers or the smelly egg. If allergies come later and defensiveness suddenly emerges, allergies appear the cause. For instance, one tactile-defensive teenager who was affectionate as an infant and not fussy became more active, touchy, and irritable by age four, when he developed allergies.

By activating the immune system, allergies weaken other systems. Today, scientists are discovering that food allergies and a weak immune system may be implicated in autism. When parents have removed milk and wheat from the diet, some of these autistic children begin to behave more normally.[5] In Chapter 13, I talk about how to treat food allergies, and in Chapter 11 how to treat airborne allergies.

Raging Hormones

During female hormonal changes, all women experience heightened sensitivity. The more heightened one's senses, the more exaggerated the sensitivity. For instance, during ovulation, a woman's sense of smell intensifies, but dulls soon after conception and throughout the first trimester of pregnancy to restrain sexual intercourse. Then smell intensifies, presumably for the protection of the developing fetus. Aversion to tobacco smoke and certain foods are pronounced. But in the sensory defensive, smell revulsion can increase to the point of nausea near food. Touch sensitivity may also increase, and the woman jumps when her two-year-old leans against her leg. In some, though, the increased pressure from the added weight attenuates tactile sensitivity.

Poor vestibular functioning and unstable hormonal fluctuation cause most moderate to severe defensives to experience panic attacks. Most panic attacks occur premenstrually, the time of the greatest hypersensitivity, when estrogen levels are low and levels of the female hormone progesterone are high. Progesterone is known to stimulate some of the same nervous system sites that are sensitive to caffeine and sodium lactate, also implicated in producing panic attacks. During pregnancy, panic disorder abates and resumes in full force after delivery—also suggesting a relationship between female hormone levels and panic attacks.

PMS is severe in the defensive, as are menopausal symptoms such as hot flashes, night sweats, and unpredictable moods. A hot flash during menopause creates an alarm reaction—essentially heat defensiveness—and leads to extreme agitation, even panic and aggression. The hormonal instability of menopause exacerbates sensory defensiveness; starting in perimenopause, the mildly defensive may become moderate, and the moderately defensive severe. Says one defensive woman, "Perimenopause makes PMS feel like a picnic."

Are hypersensitivity and overreactivity branded into the brain of the sensory defensive? Are panic attacks, anxiety, and depression inevitable, along with progressive, debilitating illness? You can't transform the structure of the nervous system: the sensory defensive will never have an easy time of it. But a proper sensory diet can buffer the nervous system so that stress becomes more manageable and dis-ease and disease less incapacitating. The next two sections outline how.

Part Three

Your Sensory Diet

The easiest step toward improving the quality of life consists in simply learning to control the body and its senses.

—MIHALY CSIKSZENTMIHALYI,
FLOW: THE PSYCHOLOGY OF OPTIMAL EXPERIENCE

7

Getting Started

Health is aliveness, spontaneity, gracefulness, and rhythm.
—ALEXANDER LOWEN, M.D.

If you're depressed, you might take an antidepressant to alleviate malaise. If you're anxious, you might take a tranquilizer to relieve angst. If you're sensory defensive, your drug of choice to relieve distress is produced within your own body. A carefully planned sensory diet, the optimum sensorimotor activities you need to feel alert and in effortless control and to perform at your peak can provide an electrochemical fix that offers short-term and long-term relief.[1]

The more you embrace the sensory diet outlined in the following chapters, the more cumulative effects will gradually change the conditions that create the defensiveness, enabling you to feel more aware of the world without feeling invaded by it, to respond to sensation not just react. As you tap into the powers of relaxation that have been drowned out by an out-of-control flight, fight, or freeze response, you will feel calmer, breathe more slowly and deeply, sleep more easily and soundly, and feel more energized, organized, and productive. "Treatment brings freedom to mild defensive-ness, choices to moderate defensiveness and opens the options of the severe," says Patricia Wilbarger.[2]

Sensory defensiveness is complex and difficult to ameliorate, and treat-ing it requires enormous commitment and effort. For a long time, you will not have known that what you were feeling had a name. Now begins a pro-cess of self-discovery. To start, you need to become an expert in under-standing sensory defensiveness, in knowing your symptoms intimately, and identifying when new symptoms arise.[3] And you must overcome defensive thinking patterns and coping strategies that present obstacles to change.

FEAR OF CHANGE

As you've spent a lifetime adjusting to your oddities, change can feel overwhelming. True, you've inhabited a tumultuous and unfriendly body, but it's the only body you know. Furthermore, the new can be overstimu-lating and disruptive and create unpredictability that undermines control.

To increase control, start your sensory diet slowly. If possible, arrange your time to free up two to three days in a row to begin your routine, such as over a weekend. Given the correct sensory diet, you should begin to see changes almost immediately—within a day or two. Once you begin to see that change is possible, you will begin to feel a greater sense of mastery.

To increase predictability, arrange the activities to be described in the following pages in a specific schedule and mentally prepare ahead of time by insuring that you have everything you need at hand. Try to engage the help of your partner in implementing the diet. Sensory adventurists, chil-dren offer much opportunity for mutual activity. Rather than watch, ride with them on the merry-go-round. Picking up, putting down, carrying, holding, or rocking an infant offers a ready-made and utterly delectable sensory plate, the "mother lode" of sensory nutrition. If you don't have an infant, try volunteering as a cuddler in a neonatal nursery if your system and schedule will tolerate it.

Once you begin a routine, the predictability and structure that you crave will quickly get you in the groove and work in your favor. If your arousal vacillates up and down and you need unpredictability to make life sizzle, you will need to vary your routine, or it will be harder to discipline yourself to do what you need to do.

DENIAL

You have learned that you are sensory defensive, that your experiences have a name and treatment offers relief. But with this knowledge is the painful recognition that something is amiss in your brain and cannot be fixed with a pill. Some part of you will feel abnormal and flawed and a deep loss for a healthy, viable self. As with any loss, you will go through a period of grieving for what you've missed—peace of mind, human affection, pleasure in the everyday, security, confidence. Life has been unfair.

As you have adapted your life around your sensitivities, mourning might start with denying that sensory defensiveness is a problem. This enables you to retain the identity that you know. And denial makes you feel as if you have more choices than perhaps your nervous system will comfortably allow.

Even if you accept that you are sensory-defensive, you might deny how much defensiveness distorts normal functioning and controls moment-to-moment decision making, how profoundly it has compromised quality of life. Instead, you chalk up your sensitivities and the idiosyncrasies used to reduce defensiveness to being "just me," not something that needs fixing.

You need to recognize that it does need fixing, or you won't commit to change.

To see the grip of sensory defensiveness on your life, note on the following chart what you will go out of your way to avoid. Use a scale of 1 to 3: 1 for sometimes, 2 for often, 3 for always.

Avoidance of Objects, People, or Situations that Stress the Senses

Social Interaction
Contact __
   Casual hug __
   Casual kiss __
   Holding hands __
   Sexual touch __
Eye contact __
Dating __
Crowds __
Restaurants __
Family gatherings __
Visiting __
   Sick people __
   Elderly __
Other __

Parenting
Hugging child __
Kissing child __
Carrying child __
Nursing an infant __
Changing diaper __
Providing care and hygiene (washing, bathing, dressing, hair brushing, etc.) __
Listening to child __
Smelling child __
Having their friends over __
Driving with child __
Visiting child's school __

Playing with child __
Other __

Recreational
Sports events __
Sport clubs __
Athletics __
Dancing __
Vacations __
Beach __
Art projects __
Amusement parks __
Movies __
Theater __
Concerts __
Mall __
Other __

Transportation
Long car trips __
Buses __
Subways __
Trains __
Airplanes __
Boats __
Bicycle __

Animals
Dogs __
Cats __
Birds __
Horses __
Other __

Appearance

Clothing __
    Textures __
    Style __
    Dressing up __
    Turtlenecks, collars __
    Elastic waistbands, cuffs __
    Socks __
    Nylons __
Shoes __
Hats __
Jewelry __

Self-care

Baths __
Showers __
Soaps __
Lotions __
Haircuts __
Shampoos __
Hair brushing __
Hair drying __
Manicures and pedicures __
Brushing teeth __
Flossing teeth __
Makeup __
    Face __
    Lipstick __
    Eyes __
Shaving __

Sleep Environment

Sheets __

Covers __

Pillow __

Partner __

Work

Environment __

Materials (computers, fax, dictaphone) __

People __

Tasks __

Study

Classrooms __

Instructor __

Transportation __

Computers __

Materials __

Self-Soothing

Massage __

Hot tub __

Sauna __

Steam __

Other

Cooking __

Cleaning __

Dentist __

Doctors __

How did you score? If it was more than 10 points, it's a wake-up call. The well-modulated enjoy a wide choice of activities and have relatively few, if any, no's in their lives. The higher your score, the more sensory defensiveness has limited your participation in life's pleasures.

As this reality hits home, you will feel angry—"Why me?" Perhaps you'll resolve this anger and move on. Or perhaps the anger will turn to depression. Despairing that nothing you do will make you normal, especially as a lifetime of having tried a myriad of self-soothing interventions has likely met with limited success, you are convinced that whatever you try won't work. This learned helplessness encourages passivity and prevents you from pursuing your goals.

Just as you learned helplessness, you can learn hope and optimism. Activity will build greater *self-efficacy*—the belief that you have some mastery over the events in your life and can better meet challenges as they arise. Remember, behavior is a reflection of the organization of your nervous system in that moment, under those conditions. As you implement your sensory diet, you modify conditions and set up your system for self-organization. As you feel less enslaved by stress and anxiety reactions, you will feel greater empowerment in general.

DISTRESS AS NORMAL

If you are exposed to stress for too long and with too little time in between to recover, tension becomes chronic and second nature. Physical symptoms like fatigue, headaches and head pressure, constricted chest, shallow breathing, nervous stomach, and tight, wadded muscles are experienced as normal. As such, you may ignore bodily symptoms until tension escalates and you feel overly stressed, depleted, ill, or disoriented—out-of-control—and you start to shut down.

To become aware of your stress barometer, you must become intimate with your body—breathing, pulse, muscular pulls, and knots. When you begin to feel tense, hurried, worried, anxious, or stressed, stop. Look at and listen to your body, using the following guide to scan for tension.

Consider copying and pinning this list next to your computer monitor, car visor, refrigerator, bathroom mirror, or wherever you spend a great deal of time.

Body Scanning for Tension

- Holding head on one side
- Head and chin jutted forward
- Jaw tight
- Shoulders raised
- Shoulders curved toward front of body
- Fists clenched, ready for a fight
- Calves tight
- Hands fiercely gripping pen, telephone, steering wheel, cup handle, computer mouse
- Stomach tight
- Chest compressed
- Breathing quick and shallow

When tension starts to escalate, you need to stop and feed your nervous system or, if marching toward shutdown, disappear to a dark, quiet place to regroup. If not, you have a recipe for disaster—a sure way of decreasing your tolerance for sensations and all the sequelae that come with it: rigid posture, shortness of temper, impulsiveness, aggression, need for control, obsessive-compulsive behavior, stress and anxiety, and psychosomatic complaints.

Once you start the sensory diet and begin to feel calmer, you will feel more of a contrast when tensing up and, before unraveling, be more likely to stop for a "sensory meal" or at least a "sensory snack."[4]

No Longer Me

If you're sensory-defensive, you have molded your identity around it. If you change, you worry whether you will still be "me."

In truth, sensory defensiveness masks one's essence. Until it's lifted, you can't truly know your nature. For instance, the body armor created by defensiveness might make you appear inhibited, arrogant, or disinterested when at heart you're not. When you begin to relax more, a different, truer sense of self will emerge. One of the many sensory-defensive children that Patricia Wilbarger has treated was a shy, clingy, fearful 4-year-old child who would stick to her mother in the mall and resist taking the escalator. Within four days of treatment, the child was running up and down the escalator, no longer fearful and cautious.[5]

Another worry is losing the exquisite sensory acuteness that allows you to be the first to smell not just the smoke but the jasmine. In fact, the defensiveness is *inhibiting* your sensory acuity and pleasurable enjoyment of the world. When overstimulated, you shut down in self-defense, fine-tune to danger, and lose your acuity. When the freshly ground pepper overwhelms your taste buds, you don't taste the steak. Shedding the defensiveness will open up the world so you can focus in on and learn from it, and appreciate its bounty. As you learn to shut out the noise, your ears will begin to pick up the full range of sounds, from running rivulets to bird songs. As you learn to ignore the glaring fluorescent, your eyes will embrace the intricate play of colors in a Van Gogh painting.

AGITATION AS DIVERSION

Another impediment to change is letting go of anxiety. Anxiety, as Freud first postulated, diverts our attention from uncomfortable and forbidden feelings. Wanting to jump out of our skin is better than feeling unlovable, flawed, murderous, or boring. Could this explain why some hyperaroused smoke? Though smoking is a stimulant that increases their heart rate and blood pressure, perhaps the increased alertness and release of endorphins that makes smoking feel pleasurable, along with oral stimulation, blocks awareness of troubling thoughts and feelings: jitteriness for angst. Similarly, you may feel overwhelmed at a party but unable to drag yourself away to an empty house.

Fortunately, a sensory diet will lower your arousal, thus widening your control and flexibility.

MISTRUST OF AUTHORITIES

For many of you, parents, friends, doctors, teachers, and mental health professionals have misunderstood your defensiveness as anxiety, neurosis, acting, a bad mood, or being temperamental. When you reached out for help, parents may have told you nothing was wrong, to stop complaining and behaving that way, encouraging denial and suppression of feelings. You may have met similar misunderstanding with professionals.

Consequently, you may have lost trust in the powers that be to advise you and learned to rely on your own devices to figure out what works for you. You may feel that seeing an occupational therapist (OT) might mean one more person to give you bad advice.

To overcome your mistrust, find an OT who is certified in sensory integration—the more training the better. Ideally, he or she should know the Wilbarger protocol and listening therapy, which I'll discuss in Chapter 9. Though an OT may not understand all the psychological repercussions of sensory defensiveness, you will find an empathetic ear for your sensory issues and relief to be *finally* understood and treated.

GREAT EXPECTATIONS?

With new choices, you don't know what the world will expect of you. If you're no longer defensive, will you have to go out to dinner with your spouse to flashy, crowded restaurants you hate? Will you have to go to

Disney World with your kids and put up with the mayhem, a noisy plane ride, and a stuffy hotel room devoid of the creature comforts that keep you sane?

This is a defensive mind-set. As your defensiveness attenuates (and hopefully even disappears), you will perceive life differently: heretofore unimaginable choices will open. "You get better and better at *being* better and better," says Patricia Oetter. This doesn't mean that you will enjoy the trip to Disney World, but it won't traumatize you. This is not an overnight process. Letting go of your old self takes a period of adjustment. Pat Holbook offers insight: "You don't suddenly become 'normal.' You have to learn and relearn how to respond in ways different than what you are used to. And you need to trust your wellness enough to even try things you could not do before. And you need to expect and accept that relapses will happen."

Hopefully, you now feel open to change and to beginning your sensory diet. Let's begin with the activities that offer the most powerful and long-lasting effect on your nervous system, those that tap into the primitive brainstem: tactile, vestibular, and proprioceptive input.

8

Priming the Pump

Those who think they have no time for bodily exercise will sooner or later have to find time for illness.

—EDWARD STANLEY, EARL OF DERBY, 1873

After a typical day at the office—a morning of chatter, beeping faxes, ringing phones, fluorescent lights—you might try to calm with positive self-talk or affirmations: "I'm strong. I can make it through this day. I will get a massage this weekend and everything will be okay." But this attempt to control stress goes from mind to body, or cortex to brain stem. It is inefficient in regulating arousal, nor can it be sustained. It is more effective to look for a solution impacting the brain stem directly, where the sensory threshold gets set, and work from the bottom up, from the body to the mind.

BOTTOM-UP PROCESSING

As the primary organizers of the nervous system, deep pressure touch, proprioception, and vestibular input offer the most powerful grounding and long-lasting results of any sensations. Sitting and watching the sunset may be calming, but the visual input is short-lived and not intense, whereas watching the sunset while you are climbing to the top of the hill and giving your muscles a workout provides a deep calm that lasts for hours.

To get a taste of the power of proprioception, get up from your chair and push hard into the wall with your arms straight until you feel some fatigue. By strongly engaging the muscles and joints—by doing "heavy work"—you are stimulating the cerebellum at the back part of your brain stem, which communicates with the reticular activating system to inhibit arousal to a normal level so you can concentrate on the task at hand. Once arousal is contained, you can think more clearly. A back rub or rocking back and forth in your chair has a similar effect.

Implementing these powerful sensations into your daily regimen will help to retrain the protective limbic system in your brain to not respond to harmless stimuli with a false alarm. As your brain switches from avoidance to approach, you will start to feel more in control of your body, mind, and emotions. And though the conventional wisdom has been that change was possible only in the young brain, we now know that the brain can be re-sculpted to some extent throughout adulthood. If you can do activity, you are not too old to change.

Push and Pull

Quickly calming and organizing, heavy work increases body awareness to help you feel more grounded—more in your body. When you are over-aroused, it calms you; when you're sluggish, it alerts you. And unlike other sensory input, heavy work rarely overloads the nervous system.

Examples of heavy work are pushing and pulling heavy loads, as in rearranging furniture, or lifting or carrying heavy objects, like a laundry basket or a child, or the resistance you feel when you walk a dog on a leash. Wearing weights on your ankles as you go about your daily business (light weights so as not to put strain on the extremities), and even while you sleep, provides traction that increases discharge from joint receptors. "I wear 2½-pound weights on my ankles during the day and night," says one woman. "It helps to feel grounded. It tells your brain, 'Your feet are right here, and you're okay!'" As the jaw is one of the main joints in our body, chewing, chomping, and sucking applies pressure to help us get it together. This is one of the primary reasons we eat when we're upset or nervous.

Here are some of the ways for the brain to receive heavy work:

Whole Body Action

- Handstands, headstands, shoulder stands, push-ups, jumping jacks, and gymnastics
- Hanging by the arms, chin-ups
- Arm wrestling
- Weight lifting
- Backpacking, or climbing stairs, or walking while wearing a weighted vest, a backpack of weights or books
- Crashing down on a trampoline
- Horseback riding
- Mountain biking
- Exercise bikes with resistance
- Rock climbing
- Contact sports: wrestling, martial arts, football
- Waterskiing, kayaking, deep-water rafting
- Swimming (the deeper under water, the more intense)

Daily Routine (Especially with Children)

- Moving furniture
- Hoeing in the garden
- Taking out the trash
- Walking the dog on a leash

- Playing tug-of-war
- Play-wrestling
- Carrying the baby
- Crawling on hands and knees up and down stairs
- Crawling through a tight space
- Rolling on the floor

Quick, Subtle Proprioceptive Activities

- Pushing hands together in a prayer position
- Pressing down with your hands on top of your head
- Lying down and pushing against a wall with your legs
- Pushing against a wall or the steering wheel of your car at a stoplight with your hands and arms outstretched
- Lying under heavy quilts, or under a weighted blanket or pillows

The effect of heavy work lasts around two hours and should be repeated during down times. The more you engage your muscles in sustained activity, versus a quick workout, the more intense the effect.

Shake, Rattle, Rock, and Roll

If you've ever ridden a roller coaster, you know the deep calm following the screaming. Psychologists say it results from the adrenaline rush and from limbic activity surviving a scary experience. But that reaction is secondary. The primary effect comes from the massive vestibular input into the brain stem, along with the deep pressure against the body from the G force, or gravity.

The vestibular receptors are the most sensitive of all sense organs and have a powerful effect on arousal, modulating the nervous system by calming those who are hyped and revving up those who are enervated. Depending on quality, intensity, and duration, this effect lasts 4 to 8 hours. Every change in head position stimulates some of the vestibular receptors in the inner ear, and you should incorporate movement in all directions into your sensory diet. When you bend your head to the side or hold it upside down, gravity pulls the calcium carbonate crystals away from their normal position in the head, changing the flow of impulses in the vestibular nerve. Spinning activates one of the canals in each ear; running and swinging move them in another direction and cause the fluid in some of the semicircular canals to back up into the sensitive receptors. The motion of a rocking chair triggers specific receptors, while riding back and forth on a glider triggers others that offer more intense input. Similarly, rolling back and forth on your belly on a large exercise ball for 15 minutes sets off a vestibular pow that has a long-lasting effect, as it replicates the rocking movement in utero. Bending upside down also provides intense vestibular stimulation, while standing, walking, and riding in a moving vehicle move the head in more subtle ways, providing milder vestibular input.

As youngsters, we get lots of vestibular input: we swing, jump on trampolines, rollerblade, dive into water, or enjoy other activities that require a quick shift from being totally vertical. This keeps our vestibular apparatus oiled. As we age, we need less intensity and "get by" with using it less and less. But the more vestibular input, the better any nervous system functions, especially one that is starved. The nervous system of the sensory defensive demands activities that offer up-and-down, side-to-side, and back-and-forth movement.

Some caution is advised. Though you can't overdose on proprioception, you can on vestibular stimulation. If you get dizzy or queasy, start out rocking, spinning, swinging, and swaying slowly, and gradually increase vestibular input. You can also modulate vestibular input by adding proprioception. Jumping on a trampoline, for instance, entails both up and down movement, and the effort to propel your body stimulates joint compressions. Bouncing up and down on a therapy ball, in contrast, does not heavily engage joint receptors.

Try some of these activities for vestibular-proprioceptive input.

- Swinging, rocking, swiveling side to side
- Jumping rope
- Tumbling
- Using a trampoline (the larger, the more input)
- Bouncing or rolling back and forth on an exercise ball, especially while lying prone
- Bike riding
- Rock climbing
- Skiing, both downhill and cross-country
- Dance, aerobics, yoga, tai chi, gymnastics, calisthenics
- Rollerblading
- Ice-skating
- Hockey
- Running, fast walking, walking on sand
- Tennis, racquetball, squash, handball
- Basketball
- Upside-down yoga postures
- Riding on a roller coaster
- Diving
- Sleeping on a waterbed

Getting in Touch

If you lack nutrients in your body, you need excess nourishment to return your system to health. If you lack touch in your life, you need excess skin stimulation to balance out your nervous system. Occupational therapists have been using terrycloth washcloths and various brushes to stimulate the skin of the tactile defensive since the 1960s. While working in a neonatal intensive care unit in the 1980s, Patricia Wilbarger tried deep-pressure skin stimulation with a nonscratching pressure brush on the infants. The results were dramatic. From this, she devised the Wilbarger protocol.[1]

The protocol entails deep-pressure skin brushing. Deep-pressure touch lies between light touch, which can scratch or tickle, and heavy

touch, which can be painful. This is followed by proprioceptive input consisting of quick compressions (push and pull) of each joint. The firm pressure to body parts and joints stimulates all the proprioceptors (the nerve
endings that give you a clear sense of your body) and helps override the
flight-or-fight reaction. And proprioception, always modulating, will balance out possible overarousal from the brushing.

Why would skin brushing be so modulating? The average human body
has around 5 million nerve endings or touch receptors. One tiny patch of
skin on the back of our hand, less than an inch square, contains:

- 9 feet of blood vessels
- 600 pain sensors
- 30 hairs
- 300 sweat glands
- 4 oil glands
- 13 yards of nerves
- 9,000 nerve endings
- 6 cold sensors
- 36 heat sensors
- 75 pressure sensors[2]

Deep-pressure touch from a thousand soft bristles at once sparks milli-
volts of electricity that stimulate many different types of tactile receptors
in the skin. The skin surges with a pleasant tingling, in my own experience, and the more often you repeat the protocol throughout the day, the
more intense and pleasurable the sensation.

The effect lasts around 2 hours. If the protocol is repeated six to eight
times a day, you can quickly stimulate millions of tactile receptors, and
your system won't have a chance to regress. Within two to three days, clinicians often report dramatic changes in defensiveness, attention, mood,
emotional stability, relating, learning, and memory. In a videotape on
sensory defensiveness, Patricia Wilbarger interviews Mary, a woman in her
thirties with pronounced tactile defensiveness. Her body is stiff, her voice

is forced, her giggle is explosive, and you get exhausted listening to her. A few days after using the Wilbarger protocol, Mary appears transformed. Her posture is less rigid, her voice has slowed down, and the pitch is within normal range. She makes eye contact more easily, her face is more relaxed, and she is not so giggly. What's more, *you* don't feel strained listening to her. More organized, Mary experienced in time profound changes in her personal relationships.[3]

In some cases, lifelong sexual dysfunction may resolve. Wilbarger closely monitors her clients and calls them a few days after they've begun the protocol. She tells of one woman who, following a week of brushing, couldn't be found. She was shacked up with her husband in a hotel, enjoying sex for the first time in her marriage!

Treatment with the intervention protocol can begin at 2 months of age. Before this time the infant's nervous system is too immature. Within two to three weeks of treatment, Wilbarger has found that defensiveness is typically substantially decreased and, in some cases, eliminated: a $2 non-scratching brush can circumvent a lifetime of misery. Furthermore, the change is permanent and occurs regardless of age. As defensive infants are often overly fussy, imagine how much child abuse, set off by incessant crying, could be prevented!

The Wilbarger protocol must be taught and monitored by a specially trained professionals, generally an occupational therapist, as both the brush and the technique are highly specific. Improper brushing will not get results and can even exacerbate defensiveness. When done properly, it has helped changed the lives of many tactile defensive sufferers, who can't envision life without it. If you are tactile defensive, it behooves you to learn it and make it a routine part of your day, like brushing your teeth. The key to success lies not in "brushing" the skin but in applying deep pressure strokes to the skin.

What are the specific mechanisms involved in such extraordinary changes from the skin brushing? Scientists are unclear. One hypothesis, proposed by the Wilbargers, relates to the pain threshold.[4] If you treat pain with acupuncture or acupressure, you stimulate endorphins. On the first visit, the effect lasts for 90 minutes or so and then the pain starts to come back slowly. But by the end of the week, patients report pain relief that extends beyond 90 minutes, without a difference in endorphin release. Brushing, augmented by joint compressions and heavy work, may create a similar release of endorphins. With repeated intervention, the protocol resets the sensory threshold.

Though several studies demonstrate the Wilbarger protocol to reduce defensiveness in children with special needs, only one study has looked at its effect on the sensory-defensive adult. A severely defensive 24-year-old woman had been admitted to an inpatient psychiatric unit for depression, panic attacks, and borderline personality traits.[5] After two weeks on the antidepressant Imipramine, her mood appeared stabilized but she remained distressed and "overwhelmed." While out on passes with her husband, she twice attempted suicide.

After six weeks, treatment began with an initial three days of skin brushing six times a day, followed by deep proprioceptive input and daily sensory-integrative treatment to treat underlying sensory inefficiencies. After the third day, a 1-hour sensorimotor treatment was added to her hospital protocol 5 days a week. After 8 weeks, her panic attacks were reduced, and she showed improvement in gravitational insecurity, body awareness, and tactile defensiveness. Before treatment, she tripped easily, wore only soft clothes, and avoided situations where she might be lightly touched. She felt easily disturbed and distracted by noise, became easily overstimulated by visual stimuli, woke up several times during the night, and she felt incompetent. After two years of treatment, her panic attacks ceased. She no longer felt accident-prone, wore clothing of varying textures, and was able to go shopping, attend church, and stand in lines. She responded normally to sound, more easily tolerated a variety of visual stimuli, seldom woke up during the night, and felt more competent. She made her sensory diet an integral part of her life, brushing one to four times a day, depending on her level of stress, and she exercised regularly.

Other Deep-Pressure Interventions

There are other ways to get skin stimulation.

Some companies sell powerful vibrators that provide a deep-pressure massage with long-lasting effects. Vibrators cause the bones to vibrate and stimulate the gravity receptors as well. Some people are calmed by leaning against a washing machine or dryer or resting their head against a train or bus window to feel the vibration. As with other interventions, vibration is integrating if you enjoy it but potentially disorganizing if you do not, so follow your body's reaction in choosing it for therapy.

Another effective means of pressure is to wear a "bear hug" vest that fits snugly next to the body, with adjustable straps and body wrap to adjust the amount of pressure as desired. For proprioceptive input, you can also add weights. At night, weighted blankets create pressure to help some sleep more restfully.

Any kind of skin stimulation will release tension, even if just briefly: loufah brushes, bath sponges, a terrycloth washcloth, a hair-brush; shower attachments that spray, needle, massage, or pulse; wooden body and foot rollers; tappers; sleeping on a terrycloth beach towel.

As part of a research study, one 22-year-old tactile defensive woman was instructed to vigorously rub her skin with a dry terrycloth washcloth and plastic bristle hairbrush for a half-hour to one hour each evening for three months.[6] Over the course of treatment, physiological parameters were measured as she was exposed to light touch, a flashing light, and a loud tone. Respiration rate, hand temperature, and skin conductance responses reflected increased relaxation and ability to tune out unpleasant stimulation over the course of the study, suggesting that the treatment helped modulate her nervous system.

Body rolling, which involves sitting on a hard ball to create pressure in specific areas of the body, offers intense deep pressure and proprioception. Like the Wilbarger protocol, the effect lasts around 2 hours. It is an inexpensive self-massage, and the ball is small enough to carry with you when traveling. You can find classes in your area or buy *Body*

Rolling, by Yamuna Zake (Healing Arts Press), and follow the instructions.

Other ways to create deep pressure include rolling across the floor, digging into the roots of your hair and yanking it and twisting it for deep pressure to your scalp, underwater swimming, and especially deep-sea diving.

Oral defensiveness is treated separately from tactile defensiveness, as the mouth is controlled by the cranial nerves. A simple technique that Patricia Wilbarger has devised that puts firm pressure against the palate is quickly effective.[7] Recall that in only two days of treatment, Serena, the girl with anorexic-like symptoms, began to eat foods she had never eaten before.

The Most Powerful Activities

The more an activity provides deep-pressure, tactile, vestibular, and proprioceptive input, the stronger and more pervasive the effect. Jumping and crashing on a large trampoline provides all these sensations at once, and, to music, auditory input as well. Martial arts, backpacking, and rock climbing offer intense heavy work. Dance, yoga, tai chi, and qigong, which I'll discuss in Chapter 15, involve movements requiring balance, coordination, weight bearing, and heavy pressure that calm, organize, and increase body awareness.

Water activities, including swimming, walking underwater, or water exercise offer resistance and pressure against the body and are excellent ways to increase body awareness. Heavy underwater pressure and a tight scuba diving suit make deep-sea diving an ultimate whole-body embrace, and the shimmering underwater pageant powerful visual stimulation. After a Sunday of scuba diving, very tactile-defensive Dave feels relaxed and less touchy for two full days.

Horseback riding is a total sensory modulation package.[8] Heat from the horse penetrates the muscles. Cantering offers deep pressure touch and vestibular stimulation, and when the horse gallops, you work hard to move up and down with the horse, intensifying deep pressure and vestibular input. As the horse trots and you bump up and down against the horse, you get proprioceptive input. Some people are also sexually aroused by the movement, which stimulates the genitals. As you change position from sitting upright to lying prone, you impact nearly every part of the body. The sheer effort of riding a horse boosts respiration, and petting the horse's smooth coat offers a pleasant tactile sensation.

Also beneficial for focus are sensory "snacks" or pick-ups. These consist of short oral motor input, like chewing or sucking, less intense movement and touch experiences, pleasing odors, interesting sights, pleasurable music, and other means of "stimming," like fidgeting, twirling hair, sighing, humming.

Evolution of a Sensory Diet

That intense tactile, vestibular, and proprioceptive sensation should be an essential part of one's sensory diet is not a notion confined to those with a disorganized nervous system. It is precisely how our bodies were designed to function.

Constantly on the go, our early ancestors hunted and foraged for food and water, walked, ran, carried children, hauled bananas and melons, fought lions and tigers, and groomed, massaged, and rubbed up against each other. Hard work, with heavy doses of deep-pressure touch and movement, was adaptive for survival, keeping bodies and minds in good working order. At the end of the day, it brought tranquility and sleep.

Movement is medication. It modulates our nervous system, creating energy, stamina, and relaxation; it improves our self-image and makes us stronger mentally and physically. Children run, jump, spin, and demand to be picked up and rocked because movement is pleasurable and helps organize the brain to do its job effectively.

Exercise purges stress chemicals. Our bodies were designed to be able to run furiously from danger or fight back with all our might, expending enormous energy and releasing stress chemicals; afterward, the person felt better. But when a flashing ambulance light, a crowded elevator, or the dentist's drill sets off alarm, there's nowhere to run to and no one to punch. You just sit and stew. Without release, these chemicals within the body become toxic. Heavy work affords an outlet.

Moreover, vigorous exercise can be the acme of pleasure. If you exercise for more than 30 to 40 minutes, your body releases endorphins, producing the runner's high. In a study of 156 severely depressed people, Duke University scientists found that three 30-minute weekly workouts brought the same relief as antidepressants.[9] And while 40 percent of those on drug treatment relapsed back into depression within six months, only 8 percent of the exercisers did. "When we are unhappy, depressed, or bored we have an easy remedy at hand: to use the body for all it's worth," asserts psychologist Mihaly Czikszentmihalyi.[10]

Exercise has both psychological and physical benefits.

The psychological benefits are as follows:

- Releases pent-up energy and frustration
- Relaxes tense muscles that contribute to feeling uptight
- Distracts us from worries
- Builds up serotonin in the brain, which diminishes anticipatory anxiety of negative sensory experiences, like being in crowded areas

The physical benefits of exercise are as follows:

- Enhances oxygenation of the blood and brain, increasing alertness and concentration
- Improves blood sugar regulation
- Lowers pH (increased acidity) of the blood, which increases energy level
- Improves circulation, digestion, and elimination
- Increases cardiorespiratory function

- Decreases cholesterol levels and blood pressure
- Improves sleep and reduces insomnia

SETTING YOUR SENSORY DIET

Setting up a sensory diet requires planning. You need to figure out a way to incorporate "sensory meals" (deep pressure, heavy work, and vestibular input) as well as "snacks" into your life according to your unique sensory needs. To set up your sensory diet:

- Evaluate your needs.
- Set up your environment.
- Gauge choice of activities by their dynamics: intensity, frequency, duration, rhythm, timing.
- Incorporate your sensory diet into your lifestyle.
- Educate others.

Evaluate Your Needs

Each person has unique sensory needs to maintain optimal arousal for the activities in question. To lower arousal into a drowsy state for sleep, one person requires silence, another listens to nature sounds, and another requires the white noise of a humming fan. Knowing your arousability helps in choosing a sport. If you are hyperaroused, fast-moving sports, such as basketball, hockey, soccer, racquetball, may be too exciting and further stress you. And competitive, confrontational sports may exhaust your nervous energy, further tensing you. Exercises that provide calm and focus, such as yoga, swimming, or dance, may be more beneficial. If, however, you jump from low to high arousal, fast-moving sports may be what you need to thrust your system into an optimal zone.

You need to schedule your activities at the right time of day for you. High-arousal introverts tend to be alert in the morning but reach their edge early and start to wind down by evening. In the morning, rock music on the car radio may increase alertness. At the end of a long day, the noise is cacaphonous.

Low-arousal extroverts, in contrast, are owls. It takes them a while to become alert and they need intensity in the morning to get going—loud music, cold water splashed on the face, jumping jacks, and caffeine—and become increasingly alert as the day goes on.

To test your arousability, squeeze a few drops of lemon on your tongue and see how much you salivate. The more you do, the greater your sensitivity and inhibition. Probably it's a sensitivity to smell that is triggering the salivation, as smell hits us faster than taste. The lemon-drop test was devised by Hans Eysenck, a psychologist at the Institute of Psychiatry in London. He was the first to look at introversion and extroversion in relation to excitation of the nervous system and the father of the biological study of personality. When Eysenck placed four drops of lemon juice on an individual's tongue for 20 seconds, extreme extroverts salivated little or not at all. Extreme introverts practically drooled, showing an increment of almost 1 gram of saliva.[11]

To figure out what gets you going, what slows you down, and what gets you over the edge, you need to be aware of the sensory qualities of daily events. Start by looking at your daily routine to see what throws off your nervous system.

Part of day you feel most organized: _____

Part of day you feel most disorganized: _____

Organizing activities: _____
_____

Disruptive activities: _____
_____

Organizing places: _____
_____

Disruptive places: _____
_____

Organizing temperature: _____

Disruptive temperature: _____

Organizing touch: _____
_____

Disruptive touch: _____
_____

Organizing sounds: _____
_____

Disruptive sounds: _____
_____

Organizing lighting: _____
_____

Disruptive lighting: _____
_____

Organizing smells: _____
_____

Disruptive smells: _____
_____

Organizing morning routine: _____
_____

Disruptive morning routine: _____
_____

Environment needed to fall asleep (dark, quiet, soft music): ____
_____

Environment needed to wake up (alarm, soft music, chitchat, sunlight): _____

Set Up Your Environment

You need to set up your environment to eliminate or reduce disruptive stimuli and enhance organizing stimuli. Subsequent chapters provide an analysis of sounds, lights, smells, temperature, and space modifications that you can easily make.

Activity Dynamics

A sensory diet consists of sensorimotor input, measured by the intensity, frequency, duration, rhythm, and timing you need to set up the conditions for self-organization.

To maintain optimal arousal, the young child needs considerable sensory input and may need to be rocked strongly (intensity) for a half-hour (duration) several times a day (frequency). As we mature, we require less input for organization, and unconsciously moving around in our seat or stretching may do the trick. But the more disorganized the nervous system, at either the high or low end, the more sensory nutrition needed to feed it. For some, that might mean as much input as for the young child— daily, ongoing, frequent, and vigorous exercise.

Intensity

Power comes from intensity. By offering deep pressure touch, the Wilbarger protocol is more powerful than a loufah brush massage. Jumping on a trampoline provides more intense vestibular input than rocking in a rocking chair. You need to learn what intensity your nervous system requires for modulation.

Frequency

To maintain optimal arousal and organization, sensorimotor activities should happen at specific intervals and throughout the day.[12] Annoying sensation, daily hassles, hurt feelings, conflict, and other stresses constantly destabilize the nervous system, and it needs to be rejuvenated. To prevent tension from escalating, incorporate into your day frequent sensory snacks: stand up and stretch; push against the wall; bend down to touch your toes.

Duration

Activities vary in time spent doing them and in length of effect. Some of the most important changes in the nervous system can come from knowing how to choose activities for their long-lasting effects. Specific treatment interventions like the Wilbarger protocol for deep-pressure touch and joint compression are short but effective for 1 to 2 hours. Others, like fidgeting in your seat or chomping on potato chips, act as brief mood changers.

You also need to know how long you need to do a particular activity. Some people get organized with 5 minutes on the trampoline; others need a half-hour of jumping and bouncing.

Rhythm

Usually, familiar, repetitive activities, which boost serotonin levels in the brain, lower arousal level, while novel or nonrhythmic activities perk you up. This is why taking a break from the computer to wash dishes or fold towels is calming. For some, however, repetition can be overly sedating. If you seesaw up and down, you may need to wash the dishes with some salsa music playing in the background lest your arousal dip too low.

Timing

In general, you should start out the day with some form of heavy work and some tactile stimulation. If you have a family to care for, you can make activities like play wrestling or jumping on a trampoline a family affair. As stress escalates, you should repeat heavy work to slough off excess stress chemicals.

Heavy work or movement activities should be repeated at noon and then again in the late afternoon or early evening. Strenuous physical activity lasts from 2 to 8 hours. If your schedule does not permit a workout during the day, early-morning vestibular input, which can last 6 to 8 hours, will sustain you. As you begin to feel tension rise during your down times, you need little pickups. The more tactile, proprioceptive, and vestibular stimulation you experience throughout the day, the more organized you will feel.

Your arousal level changes as you go through the day, necessitating a modification of the intensity, frequency, duration, and rhythm of sensori-motor input. At one point, you may need to run around the block to get organized, at another to do a few push-ups, and at another munch on a carrot. To give you some idea how events create a cumulative effect throughout the day, rate your arousal level over two days—on a work day and on a leisure day.[13]

Arousal Level

	Drowsy	Low	Optimal	Overaroused/ Overload
Wake up				
8:00				
9:00				
10:00				
11:00				
12:00				
1:00				
2:00				
3:00				
4:00				
5:00				
6:00				
7:00				
8:00				
Bedtime				

Make It a Part of Your Lifestyle

Like most adults, you probably work and care for a family. Adapting your sensory diet to such issues as time, money, and priority, and keeping it up will be challenging.

If you find exercise a drudge, especially, you will be tempted to forgo it. Don't! As the diabetic depends on insulin shots to regulate sugar level the sensory defensive depends on a daily sweat to regulate arousal level. Exercise is the fuel your body needs to operate correctly, so dislike of exercise is antibiological. It may be more of a symptom of sensory-integration dysfunction than actual desire and related to low or high muscle tone, low arousal to get going, clumsiness, uncoordinated movement, or poor balance. This is all the more reason to stimulate those movement receptors.

Enjoyment

In general, the best sensory diet is one that you enjoy and that fits in with your lifestyle so that you can keep it up. If you like to do tae-bo but the gym is overstimulating, you can punch and kick to a tape conveniently at home.

If you avoid exercise because you lack coordination, you might try taking a daily walk through a park or along a beach. Though not as intense as other exercise, walking holds many benefits for the mind as well as the body. The cross-patterned movement of our limbs—right arm and left leg, then left arm and right leg—generates electrical activity in the brain, boosting serotonin and harmonizing the nervous system. If you wear headphones and listen to music as you walk, you will add auditory input and increase coordination. If you add a weighted belt or vest or carry hand weights, you will increase weight-bearing and proprioceptive input. Walk on grass, rather than a hard surface like concrete or asphalt. A research study found that walking on a hard surface causes people unconsciously to brace their bodies by tightening their abdomens and to breathe faster and higher up into their chests, increasing arousal.[14]

Whatever you choose, weigh costs and benefits. Walking a dog is a great workout, but not if his bark startles you constantly and you can't stand his smells and licking.

Convenience

While specific activities require time and planning, there are many ways to incorporate activities into your daily routine. Here are some suggestions:

- Park farthest, rather than nearest, to the supermarket entrance and carry, rather than cart, your groceries to the car.
- Fast-walk while window shopping in the mall.
- Bend down in a gradual forward stretch while fetching something on the floor.
- Replace your electric can opener with a manual one.
- Rock or roll on a therapy ball while watching TV or working at your computer.
- Walk around the house wearing ankle weights.
- Wear a weighted vest while driving.
- Sleep with a weighted blanket.
- Sit on a movement cushion at work, at the cinema, or at lectures.
- Carry, rather than stroll, your infant.
- Replace your electric lawn mower with a manual one.

Schedule

Scheduling and preparation increase predictability, decrease disruptions, tame sensory input, and help you feel safer. If you develop consistent routines for daily activities, you will be more likely to stick to these activities.

How you start your day is crucial. If you are out of sync upon waking, you will be disorganized for a good part of the day. If family responsibilities interfere with the activities you need to start your day, try to make it a habit to get up before the rest of the family and do your morning thing.

Disruptions

Dip into your sensory survival kit to prepare for upcoming disruptive events, like your son's football game, a family dinner, or a conference.

- Wear earplugs to help drown out noise in public places.
- Do deep-pressure brushing or a dry loufah scrub before the splash and temperature change of the morning shower.
- Use a handheld hose to control pressure and spray during a shower and keep water out of the eyes.
- Wrap yourself tightly in a large terrycloth towel when getting out of the bathtub into the cool air.
- Rub your feet vigorously before walking in sand or grass.

Educate Others

For the sensory defensive, a person's voice, laugh, odor, eye contact, touch, skin feel, and movements present potentially disruptive sensory input.[15] You need to educate your significant others in ways to interact that provide appropriate sensation. For example, you might ask them to not shout or play disruptive music and to skip the aftershave.

Touch, of course, is fraught with sensation and meaning, especially between couples. You need to be open and specific about your dislike of light or unexpected touch, particularly regarding sexual matters, but also explain that at times you desperately need a firm hug. "Do hug. Don't tickle," advise Patricia and Julia Wilbarger. For those tactile defensives who have a supportive partner and can control when, where, and how someone can touch them, touch can be comfortable and even pleasurable.[16] They might ask for touch with more pressure or ask their partner to use the palm of his hand rather than the fingertips or to avoid touching a certain area. In fact, some sensory defensives feel their extreme sensitivity intensifies the pleasure of lovemaking.

Your partner needs to understand that "I can't" means you *can't*, not you *won't.* Forcing you to go to the circus will only take you into sensory overload.

If your partner, family, and friends can't understand why you are so "finicky," "sensitive," "touchy," "unreasonable," "neurotic," and so on, try to give them insight as to what your world is like with concrete examples that they can relate to. Tell them to imagine driving in their car while wearing a scratchy burlap shirt, staring into someone's blinkers ahead of them, listening to music they hate turned up to the max, all the while trying to converse with a passenger who has not bathed for a week. Explain that this is a daily reality for some sensory defensives. Or explain that you feel like they do when they're feverish or being bitten by mosquitos, and that you can feel overwhelmed and spacey like a person who has just been in a car accident.

When they do finally get it, hopefully it will change your relationship, as it did for Monica. When Monica pulled away from her husband, he took it personally and would often spiral into deep depression. Constantly anxious, she attacked him and he felt she didn't love him. "He just never understood me. He never believed that I truly loved him, no matter how many times I voiced it, because I would turn around and pick at him the next minute for crowding me."

Communication was minimal and they avoided each other. As she didn't know what was wrong with her, she felt crazy and blamed herself for their rift. When she discovered she was sensory defensive, she could explain to her husband why she withdraws and picks on him. She was able to teach him what touch felt good and what touch to avoid. "Since he has finally accepted that this 'thing' is real, it has made the biggest difference in my life. It actually feels good to know that I am not crazy. We have finally worked out a way of meeting each other's needs without the feelings of being rejected or misunderstood all the time. He understands me for the first time."

To keep your nervous system modulated, you should feed your nervous system throughout the day. Next, let's look at how to further balance your sensory diet with sound.

9

Sound Health

> Everything in the universe consists of some kind of vibrating, pulsing, rhythmic pattern.
>
> —HAZRAT INAYAT KHAN
> *RHYTHM AS PULSE, RHYTHM AS LIFE*

New Age composer Jim Oliver does a fun experiment in his workshops to illustrate the "pull," or entrainment of sound. He tells two people to stand ear to ear (one person's left ear against the other's right ear) and to use their hands to cover the other ear. He gives one person a tone to hum and the other a different, dissonant tone to hum. It is close to impossible for most people to maintain this dissonant sound for long. In a matter of minutes both are humming each other's tones, and pretty soon everyone in the room begins humming each other's tones.

Sound begins with movement that shakes up surrounding air molecules, which in turn stir other molecules, creating a ripple effect to form fields of vibrating energy. If you place a cup of water near a stereo speaker, you can watch the water dance with the musical vibration. As these vibrations hit our body, we entrain to them and they subtly alter our breath, pulse, blood pressure, muscle tension, skin temperature, brain waves, and other internal rhythms. "My objections to Wagner's music are physiological," Nietzsche said. "I breathe with difficulty as soon as Wagner's music begins to act upon me."[1]

What has entrainment got to do with the sensory defensive? Plenty.

If the tones are healing and accord to the body's natural rhythms, entrainment will influence internal rhythms and override the internal disharmony of the sensory defensive. Think of how, when you dance, the music takes over your body, which automatically adjusts to the pace, pulse, and rhythm. If the music goes against one's natural rhythms, it throws off the body's rhythms and causes discomfort.

TUNING TO THE FAST BEAT

The next time you eat in a restaurant, notice the music and how you and your fellow diners are chewing. People chew to the speed (usually fast to hurry people out) of the background music.[2] They're literally entrained to "eat to the beat." Even if eating alone, people will chew to the speed of those eating around them.

From the first moments of life, our being strives to be in harmony with our surroundings and with each other. If you videotape a parent talking to her newborn infant and then replay it in slow motion, you see an interactive synchrony between the baby's movements and the parent's speech.[3] When we feel connected, we move similarly in tandem with the other's gestures, as if on the same wavelength: He puts his hand on his cheek; unconsciously she leans her hand against her cheek. In fact, as it turns out, we *are* on the same wavelength—literally. When two friends have a harmonious conversation, their brains waves get "in sync."[4]

When relaxed, the entire body vibrates at a fundamental rate of approximately 7.8 to 8 cycles per second, matched by alpha brain waves, associated with a relaxed state, at the same frequency. Earth itself vibrates at the same fundamental frequency of 8 cycles per second. Thus, a resonance exists between the human body in a natural relaxed state and the electrically charged layers of Earth's atmosphere. Being relaxed means feeling in harmony with the world.

The fast and irregular rhythm of modern society violates this natural rhythm. While a balanced nervous system can adapt to, and to some extent override, the dissonance, and the sensation seeker feels titillated by the incongruity, the sensory defensive entrains quickly to the dissonant rhythms, and this furthers internal chaos. The loud, fast music that has become a staple of modern life—played in restaurants, department stores, banks, elevators, and even as we pump gas—contributes to their disharmony.

We even entrain unconsciously to the electrical current in our environment. In the United States and Canada, electricity operates on an alternating current of 60 cycles per second. The resonant frequency of 60-cycle electrical current relates to the B natural tone on a musical scale. In Europe the alternating electrical current is 50 cycles per second, which relates musically to G sharp. During meditation, music professor R. Murray Schafer asked American, Canadian, and German students to spontaneously sing whatever tone came naturally. For Americans and Canadians, B natural was the most frequent tone hummed. For German students it was G sharp.[5] In other words, whether we consciously hear the humming of the fan, the computer, or the refrigerator, electrical current permeates our cells, causing us to entrain to it.

TURN DOWN THE VOLUME!

Noise is a recent manmade scourge. It obscures the world, hinders the proper reception of sound, and knocks the body's rhythms out of tune, furthering dysfunction in the sensory defensive. Human hearing evolved in an environment of relative quiet, ill preparing us to endure the frequently unpredictable, uncontrollable, unwanted, and even harmful screaming, humming, buzzing, clanking, beeping sounds of modern life. At the end of the eighteenth century, when Mozart was composing, the city of Vienna was so quiet that fire alarms were delivered verbally by a shouting watchman atop St. Stephan's Cathedral. To rise above the sounds of city noise today, police car sirens are at a level of noise that reaches the threshold of pain.

As sudden and loud noises register in the brain as warning signals of danger, exposure to loud noise creates a startle response. All of us in noisy environments, and especially the sound sensitive, are prey to increased irritability, moodiness, high blood pressure, headaches, tension, hyperactivity, poor digestion, ulcers, fatigue, cardiovascular disease, decreased immunity, neurological disorders, disturbed sleep, and poor work performance. Noise can make people angry, even explosive. Crying sets off child abuse. Our noisy highways may contribute to road rage.

If loud noise is at the same frequency as the message we are trying to hear, sorting out important signals becomes difficult, and this adds to the confusion already experienced by the sensory defensive. And the defensive react not just to the noise from the street and machine noises. Even in the rustic countryside, bird cries or insect chirps can be a noisy distraction.

An alarm response to noise and bright light is so ingrained in our brain that we experience it before learning takes place: in utero. In the last trimester of pregnancy, if you shine a bright light on the mother's abdomen in the fetus's line of vision, or if you make a loud noise, the fetus will startle. If you shine a softer light or make a soft noise, the fetus actively and smoothly turns toward the stimulus, seeking it out.[6] If you play Mozart or Vivaldi toward the end of pregnancy, fetal heart rates invariably steady and kicking declines, while other music, especially rock, drives most fetuses to kick violently.

Though many noise sources are beyond our control, many things can improve our immediate sonic environments.

- Plant earth berms (mounds of dirt) and rows of thick trees or shrubs to reflect and absorb sound.
- Use the same insulation that insures greater thermal efficiency to cut down on noise: double-pane windows, weather stripping, caulking that reduces heat transfer.

- Put padding under computers, blenders, and similar machines; install refrigerators, furnaces, and washing machines on special vibration mounting; and place washer and dryer, freezer and furnace, on an isolated utility porch.
- Use soft, porous materials like carpets, upholstery, drapes, heavy textile wall hangings, and acoustic panels and tiles to reduce or dampen interior noise levels; minimize hard, nonporous surfaces such as plaster, glass, concrete, and sheet plastic that reflect sound.
- Neutralize sound through noise generators that create "white noise" to blanket or cover distracting noise and play soothing background music.
- Wear earplugs, particularly the soft foam ones, especially when flying.

MUSIC TO SOOTHE THE SOUL

If you're downhearted and one of your favorite songs pipes up from the radio, you might spontaneously jump up to boogy to the beat. If you're nervously pacing, you might feel a warm stillness take over your body—even rapture.

Music entertains us, changes our moods, soothes our souls, makes us smarter, and even heals us. For the sensory defensive, music is an important way to calm yourself when you're overwrought and rouse yourself when you've stayed in your shell for too long.

Consider music's profound effect on our minds and bodies:

- When we sing, our pupils dilate and our endorphin levels rise.
- In World War II it was discovered that even comatose patients could respond to music.
- Autistic or learning-disabled children, who find speaking an insurmountable hurdle, frequently have less trouble communicating first in song, then transferring that facility to speech.

- The tics and jerks of Parkinson patients shift to a normal ease of movement upon hearing music they like. Their EEG (brain waves) become normal and their Parkinson symptoms momentarily vanish.
- After thirty-six undergraduate students from the psychology department at the University of California in Irvine listened to 10 minutes of Mozart's "Sonata for Two Pianos in D Major," they scored 8 to 9 points higher on the Stanford-Binet spatial IQ test.
- Half an hour of listening to classical music produced the same effect as 10 milligrams of Valium in critical-care units at Saint Agnes Hospital in Baltimore.
- After listening for only 15 minutes to music they selected from four categories—New Age (selections by David Lantz, Eric Tingsan, and Nancy Rumble); mild jazz (Kenny G); classical (Mozart); or impressionist (Ravel)—subjects in a 1993 study at Michigan State University showed increased levels of interleukin-1 (IL-1) in the blood by 12.5 to 14 percent, indicating enhanced immune functioning, along with up to 25 percent decreased levels of cortisol.[7]

Nourishing Sounds

As we listen to music, our heart rate responds to musical variables such as frequency, tempo, and volume and tends to speed up and slow down to match, or entrain, to the rhythm of a sound. Music that replicates the resting and relaxed human heart rate of 1 beat per second (60 beats per minute) is the most calming and healing, as it will slow down the heart beat. Music that goes against this basic rhythm will accelerate heart beat and can excite us to the point of agitation. According to New Age composer Steven Halpern, most music that we know in the West "dominates and overrides the natural rhythm of your heart by entraining it to the rhythm of the drummer (or these days, more likely a drum machine)."[8]

When we are stressed, calming music unconsciously helps us breathe slower and deeper. And it slows down and stabilizes brain waves. The fastest brain waves are beta waves, which occur during ordinary consciousness as we focus our attention and when we experience strong negative emotions. Somewhat slower alpha waves occur during an awake, relaxed state, heightened awareness, as during meditation, and just before nodding off. Theta waves, even slower, occur during periods of peak creativity, meditation, and sleep, while delta waves, the slowest, occur during deep sleep, deep meditation, and unconsciousness. The slower the brain waves, the more relaxed, contented, and peaceful we feel. Certain baroque and New Age music can shift consciousness from the beta toward the alpha range, enhancing alertness and overall well-being. Shamanic drumming can take the listener into the theta range and induce altered states of consciousness.

Music also influences blood pressure, blood circulation, temperature control, and sweating. For example, a 1989 study showed that Don Campbell's album *Essence: Crystal Meditations*, which pulses simultaneously at both alpha and theta rhythms, and Daniel Kobialka's *Timeless Lullaby* significantly reduced blood pressure in all nine subjects.[9]

Listening Wisely

Any music that moves you, literally and figuratively, is emotionally therapeutic. Joyful and emotionally rich music can cause shivers of delight, even euphoria. Imagine movies without the background music to carry the moment!

Most music, however, is not consciously composed for the relaxing or healing needed by the sensory defensive, and in choosing music you need to know its effect on your body. When overstimulated, you need music to help you calm. But you also need music to get your body moving, especially when you feel sluggish.

Rock music can stir you when you are in the mood for excitement, but it can also create tension, dissonance, stress, and physical pain when you are already hyped. Opposing the natural beat of the heart and contrary to the rhythm of the arterial pulsations, the short-short-long-pause rhythm of the rock music (stopped-anapestic rhythm) overpowers the internal rhythm of the body, confusing heart and body.[10] Behavioral kinesiologist John Diamond found that, even at harmless volumes, the standard rhythms of some rock music weaken the muscles by as much as two-thirds in 90 percent of those tested.[11] And while the person with a normal nervous system will return to a relaxed baseline, the sensory defensive may remain in an overly excited state.

When we are in the doldrums and feeling emotionally numb, romantic music like Tchaikovsky, Schubert, Schumann, Chopin, and Liszt evoke fierce emotions. But if we feel overloaded, this music can quicken our heart beat and hike up tension.

Gregorian chant, which uses the rhythms of natural breathing to create a sense of relaxed spaciousness, acts as a good stress reducer, and though the repetitious chanting makes it boring for active listening, it serves well for quiet study and meditation. Some baroque music (Bach or Pachelbel) pulses at around 60 beats per minute and has a predictable rhythm that integrates easily with inner speech and thought. Classical music (Mozart or Haydn) has continuity, clarity, and an order within its sound, but greater changes in rhythm, tone, and color. It is good music for mental organization. New Age music (for example, the music of Steven Halpern or Brian Eno) has no dominant rhythm and helps to unwind. It elongates our sense of space and time, induces a state of relaxed alertness, and is excellent as ambient music, to slowly move or fall asleep to. When you are too much in your head, New Age music, as well as romantic music and jazz, help to shift awareness from your left to right hemisphere.[12]

Vary your selections. After about twenty minutes, the brain begins to tune out the no longer novel tune, and tedium creates irritability.

Though the sensory defensive generally need calming music, it is not a good choice if you feel depressed and your arousal level is too low. In a compelling 10-week experiment, the Florida Protective Services System Abuse Registry Hot Line played different types of music over the telephone—classical, popular, relaxation and nature sounds, country, and contemporary jazz—while callers waited for counselors to come on the line.[13] The smallest number of hang-ups during the wait happened during uplifting jazz sessions, which featured selections from Miles Davis, Art Farmer, John McLaughlin, and Esther Phillips. Relaxation, nature music, and the Pachelbel Canon yielded the most hang-ups.

Moving

We listen to music with our bodies. When listening to disco music, who can stop their foot from tapping or their body from gyrating? Go with the beat. Moving to music will help you get in touch with your inner rhythms, and it will make you feel more grounded in space, increasing body awareness. And it feels good! But don't choreograph your movements—express them freely by letting your body unwind to the music as it desires and go with the flow.

The best way to choose music with the right rhythmic pattern for your body is to play it and see what your body does. When you need your body to get going and release tension, big band, pop, and country-western can spur light to moderate movement, while music by the Rolling Stones, Stevie Wonder, or Michael Jackson can set your body shaking. The lively rhythm of Latin American music like salsa and marenga inspires your body to move briskly and rhythmically, while samba, notes music therapist Don Campbell, has the rare ability to soothe and awaken at the same time.

All known drum rhythms have one to two basic patterns—either the rapid tap, tap of animal hooves from our past as hunters or the measured beat of the human heart, the throb of life. The vibration from drums taps bone conduction and penetrates the body's core. When it is played in sync with the body's rhythms, it gets you moving and provides intensity that is at the same time organizing, calming, and grounding.[14] Does the drum have to be at 60 times per minute? Not at all. Not every sound we hear fully entrains the body. Actually, drums that beat 120 times per minute, double the heart's resting rate, only increase the heartbeat somewhat and, after about five minutes, paradoxically deeply calm the body. In the womb, after all, the mother's heartbeat accelerated in an energized state, as during exercise or sex, followed by de-acceleration and calm. What's important is the actual rhythm.

Moving to some New Age music allows your body to unfold slowly, and when it's just right, your body will spontaneously undulate, twist, turn, pulse, and open up at its own pace and rhythm.

The body wants to rock, begging for vestibular input, though these days in our urban world it's generally not socially acceptable unless we're holding a baby, embraced in a lover's arms, or in sorrow. Throughout much of the world, people spend their day in rhythmic movement: pounding rice, kneading bread, baling hay, lying and sleeping in a hammock, and holding and swaying with their babies. Getting into the habit of allowing your body to rock or sway to music—or otherwise—affords strong sensory nourishment.

Vocal Power

In the late 1960s, Alfred Tomatis, a French ENT doctor, was called in to investigate a curious, unexplained melancholy and listlessness in an order of Benedictine monks in the south of France. He found seventy of the ninety monks "slumped in their cells like wet dishrags." His diagnosis? The monks suffered from a lack of Gregorian chant that had been part of their daily routine. Once the chanting was reinstated, within six months the monks were again vigorous, enthusiastic, and healthy.[15] Perhaps it's not so curious that in the early 1990s Gregorian chant by the Benedictine monks of Santa Domingo de Silos in Spain rose to the top of the classical and pop music charts in Europe and the United States.

Listening to music is not the only way to experience healing power. Just as you can entrain to external rhythms produced from sounds coming from outside, you can also benefit from the healing power of your own voice. When you chant, hum, or sing, you create vibration in the upper body that feels like an inner massage: breathing deepens, jaw and throat relax, tension releases.

If you chant emphasizing vowel sounds, a practice that appears in religious, spiritual, and healing practices throughout the world, you boost serotonin level and release endorphins in the brain. At the same time, the mental concentration allows the right and left hemispheres to get in sync, while the inner white noise that chanting creates blots extraneous noises, making it conducive to a meditative state. In India, ritual chanting creates such powerfully altered states that people who allow themselves to be intentionally bitten by cobras somehow don't become ill.

As you chant, different pitches vibrate differently on the body. Most find that low notes (vowels "uh" and "oo") resonate in the lower parts of their bodies. Middle notes (vowels "oh," "ah," and "eye") open up the chest cavity and massage the throat. Five minutes of repeating "oh" can change the skin temperature, muscle tension, brain waves, and breath and heart rates and is a great sensory tune-up during down times. A minute or so of the "ah" sound, which you produce when you yawn, will relax your jaw and open up your breathing. High notes (vowels "aye" and "ee") localize in the sinus cavities and skull and wake up the body. Three to five minutes of "ee" will keep you alert when you're sluggish.

A simple, powerful common chant is repeating "Om" (you start with the lips shaping the "ah" sound, slowly changing to the "o" sound, and ending with the closed-lips, "mmm" humming sound). Even a few minutes appears to transform one's energy state, while continuing for 10 minutes or longer slows down brain waves to a deep state of consciousness. Afterward, you feel as if you've had an aerobic workout. Often people chant one word, like peace, love, God, Allah, Jesus, or hallelujah. You can find chants from Christian, Jewish, Sufi, Hindu, and Buddhist traditions, and those of the various Indian tribes.

Many religious practices repeat a phrase or mantra while moving rhythmically. This elicits a trancelike state that makes worshippers feel close to their god. Religious Jews start their day by fervently chanting prayers as they bob their heads and sway back and forth.

THERAPEUTIC LISTENING

As sound vibrates the inner ear, it stimulates the vestibular sense, the conductor of the entire nervous system—"the background beat that lays the rhythm for all learning," as OT Sheila Frick, who conducts workshops on the use of therapeutic listening in occupational therapy, describes it.[16] This close connection between the auditory and vestibular systems makes listening to music a powerful conduit for directly impacting the vestibular system and enhancing sensory integration. For instance, the reticular activating system, which orchestrates alertness, and therefore sensory modulation, receives input from both the auditory and vestibular systems. This is why music so quickly revs us up and calms us down. In addition, through the vagus nerve, the inner ear connects with the larynx, heart, lungs, stomach, liver, bladder, kidneys, and small and large intestine, suggesting that auditory vibrations impact the regulation and control of all the major organs of the body. Little wonder listening to music has such healing power!

To release all this power from sound requires that you listen very well. And this takes more than a love of music and supersonic sound speakers. It requires specially electronically altered music that filters in and muffles certain sounds, creating dissonance. As you listen to specifically selected compact discs through headphones, the unexpected sounds wake up the brain and force it to listen and process the music.

The alteration also causes the stapedius muscle in the middle ear to contract and then relax, teaching the brain how to tune out aversive sound and help attenuate auditory defensiveness and gravitational insecurity. Each CD is modified for different purposes, such as for self-regulation, body awareness, auditory processing, and cognitive skills. To lightly draw the listener in, the music is generally played softly.

If your therapeutic listening program is right, you experience greater internal harmony. Breathing slows, sleep is more restful, focus and concentration are better, coordination and balance improve, even handwriting is better, and you feel less overaroused and sensory defensive to sound, touch, movement, and so on.

The trailblazer of therapeutic listening is Alfred Tomatis.[17] Using primarily music by Mozart, specifically the violin concertos, which he felt had the greatest healing effect on the human body, and the mother's voice and Gregorian chant, Tomatis developed specific techniques using modified sound and music for enhanced therapeutic effects. His method is based on filtered sound and the effects of high frequency on the whole nervous system. He believes that high-frequency sounds (3,000 to 8,000 hertz or more) generally resonate in the brain and affect mental functions, such as thinking, spatial perception, and memory. Middle-frequency sounds (750 to 3,000 hertz), as in the human voice, tend to stimulate the heart, lungs, and emotions. Low sounds (125 to 750 hertz) affect physical movement: a low drone sound, like a fan, tends to make us groggy, while a low, fast rhythm, like a drumbeat, makes it difficult to concentrate or be still; few listen to a drumbeat as background music for working. By progressively filtering out low-sound frequency sounds for varying lengths of time, Tomatis has been immensely successful and influential in treating developmental problems, including challenges with social interaction, voice development, speech impediments, and autism. In his newsletter *Self-Healing,* Dr. Andrew Weil lists the Tomatis method as a noninvasive, safe alternative to Ritalin in adults and children suffering from attention-deficit and hyperactivity disorders.

Believing the Tomatis method too lengthy, Dr. Guy Berard, a French medical doctor who trained with Tomatis, developed auditory integration training (AIT). The Berard method, which utilizes all types of music—classical, jazz, instrumental, etc.—distorts sound frequencies and modulates them at random intervals for random periods of time. AIT gained worldwide fame in 1990 with the publication of Annabel Stehli's biography of her severely autistic daughter Georgie (*The Sound of a Miracle*), who shed most, if not all, of her autistic behaviors after a course of twenty AIT treatments in Berard's clinic.

Another therapeutic listening program is the SAMONAS method, developed by Tomatis-trained Ingo Steinback, a German sound engineer with an extensive background in music and physics and an interest in psychiatric problems. Feeling clarity was an important component in the healing process, he endeavored to make recordings as realistic and spatially expansive as the sounds heard in a concert hall. By heightening his attention to the structural elements contained in all natural sounds, and capturing them in his recordings, he noticed that the listener immediately perked up even to unfiltered music. Using classical music (mostly Mozart) and nature sounds, he developed special technology to capture music as sound in space, so you feel that you are sitting in a concert hall or out in nature, and combined it with the Tomatis method of filtering.

While both the Tomatis and Berard methods are costly and dependent on a treatment facility, the SAMONAS method is available on compact discs that can be played on relatively inexpensive disc players with good-quality headphones and can be listened to in a treatment facility or home. I use SAMONAS discs for my home listening program. One is a nature tape divided into two half-hour tracks for relaxation. The first track creates alpha waves, while the second creates theta waves; within seconds I feel transported into a trancelike state. Amid ocean surf and music of Tibetan bowls, my hands unfist, my fingers unfurl and spread out wide, and my arms straighten out, as energy infuses my body and opens up blocked energy channels. Another is a Mozart tape for thinking, and I listen to it while writing at the computer. On one part of the track, I hear ordinary melodious Mozart, while on other parts I hear high-pitched sounds so distorted that they seem like scratches. At first I thought the CD was flawed. But it wasn't, and it works.

Now that we've set up a sensory diet of healing touch, movement, and sound, let's explore how to expand your menu to encompass the healing power of light.

10

Seeing the Whole Picture

These fluorescent lights are sucking the life out of me.

—FROM THE FILM *JOE VS. THE VOLCANO*

To control what touches your skin is hard: light touch is unavoidable, even if it is only from the movement of your clothes. To control what bounces off your eardrum is difficult: something is always humming, whirring, or sending out electrical current. To control what hits your nasal passage is nigh impossible: whiffs from miles away can awaken you from sleep. But you *can* control what light hits your iris, at least in your home. Which source of light is modulating? Which is disorganizing? This is important information for the sensory defensive.

All of life is energy and vibration, electromagnetic waves of light, color, and sound. As yogi and spiritual leader Paramahansa Yogananda sums up, "If our senses conveyed the whole truth to us, we would see the earth as rivers and glaciers of electrons, each speck of dust as a rolling mass of light." The frequency of vibrating energy contained in each color, whether from a tree, a lightbulb, or the shirt covering us, intertwines with other life energies to affect us continually.

The human body too is an expression of energy and vibration, affected and nourished by light. Light therapy pioneer and photobiologist John Ott describes light as a nutrient much like food. The right kind is medicine and helps regulate our internal biological clock, which controls most body functions, including heart rate, breathing, digestion, and brain waves. The wrong kind is poison and further disrupts the daily, monthly, and annual rhythms of the sensory defensive, contributing to their fatigue, depression, and compromised immune system.

NIGHT AND DAY

Sustaining all life on Earth and our source of light, warmth, and energy is the sun. At the dawn of civilization, its warm yellow rays woke up the world and we became active and alert. As the sun folded back into the sky in a brilliant display of orange, red, and yellow and gradually into the dark blue of night, the first humans slowly wound down into rest and then sleep. From cave dweller to farmer, this pattern has repeated daily and seasonally, enabling us to synchronize our biological rhythms according to fluctuations in light and temperature, with predictable biochemical and behavioral changes.

Then about a hundred years ago, a lightbulb lit up the world and drew us indoors: night became day. Confused by this sudden extension of light, our natural 24-hour night-day cycles, or circadian rhythms, which depend on the spectral light of the sun, jolted out of their track. Because our bodies were designed to coincide with Earth's rhythms, this was no small event. These circadian rhythms are our body's timekeeper and fundamental to its functioning; our hormones, immune system, sexual development, and nervous system are all guided by this internal clock. "Where the sun does not enter, the doctor does," says an Italian proverb.

Everyone's body is affected by changes in the day-night cycle, as anyone who has experienced jet lag knows. When internal rhythms are already off, your body is more dependent on external regulators, and therefore more thrown by changing rhythms. This is why sleep problems and PMS are rampant in the sensory defensive.

Deep within our brain sits the pineal organ, our light meter. Receiving light-activated information from the eyes, by way of the hypothalamus, it sends out, via its neurotransmitter melatonin, hormonal messages throughout the body to regulate our daily sleep cycles. What effect might artificial light have on its functioning, both biologically and behaviorally? One change might be the earlier onset of menses. Coinciding with the invention of electricity, its onset has lowered from an average age of 15 or so a hundred years ago to age 12 in places in the world that use the greatest amount of artificial light. Girls in Rio de Janeiro may begin menstruating at age 12, while native girls in the Amazon rain forest begin at age 16. High levels of melatonin, usually associated with shorter days, decrease sex hormones and slow sexual maturation, while low levels of melatonin, usually associated with longer days, have the opposite effect. Extended indoor light might have manipulated the level of melatonin, triggering an earlier onset of menses.

LET THERE BE LIGHT

Only a speck of the sun's energy reaches us and we perceive even less with the naked eye—only a rainbow of rays from violet to indigo, blue, green, yellow, orange, and red.

Sunlight consists of a fairly balanced spectrum of visible color, with its energy peaking slightly in the blue-green area. To keep the body's systems in balance, we need a balance of the seven colors. But unnatural lighting offers only a portion of the full spectrum of the sun's light. Lacking in the green, blue, and violet wavelength, incandescent bulbs emit much more red and yellow light than normal daylight—thus lamp light appears yellow—and produce more infrared heat than they do light. Traditional fluorescent tubes, such as cool white, warm white, and soft pink, overrepresent certain yellow-orange colors and are deficient in red and blue-violet, where the sun's emission is the strongest.

Fluorescent lights also send out pulsing vibrations that, though not easily noticeable, become so when older lights hum and flicker. These pulsations can interfere with your own vibrations and, along with an elevation in the yellow range, make you hyperactive and irritable, dizzy and even faint. A sensory-defensive man said they made him feel "thirsty." A defensive woman with an IQ of 157 believes that as a child, she failed some classes in grade school because the fluorescent lighting made her dopey. Some defensives panic from intense overhead fluorescent lighting, like that found in supermarkets. "People seem one hundred miles away and I want to tell people to get out of my space," said one woman. Further, fluorescent lights emit mercury vapor that creates blatant distortions of the light spectrum. John Ott believes that these lights should come with a warning label: mercury vapor can cause food allergies. Ott also believes that the cathode ends of fluorescent lights emit low levels of X rays. When he placed geranium plants near the ends of the tubes, they wilted, but they flourished when he covered the ends with lead foil to absorb the suspected X rays.[1]

As light is a source of information, distortions of the visible light spectrum impact our well-being. Most indoor lighting looks yellowish and dingy. Bright light makes our surroundings look flat, and unnaturally colored light sources cause vague uneasiness: Under bluish white light, people appear unwell.

For our body to absorb nutrients and thrive, we require the sun's full spectrum of solar radiation—the infrared (heat just beyond red that we feel when sunburned), the visible color spectrum, *and* the ultraviolet (UV) wavelengths (just beyond violet). But UV light has gotten much bad press as a cause of skin cancer. People are encouraged to avoid the sun altogether and, when outside, to coat their skin with sunblock and cover their eyes with sunglasses. Is it possible that in a classic case of throwing out the baby with the bath water, we may be avoiding the sun's harmful rays at the expense of its essential life force?

When UV rays from the sun penetrate the skin's surface they stimulate blood circulation, increase white blood cells, lower blood pressure, increase protein metabolism, lessen fatigue, and increase the release of endorphins. Until the advent of antibiotics in the late 1930s, basking in the sun was the treatment for tuberculosis. Making possible the production of vitamin D, UV light increases absorption of calcium into our bones.

As UV light is virtually absent from incandescent lighting (lightbulbs), shielded in standard fluorescent bulbs, and blocked by normal window glass, including that on our automobiles and eyeglasses, we receive an inadequate supply. And while creating daylight might seem as easy as turning on a switch, it is brighter outside even on a rainy morning than inside with the lights on. Sixteen hours indoors provides dramatically less light than that received from a single hour outdoors. Light-deprived, we literally live in the twilight zone. With our modern indoor lifestyle and our habit of covering up when outdoors, we synthesize only a tiny proportion of the vitamin D that a naked hunter on the African savannah would absorb, and this may be vastly inadequate for our metabolic needs.

Few know more about the quality of light and its effect on our health than John Ott. While doing some time-lapse photography for Walt Disney, he observed that under fluorescent lights pumpkin-seed sprouts would not fully mature, but they flourished with the addition of ultraviolet light.[2] In later experiments during the 1950s and 1960s, he found that wavelengths of light in the orange-red-pink range—not too far from the wavelength peaks of lightbulbs—caused laboratory animals to lose their hair, show excessive calcium deposits in their hearts, and develop large, fast-growing tumors.[3]

Concluding that natural light is as crucial to the life and health of animals as it is to plants, Ott recommended to Duro-Test Corporation that it modify one of its fluorescent tubes to more closely replicate the full spectrum of sunlight. In 1973, Ott and the Environmental Health Research Institute conducted a study comparing the performance of four first-grade, windowless classrooms in Sarasota, Florida, under full-spectrum, radiation-shielded fluorescent light fixtures or the standard cool-white fluorescent.[4] Under the cool-white fluorescent lighting, some students demonstrated hyperactivity, fatigue, irritability, and attention deficits. Under exposure to full-spectrum lighting for one month, their behavior, classroom performance, and overall academic achievement improved markedly. Several learning-disabled children with extreme hyperactivity calmed down and seemed to overcome some of their learning and reading problems.

Additionally, children in rooms with full-spectrum lighting developed one-third the number of cavities. Sharon, Feller, and Burney reported similar results on the development of cavities.[5] Given that the full color spectrum of the sun's rays increases calcium absorption, it is not a surprise that one would get fewer cavities after exposure to full-spectrum lighting.

Additionally, experiments with fluorescent lights that offer the full color spectrum of the sun's rays show people to have less visual and bodily fatigue and improved visual acuity. Yellowish light on white paper creates a glare, causing squinting and eyestrain, while full-spectrum fluorescent light absorbs into the white paper with no resulting glare, and the letters stand out clearly. When Control Data Corporation installed full-spectrum fluorescent tubes in their workstations, the data input error rate dropped dramatically and the company saved more than $235,000 per year.[6]

How much sun exposure do we need to optimize health? John Ott recommends 6 hours a day of natural daylight, while avoiding direct sunlight between 10 A.M. and 2 P.M. (If you have to tip your head back to face directly into the sun, it is in the danger zone.) Though impractical for most, approximately 1½ to 2 hours a day of gentle morning or late-afternoon sun is the recommended minimum daily requirement (MDR). The bare minimum sunlight to produce adequate daily vitamin D levels is 30 minutes of exposure to spring or summer sun. Without the MDR, your body will begin to compensate for lack of sufficient nutrition. Some possible effects include decrease in energy; cravings for carbohydrates, sugar, and caffeine; need for more sleep; decreased desire for sex and other pleasurable activities; decreased attention span; and mood disturbances.

We can increase daily exposure to the sun's warm rays by prudent indirect exposure, unfiltered by windows or eyeglasses, and minimize the risk for skin cancer by avoiding prolonged sun exposure or burning. We can increase outdoor activities, like a daily walk, and take greater advantage of our backyards and porches. City dwellers can bring UV radiation into their homes by using windows made of UV-admitting plastic or fluorescent lights that include a UV component. Full-spectrum lighting, the nearest thing to sunlight in terms of spectral distribution and brightness, and without heat and glare, is available in most lighting stores both in a lightbulb and in fluorescent lighting, which perhaps yields the closest solar match in commercial lighting. Eliminating much of the glare that sets off a defensive response to light, full-spectrum lighting facilitates internal organization, and defensives should utilize it throughout their indoor space. An Ott light for computer work enables you to see the screen more clearly and accurately and provides the benefit of sunlight while working. And the snow-white illumination is uplifting. If you work in an office with overhead fluorescent lights, install full-spectrum fluorescents over your desk or bring your own Ott desk light or floor lamp. Installing full-spectrum lighting in your bathroom will help wake you up in the morning, and your body will receive the same effect as natural sunlight. And the whiteness of the light makes you look more natural, as you do in sunlight.

SEEING THROUGH A HOLE

At the turn of the century, a New York opthalmologist named William Bates declared that mental tension was at the root of all vision problems. Sight could be naturally restored through relaxation and retraining of visual skills and habits. His ideas paved the way for a new approach to vision.

Field of vision is our ability to perceive things peripherally while simultaneously looking straight ahead. Peripheral vision functions to perceive movement, rather than detail, so we are at all times aware of surrounding danger. Under stress, an individual's perceptual fields constrict, restricting the flow of information between the eyes and brain.[7] When this happens, declares optometrist Jacob Liberman, author of *Light: Medicine of the Future*, we "perceive less and less and eventually look at the world through a 'hole,' rather than perceiving it as a 'whole.'"[8] In addition to light sensitivity, the sensory defensive commonly display problems with visual processing, such as focusing the eyes for binocular control (the ability to form a single visual image from two images that the eyes record separately).

When the visual field is open, explains Liberman, you are aware "where you were looking before, and where you will be looking next." When the visual field collapses and you perceive only a small piece of the present, you have a limited view of where you are and where you are moving. You feel "lost in space," a common complaint of the sensory defensive. Trish, as we recall, suffered dissociation as a result of needing to shut out the pressure of her glasses against her face and in response to limited peripheral vision, which diminished her ability to search out danger.

At any point in time, our visual fields expand and contract in relation to our consciousness and quality of breathing. To appreciate the relationship between eye tension and physical tension, do this exercise and observe the change in breath when your field of vision is narrowed. Place your hands just underneath the tip of your sternum and note the movement of your diaphragm as you breathe. Focus your eyes on one point and squint slightly. Note how as you restricted your field of vision, your breathing became shallow and your diaphragm tightened. Now, open up your peripheral vision so you can sense what's at your sides. You will feel yourself spontaneously breathe in and your diaphragm widen.

EYES WIDE OPEN

We think we have eyes for sight. Yet this is only a small part of what our eyes do. Light through the eyes goes directly from the visual cortex into two different pathways into the brain, the cerebral cortex and the hypo-thalamus in the limbic system, and affects every cell of the body.[9]

Containing 70 percent of the body's sense receptors, the eyes are the first register of approximately 90 percent of all the information from the environment into the body, making it the primary way in which we evalu-ate and understand the world. Closing this channel of communication impacts our ability to acquire and process information. But if you open up the visual fields so that more light enters the brain, all brain functions are enhanced, and things begin to make more sense.

How do you do this? With light therapy.

When different portions of intense colored light are flashed into your eyes, each with a specific effect on the brain and the nervous system, syn-tonic (from "syntony," which means to bring into balance) phototherapy reestablishes the body's rhythms and puts your body into balance. Light therapy raises endorphin levels; stabilizes brain waves; lowers heart rate, respiration, and blood pressure; strengthens the immune system; and expands the visual field. Clinical depression, stress, light sensitivity and visual problems, premenstrual syndrome, sexual dysfunction, chronic fatigue, thyroid problems, migraines, and jet lag are among the conditions improved by light therapy. A pioneer in holistic treatment for pain, depression, and stress-related disorders, clinician Norman Shealy discov-ered that oxytocin, the relaxation and nurturing hormone, was raised in his patients as much by the red light of a Lumatron phototherapy device as it was by having sex![10] Given that light travels through the hypothalamus, the master controller of autonomic functioning, the stress response, hunger, thirst, and sex, these results are not surprising.

As higher learning rests on the integrity of sensory processing, the more light your eyes gulp in, the better cognitive processes like memory and concentration should be. This truth is precisely what Jacob Liberman found in conducting a study of the effects of syntonic colored light therapy on visual-field size, memory, speed, and accuracy of eye movements in chil-dren with learning problems.[11] He prescribed frequencies of light for 20-minute periods, four times per week for 6 weeks. The visual field for the experimental group was 208 times greater than for the control group, visual attention span almost four times greater, and visual memory seven times greater. Auditory memory enhanced as well, though not significantly so. Fully 75 percent of the children reported improvements in schoolwork, and handwriting improved in 40 percent. Withdrawn children came out of their shell, hyperactive ones calmed down. Additionally, the two children on Ritalin were able to totally eliminate daily use.

Others experimenting with color filters have found equally impressive results. When dyslexic children read through blue plastic filters, they read better. Apparently when enough of the red is removed, dyslexics' eyes work more normally.[12]

As the senses work synergistically, changes will occur simultaneously in other sensory modalities. Optometrist John Downing, the inventor of the Lumatron phototherapy device and a light therapy practitioner for over 30 years, treated a woman who had lost her sense of smell four years prior to treatment. She regained her sense of smell after only one treatment of light therapy, and it returned more completely than ever before.[13]

Each color of light is a different wavelength, or frequency, and sends a different vibration into the energy system. One color excites, while another calms; one shocks, while the other uplifts.[14] The red end of the light spectrum has the longest wavelength and slowest frequency of vibration. Like the sun's fiery glow, its magnetic energy is warming and stimulating, raising blood pressure, respiration rate, heartbeat, muscle activity, and brain waves. In a study done at the University of Texas, subjects watched colored lights as their hand-grip strength was measured. When looking at red light, their grip became 13.5 percent stronger.[15]

In the middle of the spectrum, green subdues tension and is good for concentration and meditation. On the cool end of the spectrum, blue lowers internal rhythms and sedates. In a study in which hospital patients with tremors watched blue light, their tremors lessened.[16] Violet, with the shortest wavelength and the quickest vibration, is the most cooling. It has been used to soothe mental conditions, calm the high-strung, and induce a deep, relaxed sleep. It counteracts and balances the color red.

For greater effect, syntonic phototherapy often combines colors as follows:

Red-orange: strong stimulant; excites senses

Lemon: chronic equalizer; detoxifier

Turquoise: acute equilibrator; anti-inflammatory; for fever, infection, edema, and head trauma

Indigo: strong depressant; for pain, headaches, and twitches, and to shrink masses

Scarlet: increases functions of heart, emotions, reproduction, and vascular system

Magenta: balances functions of heart, emotions, reproduction, and vascular system

Purple: decreases functions of heart, emotions, reproduction, and vascular system; induces relaxation and sleep; lowers body temperature; and decreases sensitivity to pain.

Red, orange, and yellow generally tend to activate the sympathetic nervous system, while colors above that point—yellow-green (lemon), green, blue-green (turquoise), blue, indigo and violet—tend to activate the parasympathetic nervous system. However, this response varies greatly with each individual, and it is up to the doctor—usually an optometrist, physician, psychiatrist, psychologist, or chiropractor—to determine the appropriate colors for each patient. Incorrectly used, red can produce tension, while blue can produce depression, and each shut down the visual field.

Initially, it might seem that the overaroused sensory defensive would benefit from blue. Yet the arousal of some sensory defensives vacillates unpredictably and in overload the person can feel at once depleted and charged. Thus, deciding the best color or colors takes clinical experience by a trained professional.

A typical protocol of light therapy involves twenty 20-minute daily sessions of exposure to colored lenses. Some clinicians treat with light flicking at varying rates, to better wake up the brain. According to John Downing, the warmer the color, the higher the flicker rate (ranging from red, at 15 Hz, to blue, at 9 Hz, to violet, at 1 Hz flash rate), though the flickering should be set to meet individual comfort.[17] Like the hypnotic effect of staring at a wavering candle flame, flickering induces entrainment or trance in about 60 percent of subjects, who can then be easily hypnotized. Not everyone can tolerate flickering. Most require a steady light. Downing cautions that the use of flashing lights can induce seizures in those prone to photoconvulsive epilepsy (approximately 1 in 2,850 patients).

Though light therapy is most intense with a light-therapy device, these are costly. There are, however, some less powerful home devices that have become available. *Let There Be Light*, by Darius Dinshah, outlines how to use different colored filters directly on the body to alleviate disease. Color-therapy eyewear is also helpful.

How well does syntonic phototherapy work in eliminating visual defensiveness? Though little systematic research has been done, clinical reports demonstrate good success. Here is Anna's experience.

For a period of 24 days, she underwent twenty sessions consisting of 10 minutes peering at red-indigo light and 10 minutes peering at green-yellow light. Initially, she felt no change in light sensitivity, but by the seventh session, she felt somewhat more able to tolerate blinking car lights and not cover her eyes. Previously unable to tolerate the tint in sunglasses, she found she could now wear gray-tinted Ott sunglasses.

During her thirteenth session, she focused continually on the red without constantly blinking, as she had been. The red seemed lighter and brighter. She thought the color filter had been changed, but it had not. As she looked into the light, she felt a pressure in her chest but at the same time wanted to look at the red forever.

Five minutes after completing the 20-minute session, she began to feel extreme head pressure, as if she had a vice slightly above her eyes by the temples. "I wasn't afraid. I knew that something in my brain was actively reworking and I felt this was a good sign." Eyes closed, she sat in her car for about 20 minutes as the pressure slowly subsided.

She started to drive. Her whole being felt in slow motion. It was night, and, after a few blocks, she realized that rear car lights looked bright red. Fascinated, she stared at their luminosity. Next she noticed the intensity of the green traffic light and again stared, as if seeing the world anew, suddenly lit like a Christmas tree, all red and green. She realized that her eyes were wide open, no longer slits. She had spent years walking around in a haze, blinded by glare, with her brain taking in only a sliver of light. By the twentieth session, her eyes opened so wide that she felt bug-eyed. Upon evaluation, the optometrist discovered that Anna's field of vision had opened to normal and that the visual defensiveness had greatly subsided.

Unleashing Memories

When light hits the cerebral cortex, we think about it, organize it, and make sense of it. When it hits the limbic system, it jars our emotions, and old painful memories literally gush out, and are often accompanied by the bodily symptoms associated with the original experience.

Memories are recorded verbally as a story and physiologically as sensation. During times of emotional and physical stress, memory gets encoded at deeper psychophysiological levels by the release of hormones and messenger molecules, or neurotransmitters, all the way down to the cellular level. The memory, however, becomes bound to that specific psychophysiological state of stress, and frequently is inaccessible at the verbal level. Contrary to talk therapy, in which you *recall* the memory, light therapy and, as we'll see later, some body work and hypnotherapy, dig inside the tissues and sinew and jiggle loose memories at a psychophysiological level, causing you to *relive* the full impact of the experience.

Following her fourth session of therapy, Anna curled up like a tiny infant in her crib. Whimpering like a baby, she peered out, terrified, at the world. She felt a powerful urge to slash her body and dug her fingernails into her arm. Powerless to control the intensity of the experience, she felt crazy. Her terror continued for an agonizing 20 minutes, and then the feelings started to subside. All night, she mourned the frightened and unloved infant inside.

After the sixth session, her face involuntarily began to furiously flick to the left, again and again, and she filled with dread. Suddenly, the memory came to her. She was around 15 and sitting at the dinner table, when her raging father unjustly slapped her across the face, stunning her. Again, the intensity of the experience lasted for about 20 minutes, and then she felt peaceful, as if the memory had been burned out of her brain. She had never experienced anything this powerful in psychotherapy, and, initially, the experience consumed and terrified her. When she realized that the feelings were short-lived and cathartic, she welcomed the cleansing.

Her experience is not unusual. Many have found light therapy to invoke traumatic memories, which is why it should be administered in conjunction with psychotherapy. As sensory defensiveness creates traumatic memories, light therapy may be a useful tool for unblocking some of these somatic memories and offer relief from ongoing suffering.

SAD

Once at a friend's house for dinner in the company of people I greatly enjoyed, I couldn't wait for the evening to end. The house was brightly lit, and my extremely sensitive eyes were in a perpetual squint, as the glare steadily wore down my ability to take in the titillating conversation. While the lights were making my life miserable, they were keeping my friend from depression. She has a syndrome called seasonal affective disorder (SAD), a cyclical depression that occurs from lack of sufficient light exposure.[18]

Light's profound input in bodily functions and behavior becomes most evident when we lack it. As winter approaches and the hours of daylight lessen, we begin to show signs of hibernation: eating more, storing more fat, becoming lethargic, sleeping more, and, as dark approaches, returning quickly to our caves. Along with this dampened activity comes, for most, some degree of winter blues, possibly due to an increased production at night of the sedating hormone melatonin. "Lethargics are to be laid in the light and exposed to the rays of the sun, for the disease is gloom," observed Artaeus in the second century A.D. As the sensory defensive can be light-sensitive and highly reactive to extreme temperatures with seasonal changes, the blues can hit hard.

There is help: daily exposure to a full-spectrum lightbox screen that delivers between 2,500 and 10,000 units of illumination (lux) of light energy, twenty times brighter than that of average indoor lighting, for about half an hour each morning. This is considered the antidepressant of choice for SAD sufferers. Two hours of bright light in the mornings or evenings with an Ott-Lite, a full-spectrum fluorescent lightbox, and dim red light also works wonders on reversing PMS symptoms. Morning bright light also eliminates menopausal hot flashes.

COMBINING THE SENSES

In life, we use the senses synergistically. As such, combining sensation enhances healing. There are devices where you can listen to specifically composed music through headphones while watching colored lights through goggles. Mary Bolles, an education specialist in Boulder, Colorado, combines concurrent movement on a motion table, auditory integration sound therapy through headphones, and light therapy to treat learning-disabled children. As the table moves in circles, the vestibular movement makes the fluid in the inner-ear canals move, exciting the brain stem. That spurs the firing of information, including the visual, and learning. "Some of these kids just can't get a whole sentence together or can't remember the names of their playmates. However, when they're under the light, and they're moving, they say everything perfectly."[19]

Now that we've explored a sensory diet of modulating touch, movement, sound, and light, let's look at how we can spice it up further by paying attention to the air that we breathe.

11

Air Control

> The Lord hath created medicines out of the earth, and he that
> is wise will not abhor them.
>
> —ECCLESIASTES 38:4

We can sit in a room painted in a color we hate, while listening to music
we despise. But we can't sit in a room with a noxious odor without fleeing
or pinching our nose closed. While touch, sight, and hearing arrive at the
limbic system through several electrical pathways, smell involves only a
few synapses to hit the amygdala, and we cannot tune it out. That is its
intent—so we can protect ourselves from dangers like fire.

As with sound and light, odors that oppose the body's natural rhythms,
specifically the synthetic chemical odors of modern society, might be
pushing the sensory defensive further over the edge. Nature's scents, in
contrast, balance us and counteract the ill effect of the chemicals that permeate our lives.

CHEMICALS EVERYWHERE

Since she was a child, Carolyne, now 54 years old, has suffered three plagues: noise, fluorescent lights, and chemicals. Plastic or rubber products, pantyhose, or anything elasticized make her itch like crazy, perspire profusely, and break out in a rash. Allergic to hair spray fumes, nail polish, and a host of shampoos, she has a hard time breathing when she walks into a beauty parlor and gets depressed. Walking into a fabric store sent her head reeling, as she was allergic to the formaldehyde in the synthetic fabrics.

She discovered her allergy to formaldehyde in the late 1970s. Some underwear with little sparkles in it ate her skin away almost to the bone where the fabric rubbed her thighs. Another time, after rolling with her boyfriend on newly carpeted floor—a prime source of formaldehyde and other chemicals—she found her skin was eaten through wherever his beard had caused little scratch marks. Bleeding all over and requiring massive doses of cortisone, she was wrapped in bandages for weeks and almost lost her eyesight.

And it wasn't only formaldehyde. One day she passed out in a store that had just been sprayed with pesticides. And she got intense headaches from MSG, commonly used in Chinese cooking.

The perfumes and makeup we use, the clothing we wear (especially when dry-cleaned), the food we eat, the carpets we walk on, the paint covering our walls, and the air that comes into our buildings contain over 150 different chemicals. The National Academy of Sciences has suggested that as many as 37 million people may experience "increased allergic sensitivity" to a multitude of these chemicals.[1]

Could this relate to sensory defensiveness? In fact, chemical sensitivity *is* olfactory defensiveness: odors others are able to ignore set off alarm. On the other hand, chemicals are not "harmless" routine sensations. The more fragile nervous and immune systems of the sensory defensive are more vulnerable to toxins in the environment. But anyone who experiences chronic exposure can become chemically sensitive.

In sick building syndrome, whole groups of people report chemical sensitivities.[2] Shortly after remodeling and installing new carpeting in Waterside Mall, the Washington, D.C., headquarters of the Environmental Protection Agency (EPA), hundreds of employees began experiencing headaches, fatigue, dizziness, nausea, and respiratory problems. Around seventy-five people were forced to work at home. A survey in 1991 by the EPA found that approximately one-third of inhabitants of sealed buildings reported sensitivity to one or more chemicals.

As a result of repeated exposure or one huge dose, some individuals are unable to tolerate almost any chemical product, a syndrome called multiple chemical sensitivity (MCS). Allergic to the twentieth and twenty-first centuries, these people live isolated within sterile self-made prisons. Marcel Proust, Florence Nightingale, and William James all complained of the vague, unsubstantiated illness now known as MCS. Proust encased himself in a cork-lined room for the last years of his life to protect himself from the outside environment and implored friends to refrain from wearing perfume in his presence.

The American Medical Association denies MCS as a clinical entity, and the government long denied the reality of Gulf War syndrome, which affects some 80,000 vets with symptoms virtually identical to MCS—fatigue, joint pain, loss of motivation, muscle aches, memory difficulties, diarrhea, headache, abdominal pain, stiffness, tingling fingers and toes. Since both MCS and Gulf War syndrome cover an array of symptoms that do not have a definitive physiological marker, like a proliferation of white blood cells, both are considered to be psychogenic. Many psychologists concur, describing many MCS sufferers as emotionally unstable.

This stance begs the mind-body question. Nothing is ever all in the head or all in the body; body and mind continually interact. That some individuals demonstrate these physical symptoms while others equally exposed don't may relate to amount of exposure or to a difference in physiological vulnerability. When that vulnerability involves the senses, in this case the olfactory, the red flag of sensory defensiveness should wave—it may very well be a contributing factor to that vulnerability. In fact, many

MCS sufferers exhibit defensive reactions in other senses. The constitutionally hypersensitive and reactive are notoriously allergic. When a shy person enters a dusty, unfamiliar room, he's likelier than others to have an allergic reaction. As stress wears down the body's systems, including the immune system, the body's ability to fight foreign agents diminishes. MCS may be one of the extreme consequences of sensory defensiveness for some sufferers. In others, toxic overload unbalances the body's systems and puts the senses on the defensive.

Removing Toxins

The first advice to the chemically sensitive is avoidance. Clothing, furniture, carpets, paints, cleaning products, self-care—all should be as chemically free as possible. Many health food stores sell cleaning agents and cosmetics without synthetic fragrance or harsh chemicals. Unbleached clothing made of organic cotton fabric can be bought from some specialized clothing manufacturers.

The air and water must be as free of allergens and toxins as possible. Sunlight is a natural killer of toxins. Opening your windows to natural sunlight can destroy many of these noxious chemicals. Some MCS sufferers sleep best outdoors, regardless of the temperature.

An electrostatic air cleaner removes indoor allergens, as does an ionizer. An ionizer (a silent ionizer is now available, though it is more costly than others) releases negative ions into the air and boosts mood by releasing more of the brain chemical serotonin. It is the release of negative ions that makes us feel uplifted in a thunderstorm, a visit to the seashore, or a mountain stream.

Another way to clean indoor air and neutralize noxious chemicals is to bring nature into the house or office. Houseplants breathe during the day, giving off fresh oxygen and purifying the air. According to the experts, just one plant in every 100 square feet of floor space can make a difference in the air you breathe. The following table lists plants that, according to research by NASA, reduce the effects of certain pollutants.

Best Plants	Source of Pollutants
Areca palm, Boston fern, Spider plant, Azalea	Formaldehyde and foam insulation
Dieffenbachia	Plywood
Philodendron	Particle board
Spider plant	Clothing
Golden pothos	Carpeting
Chrysanthemum	Household cleaner
Bamboo plant	Furniture
Corn plant	Paper goods
Mother-in-law tongue	Water repellents
English ivy	Tobacco smoke
Marginata dracaena	Gasoline and lacquers
Janet Craig dracaena	Synthetic fibers
Chrysanthemum	Plastics
Gerbera daisy	Inks
Warneckeii dracaena	Oils and varnishes
Peace lily	Detergents
Peace lily	Paints

SMELL THE ROSES

Plants help clean the air in another way—through their essential oils.

Why is sniffing a rose so delightfully transporting? Why do we perk up to the odor of peppermint? It is the transcending power of their essential oils released into the air.

Contained in this fragrance are the plant's therapeutic and nutritional properties, photosynthesized from vital solar energy. Their oxygenating molecules carry nutrients and powerful phytochemicals to the cells, bringing life to the plants, destroying infections, staving off illness, spurring growth, and stimulating healing. When concentrated, these essential oils are potent—one drop of chamomile essential oil equals about 30 cups of chamomile herbal tea and may contain as many as 200 to 800 healing constituents.

This power forms the basis for aromatherapy, the uses of aromatics and essential oils from plants to heal body and psyche. As essential oils hit the air, oxygenating molecules as well as negative ions are released, killing microbes in the air and making them an excellent air-detoxifying agent and air deodorizer. Synthetic scents, in contrast, mask unwanted odors and add more chemical toxins. As essential oils hit our nasal passages and skin, they rapidly work physical, emotional, and psychological wonders that make them vital to one's sensory diet.

When we inhale essential oils, some of the odor molecules travel to the lungs and some to the brain. From the lungs, they enter the bloodstream, similarly to when they are absorbed through the skin, and circulate to tissues, glands, and organs for up to 24 hours, eventually being eliminated through sweat, breathing, and other bodily excretions. If you rub a fresh garlic clove on the sole of your foot, you will detect a garlic odor on your breath within 15 to 30 minutes. Unlike chemical drugs that remain in the body, essential oils leave no toxins behind. As odor molecules hit the olfactory bulbs at the base of the brain, the nerve impulses get routed directly to the creative, right side of the cortex and to the limbic system, where they stir our emotions, set our mood, alter stress and energy levels, and enhance sensuality.

The practice of concentrating the essence of various flowers, fruits, herbs, and plants for therapeutic use has been around at least since the time of the pharaohs. Ancient Egyptians used herbal oils as skin conditioners and employed floral aromas to calm the mind and improve the function of various glands.

In modern times, the products of perfume and chemical companies dominate our scent preferences. Yet are these imitations truly therapeutic to our bodies or our minds? Though enticing, the popular perfumes that we spray and dab on our skin contain synthetic components or chemicals, some of which can be harmful. Some people, particularly those who have suffered head trauma, are so allergic to fragrance that they wear a surgical mask in public. Says one woman, "Perfumes of any kind, even from clothes washed in laundry soap, shampoos, and deodorants, make me feel faint, dizzy, confused and gasping for breath. And I even detect a masking fragrance with the supposedly 'unscented.'"

In the United States, some chemically sensitive groups are trying to enact "fragrance-free zones," where personal perfumes or scented cosmetics are prohibited. Though it's virtually impossible to ban people from wearing or spraying their favorite synthetic scents, the use of aromatherapy is gaining ground. For over a century, research has been documenting the power of nature's scents. A study at the Old Manor Hospital in Salisbury, England, found that diffused lavender essential oil could successfully replace medication to relieve insomnia. At the Royal Shrewsbury Hospital in England, a combination of lavender, jasmine, and ylang-ylang essential oils, diffused throughout the coronary care ward, showed a 71 percent reduction in anxiety levels as opposed to a 25 percent reduction for the control group.

The Japanese have long been sniffing out nature's healing properties. Professor Shizuo Torii and his colleagues at Toho University in Tokyo found jasmine to increase alertness and attention by stimulating beta brain wave activity. Based upon his research, Japan's largest Japanese construction firms are enhancing efficiency and reducing stress among office workers by pumping essential oils through air-conditioning systems.

Would the sensory defensive find this stressful? Actually, they might. Natural or chemical, fragrance preference is deeply personal: one person's rose is another's rotten egg. And though chemical sensitivity or olfactory defensiveness occurs largely in response to the chemicals in synthetically produced scents, one can be aversive to nature's scents. Some autistic children have become agitated even by lavender, considered the most universally benign essential oil.

In general, though, the defensive not only tolerate nature's scents but find them indispensable for self-calming. At the Atlantic Institute of Aromatherapy in Tampa, Florida, researchers are exploring the use of aromatherapy as a reward for a child's compliance to her sensory diet.[3] Alli is a 7-year-old child with extreme tactile defensiveness and a diagnosis of oppositional defiant disorder. When she was 3, she complained that clothing hurt, and by 5 she refused to get dressed. If Alli initiated exercises that included jumping on her bed and bouncing around on the floor, and if her crying, whining, and complaining were minimal, she was allowed a "smell strip" with her preferred blends of orange, clary sage, and sandalwood on the way to school in the car. Since instituting this aroma motivation procedure, Alli has been consistently completing her exercises without problems and is less agitated when she leaves for school.

The effect of essential oils ranges from subtle to intense, from euphoria to disgust, from calming to energizing. Some essential oils are sedating (lavender, geranium, chamomile), while others are stimulating (lemon, peppermint, patchouli). Yet as the nervous system of the sensory defensive is unstable and, in some, can quickly vacillate from low to high arousal, you need to determine the effect of an individual oil or combination thereof on your system. For example, geranium, pine, angelica, rosemary, and thyme each act directly upon the adrenals, but in different ways.

Buy only pure, natural essential oils from reputable manufacturers. To judge the quality of the oil, place one drop into the palm of your hand. The oil should be absorbed, and the area where you poured it should feel dry. A slight oily film on your skin indicates the oil has been diluted with synthetics.

From Bottle to Brain

Inhaling oils released into the air will immediately stimulate and oxygenate your brain. For quick inhalation, place 2 to 5 drops of essential oil into the palms of your hands, cup over your mouth, and breathe deeply. Or apply oils to a clean tissue or handkerchief and inhale.

The most effective way to finely vaporize oils without harming or altering their vital components and valuable properties is with a diffusor, a special air-pump device uniquely designed to dispense essential oils into the atmosphere. Or you can place 5 to 10 drops of essential oil onto an absorbent pad (found in the aromatherapy section of health food stores) and secure it with a paper clip onto the outside of a fan, air conditioner, or air filter. As the air blows, it disperses the oils. Similarly, you can throw in 1 to 2 drops of peppermint, lemon, or frankincense oil in a cold-water humidifier-vaporizer. Adding honey, sea salt, or bath salt to the water will emulsify the oils. As heat destroys some of the healing properties of the oils, heat sources for releasing the oils into the air, like a lamp ring over a lightbulb or an aroma lamp (a small dish on top and a candle underneath), are not recommended. For a special delight, try throwing 10 drops of your favorite oil on your towels, linens, and clothing, especially underwear, during a cold-water wash.

For aromatherapy transdermally, add 5 to 10 drops of pure essential oils per 1 ounce of a carrier oil, such as sweet almond, jojoba, canola, grapeseed, or apricot, and apply it to the skin. Always skin-test an essential oil before using it by applying a drop of the oil to a small area first. The only essential oil safe enough to apply undiluted is lavender, as few people are allergic. For a skin tonic spritzer, mix 4 ounces of distilled water with 20 to 30 drops of pure essential oil. Shake well before each use and avoid spraying directly into eyes. Keep spritzer refrigerated to enhance its refreshing effect.

The ultimate in relaxation and rejuvenation is the aromatherapy massage. It restores, rejuvenates, and nourishes the skin, liberates toxins from the muscles, opens congested nerves, increases blood and lymph flow, and calms the nervous system.

There are many ways to surround your day and night with natural fragrance. To avoid startling awake to the sound of an alarm clock, try waking to a diffuser with a timer. Invented by Japanese, it sprays a whiff of refreshing lemon grass and mandarin to gently arouse you. For the shower, try putting 2 to 3 drops of essential oil on the floor in front of your feet, and shower with soap, shampoo, and conditioners made with essential oils. If you feel drowsy in the morning, try more stimulating fragrances, like orange, rosemary, eucalyptus, lemon, lime, or pine. If you awake hyped, try calming scents, like jasmine, geranium, rose, or lavender.

When you rise, a glass of water squeezed with a fresh lemon will help you feel more energized and clean out your digestive system. An aromatic tea like peppermint will help you get going in the morning. If you need relaxing, try Earl Grey, which contains oil of bergamot. In the evening, chamomile tea will help you wind down to sleep.

In the morning, diffuse the car with lavender, which will both calm and energize, setting up body and mind for the day. The most useful and versatile of all essential oils, lavender increases restful, meditative states, alpha brain wave activity, mental concentration, and cerebral blood circulation.

Diffusing rosemary aids concentration. A combination of lavender and rosemary will help you concentrate in a relaxed way. (However, don't use rosemary during pregnancy or if you have high blood pressure.) Other oils to enhance mental clarity and acuity include jasmine, patchouli, lemon grass, or invigorating pine (think of walking in a pine forest). During down times, peppermint or eucalyptus will refresh and energize. The Tokyo Stock Exchange fragrances its inside air each afternoon with peppermint.

As you start marching up into overload or need to combat stressful situations like a traffic jam, try diffusing soothing scented geranium (from the species *Pelargonium*), which mixes well with lavender, or rub some sedating neroli (from orange blossoms) on your wrists and inhale. To relieve menopausal or PMS symptoms, try lavender, chamomile, neroli, or clary sage. (A note of caution: Overuse of clary sage might produce headache and may actually raise blood pressure and cause dizziness, rather than alleviate those conditions.) A combination of geranium and frankincense or rose, a gently euphoric antidepressant, will boost low spirits.

After an especially stressful day, soaking in an aroma bath and inhaling the fragrance harmonizes the body, skin, and mind. As the oils evaporate quickly, wait until the bath is full and then swirl 4 to 5 drops of essential oil into the bath water. Lie back, breathe in, soak for 20 minutes or so, and rest for a half-hour. For the ultimate in relaxing the body and uplifting the spirit, try mixing lavender, geranium, and rose into the bath water, or lavender, ylang-ylang, and patchouli. For cleansing and detoxifying, throw eucalyptus, tea tree, or pine oil in water onto the heat source of a sauna or the steam source in a steam bath. Add a few drops of lemon or peppermint oil to dishwater, the washing machine, or the dishwasher to disinfect and purify.

After dinner, a little jasmine helps to relax and get ready for sleep. To help you fall asleep, spray your bed linens and your pillow with some lavender or with a futon dryer invented by the Japanese that spreads a floral fragrance over the bedding. Rubbing some lavender on the bottom of your feet before nodding off will distribute the oil to every cell in your body in approximately 20 minutes. If you are in the mood for sex, neroli is a hypnotic aphrodisiac that can help diffuse sexual tension. This is why the orange blossom has been the traditional flower of bridal bouquets for generations. Other reputed aphrodisiacs are sandalwood and ylang-ylang.

Of course you don't need essential oils to reap nature's scent pharmacy. Taking a walk among trees and flowers relaxes and re-energizes—a nice lunch break for the stressed—as does keeping cut flowers with fragrance, like rose or jasmine, in your home and office.

Our sensory diet now includes modulating touch, movement, sound, light, and odors. All is experienced in space. Let's look at how the sensory defensive conceive of the space they inhabit and how to enhance it.

12

A Harmonious Space

The environment is the extended body. It must be peaceful.

—DEEPAK CHOPRA

Think back on the world in which we evolved—the sounds, sights, and smells. Brightness came from a star-filled sky or a sun-drenched day, filled with nature's scents. Lives were daily entwined with the sun, wind, rain, soil, fire, plants, and animals. Surrounded by sounds, odors, and light that cued them into day-night, summer-winter, solstice-equinox, humans cycled in and out of the seasons according to inborn biological rhythms.

And then came electricity. We now seal ourselves within refrigerated boxes in hot climates and heated boxes in cold climates that leave us to breathe contaminated air, listen to the unwanted whirring of machines, and eat, converse, and work under a blanket of artificial and impoverished solar radiation—all at once sensorily overstimulating and understimulating.[1]

Does it matter?

Indeed.

Where we are helps define who we are. Emotional chameleons, people become crabby in the humidity, blue in the cold, giddy high up in the Andes, edgy in a crowd. People are more likely to help when the sun is shining. Criminals show less aggression incarcerated in a pink room.[2]

Yet though biology sets basic rules for survival, environmental demand and cultural mores refine our responses. The Peruvians don't get light-headed in the altiplano, 13,500 feet above sea level, and the Japanese move comfortably in crowds.

We each inhabit entirely different sensory worlds. The adaptable can stretch the biological envelope considerably. Some hardy folk can skinny-dip in ice water without becoming hypothermic. Adventurers from all over the map have climbed dangerously air-thin Mount Everest without the use of oxygen!

But for the poorly adaptable sensory defensive, biology is exaggerated, and they are the first to get hot or cold and reel from even a mild change in elevation. A comfortably designed environment is an imperative.

OUR BUBBLE OF SPACE

We experience our bodies in dynamic space and time. As much a psychological as a physical phenomenon, boundaries of the self extend beyond the body into an invisible bubble of space—*our* territory. We sense people as close or distant and maintain a uniform distance from each other. Wrote poet W. H. Auden in "Prologue: The Birth of Architecture,"

> *Some thirty inches from my nose*
> *The frontier of my Person goes,*
> *And all the untilled air between*
> *Is private pagus or demesne.*
> *Stranger, unless with bedroom eyes*
> *I beckon you to fraternize,*

Beware of rudely crossing it:
I have no gun but I can spit.

An essential part of self is making these boundaries explicit. How that gets played out varies from society to society.

In low-touch cultures, like Germany, the United States, and Great Britain, where babies spend most of the day in cribs and other containers, people live surrounded by a broad invisible bubble and need space from another. "Waiting for a bus," observed Ashley Montagu, "Americans will space themselves like sparrows on a telephone wire, in contrast to Mediterranean peoples, who will push the crowd together."[3]

Anthropologist Edward Hall extensively studied personal space.[4] For the average American, "intimate space" is about 18 inches around the head. Only pets and intimates dare venture this close, where you feel the other's body and warmth, smell their breath and body odors, and speak softly or whisper. In social settings, you maintain elbow space by leaning back, holding a drink or a cigarette. When a stranger violates this space, as on a crowded subway or bus, you become as immobile as possible, tensing up and withdrawing into your body, hands to your side, staring into empty space.

"Personal space," the 2 to 4 feet surrounding you, is just outside of touching distance and constitutes the protective bubble between you and others. At this distance, you cannot feel another's body heat, and odors are not readily apparent unless someone has offensive breath or their cologne intrudes upon your space. Looking and chatting are the tools for communication. "Social space" is 4 to 8 feet, appropriate during work and social gatherings. No one expects to be touched. "Public space" is areas beyond 9 to 10 feet.

In high-touch cultures like France and Japan, the bubble narrows and bodies more comfortably commingle. In Japan, where mothers continually keep their babies close (the mother-baby relationship is referred to as "skinship,") this early, intense closeness paves the way for later intimacy with others. Japanese has no word for "privacy," and crowding together is a sign of warm and pleasant intimacy. In France, men and women traditionally greet each other with kisses and embraces.

Yet culture only sets a norm for personal and social space. Whether you live in England or in Japan, how wide a fence you need around you to feel contained and safe and who can open the gate and enter ultimately rests on individual comfort with physical intimacy.

Those comfortable with touch feel connected to their body and grounded in space. They live more closely knit and in the moment: time and space broaden. When American golfer Tiger Woods fell sobbing into his father's safe arms after winning the Masters, it was all the more poignant for its rarity in a touch-inhibited culture.

Those uncomfortable with touch feel a poor connection to their body, panic if they are approached too closely, and are in constant flight-fight mode. For them, time and space narrow. Sensory defensives feel uncomfortable talking to someone who stands too close or touches them when they talk.[5] In fact, what most consider safe social space feels heavy with the *possibility* of someone encroaching on personal space. Even public space feels threatening. As one sensory-defensive woman said, "I can't work, read, or even watch TV if anyone in my family is awake." Intimate space is closed most of the time even to intimates and, if violated, can provoke fight in a flash. The need to stay tightly contained in your bubble manifests itself in body language or a soft-spoken voice that suggests your unwillingness to extend yourself beyond your space.

As walking out the door places you at the mercy of all sorts of sensory mischief, the further you are from home, the more space shrinks. If you are uncoordinated or unbalanced, space takes on additional danger as you negotiate elevators, stairs, escalators, and so on. Fear resurrects the flight reaction, creating an explosive need for space. Fear, plus crowding, can produce panic. Home becomes your sanctuary.

NURTURING ENVIRONMENTS

Cluttered or sparse, messy or neat, your home mirrors your state of mind and influences it. The more sensitive your senses, the more ambience influences your well-being. Carefully designing your exterior landscape will help modify and organize your interior one.

To relax, your environment must be beautiful, orderly, and nontoxic. It should have peaceful sounds, soothing colors, healing scents, proper lighting for the task at hand, comfortable furniture, a pleasant view, private nooks and crannies, warmth, and freedom from interruption.

And it should have variety. Humans thrive on change, as the brain turns off to sameness. The modern indoor environment, including the sealed metal-and-glass cocoons in which we drive, has unchanging temperature, static noise, and uniform lighting that create exhausting sensory monotony.

Energy Flow

One way to create spatial order and harmony is through the Chinese design rage *feng shui*. Combining a bit of superstition and a lot of common sense, *feng shui*, or "wind and water," loosely translated as ambience, is an ancient system in which furniture and objects are placed to encourage the natural flow of vital energy, or *chi*. Balancing yin and yang (female and male), earth and sky, boredom and anxious overexitement, a "just right" space keeps you relaxed and stimulated. If you are drawn toward a particular corner of the den, this space flows with good energy, creating balance and harmony and insuring good *feng shui*. If thinking is laborious at your desk, the *feng shui* philosophy would deem it an unhealthy space that sucks the energy out of your body.

Central to *feng shui* is removing visual distraction, or clutter. Clutter creates stagnant energy, constricting energy flow and compounding chaos. Knowing this instinctively, many sensory defensives are neat-freaks. This does not mean your space has good *feng shui*, just that every object, essential or not, is in its place. Other defensives feel too depleted to clean or put things away and, though craving order, live in a jumbled mess and particularly if they have children.

Think of uncluttering as a constant process. On more energetic days, put away objects not used on a regular basis, including kitchen utensils or garden tools. A chair in your bedroom that you don't use, or files on your desk that you don't look at frequently, or a book sitting on your night-stand that you don't intend to read for a while create clutter. When moving, throw out or give away what you haven't worn or used for the last year. Surround yourself with objects that you absolutely love and remove the rest. Hang artwork at eye level where you can see it so it can uplift your mood.

Place furniture to create clean lines and redirect the flow of energy. Keep traffic lanes, passageways, doors, and windows unblocked. Position the most important piece of furniture first—the bed in the bedroom, the sofa in the living room—and arrange everything else around it. If a space is stuffed with furniture, it constricts energy. If a space is too large or too open, it loses a sense of intimacy and protection. But allow some open spaces rather than filling each corner with furniture.

Nature's shapes curve and undulate. The unnatural straight and flat boxes that we inhabit can feel confining. Furniture with rounded, flowing lines balance the geometry of our homes. An archway or arched or rounded window frames a view and imparts a warm, inviting feeling. Plants with rounded leaves, paintings with flowing lines, vases, mirrors, picture frames, and ceramic bowls in rounded form create symmetry and connect us to more natural forms.

The walls of the room are protective barriers. Put chairs against solid walls to feel better protected and less vulnerable. Position your chair so that your back is not against a window, as this leaves your back unprotected. Place your bed, desk, or table to face the room's entrance so that you won't be startled by what comes in. If this is not possible, a mirror should reflect the doorway. Mirrors help all around, enlarging the room, bringing good views, light, space, and extra vantage points. A mirror at the entrance will make guests feel comfortable, as they can stop and adjust their appearance.

Design your space so that no one will bump into you and increase your anxiety, especially kitchen space. Convenience is essential. Right-handed people should place their desk phone on the right so they don't have to twist uncomfortably to answer it. Anything that organizes and creates shortcuts helps the constantly exhausted sensory defensive cope better.

Maintain your space. A leaky roof, stuck or hard-to-open doors, chipped paint on walls or furniture, anything broken or not working, and especially leaking faucets or toilets, drain energy and further distress you.

Rely on nature to restore your nerves and enrich your environment. Fill your home and office with live plants, both for nature's tranquilizing presence and as an air detoxifier. Open windows to let in fresh air. Add the cooling presence of water with a cascading waterfall, an aquarium, or a bowl of water with floating flowers. Place wind chimes outside a door to create a pleasant, rejuvenating sound; both wind chimes and water fountains help drown out ambient noise. To help get your daily ration of sunlight, maximize window light and illuminate dark gloomy corners with full-spectrum lighting. Nontinted skylights or windows bring in more sunlight.

Play with your senses. Hang crystal pendants in a window to refract natural light into prismatic colors. Beam accent lighting on art objects. Use blue or violet lightbulbs to create peace and tranquility. Place shimmering, luminous lamps or an undulating lava lamp in a relaxing area, where you can recline and gaze. Hang stained glass in front of windows. Dangle a mobile from the ceiling—the movement is reminiscent of trees in the breeze and helps move stagnant air and capture the eye.

Color

In a room painted black, the color closest to the dead of night, we feel closed in. In a room painted soft yellow, the color closest to sunshine, the room feels expansive and uplifting. Most people's mood shifts according to the colors that surround them. Before going on stage or TV, performers and speakers wait in the "green room," as green has a restful effect. Schoolrooms painted blue settle down hyperactive children.

Color is power. It is an affordable and fun means to transform your surroundings to help you better cope with stress. If a beige wall further saps your energy, paint it a color that will energize your spirit and delight your eye. Painful or drab colors weaken inner balance and must go.

While color preference reflects one's unique sensitivities, and one's cultural influence—think of the red/black ambience in a Chinese restaurant and the earth tones in a Mexican one—color in general affects people fairly uniformly. "Warm" colors—red, yellow, peach, pink, and orange— seem to force our focus outward. The "cool" colors—blues, greens, and purples—seem to foster inward orientation. Calm but too-cool gray, black, and white so understimulate as to invite depression.

These effects come from an energy that goes beyond sight. Picking up color vibrations, many blind people can differentiate colors by pressing their fingers or hands over an object: some colors feel hot; some feel cool. Sighted subjects wearing blindfolds respond differently to different colors as well.

To calm the sensory defensive, "color therapists" would encourage decorating in cool colors. But the complicated human nervous system rarely follows simple rules—especially an unstable one. Some sensory defensives need ongoing calming, while others vacillate up and down and rely on colors to energize. Blue might calm one excitable person and plunge another down depression's black hole. Likewise, bright colors may overexcite and force the defensive to retreat further inside their sensitive skin. In others, bright red and orange walls get their starved nervous system going. Pink might stimulate in a relaxing way, which is why it reduces aggression in prisoners.

Color preference relies as well on the defensive's light tolerance. Our eyes are most comfortably adjusted by neutral, nondistracting, cool colors. Too much white causes glare and constricts the pupil. Too much blue tires the eyes because reflected or direct blue light makes focusing difficult. Bright colors and high contrast can produce eye fatigue. If defensive eyes shut out light, red might be almost painful to look at and a black-and-white checkerboard pattern distracting.

The best colors are those you like the most. Your gut reaction will tell you which colors feel pleasant, exciting, healing, suffocating, and dull. On the other hand, some general rules apply in selecting a color scheme.

Is the room dark or sunny, large or small, cold or warm? Light enters through doors and windows and is reflected off walls and furnishings. Light-colored walls reflect more light and create the illusion of space, making a smaller room look larger and a darker room brighter, while black and dark colors generally narrow space. Rich, vibrant colors, like yellow, will make a large room feel more intimate. Greens and blues create large, cool, airy spaces, as does white. Highlights of reds, oranges, or yellows will make a dim, cool room noticeably warmer. A blue room feels cooler than a warm-colored or neutral room at the same temperature, making blues and mauves best suited for smaller, sunnier rooms.

The main color of a room should reflect the room's function. While blue works well in a bedroom, in a living or dining room it might direct attention inward and suppress conversation. Reds and oranges in a work area will distract and tire the eyes, while purple, blues, and greens will help relax the eyes.

As the brain thrives on variety, each area should contain some contrasts of dark and light, warm and cool. Trendy faux walls incorporate different hues and shades of the same color or washes of different colors that combine to create a feeling of light and movement that changes subtly throughout the day. This gives them an ethereal quality. The popular monochromatic painted wall is more passive and static.

Why is it that you can decorate a room in your favorite colors and not be drawn to it? Something about the color scheme is unbalanced. To create harmony, colors must reflect nature's color design. Neighboring colors on the color wheel (red, orange, yellow, green, blue, and purple arranged in a circle) support and enhance each other. Think of the red-orange of the autumn leaf or the blue-green of the ocean's waters.

Contrasting colors are opposites on the color wheel, balancing and exciting each other: Green is complementary to red, orange to blue, yellow to violet. In nature, we often find violet flowers with yellow centers and blue birds with yellow-orange highlights in their wings. Use of contrasting colors balances the warm and the cool. Some energizing yellow in a room painted blue can combat blue's sometime depressing effect.

Temperature

The most organized, aesthetically colorful environment will debilitate if the temperature is too warm, too cold, too dry, or too stuffy.

Everyone has a different optimum temperature level. Also, the thermal environment consists of not only temperature but of humidity and air motion. Ninety degrees, high humidity, and still air distress most people, while the same temperature at reduced humidity and a nice breeze can feel pleasant.

The indoor, recycled air created by heating and air-conditioning can feel too cold in the summer and too hot and dry in the winter, making us drowsy, sluggish, and irritable. Even if the indoor air feels comfortable, the quick temperature change of walking out of a chilled building into the humid outdoors is wearing.

The poorly adaptable sensory defensive must have a proper thermal environment. And not only for comfort—in a humid atmosphere with high pollen counts, many suffer allergies and hay fever. Heat or cold also can produce an allergic response.

To combat dry winter air, use a humidifier. Rather than maintaining central air at a constant high and sucking moisture out of the air, consider cooler temperatures and the use of space heaters. In the hot summer months, dehumidifiers and air-conditioning lower humidity. Clean out the central air ducts, which carry molds that cause endless misery to the often-allergic sensory defensive.

As much as possible, manipulate your thermal environment naturally to connect your body to the natural rhythms for which it was designed. Air-conditioning may not allow your body to adapt to heat. Opening your windows during the warm months and using natural cooling techniques, such as shading and fans to create air motion, keep you more in touch with seasonal changes, while plants add moisture to the air naturally.

Rejuvenation Room

Whether it's the corner of a closet, a nook in the bedroom hidden by a beautifully colored screen, or an area up in the attic, the sensory defensive need private space—a hideaway from sensory overload and the demands of others. It should be small enough to allow you to feel contained and safe, softly colored and textured to encourage relaxation, and quiet. You should be able to darken the space for meditation or light therapy. It should include something that moves, rocks, or sways such as a rocking chair, hanging hammock, or movement cushion.

Every aspect should be beautiful and allow for self-expression, with reminders of things that make you happy. Eliminate anything that will do you harm—toxic materials, stressful lighting, and unnerving noise, like a ticking clock.

ESCAPE TO NATURE

An ideal way to escape sensory overload is to retreat into the wilderness from time to time. The "distant calls, echoes, stealthy rustlings, and the lapping of waves" heard in the African bush at twilight, noted Alfred Tomatis in his autobiography *The Conscious Ear,* uncannily reverberate with the internal sounds of the womb.

Many sensory defensives only feel truly at home in the country. For Swedish film director Ingmar Bergman, that place is Farö, a flat, wind-swept island in the Baltic Sea. Constantly tense and anxious in Stockholm, everything bothers him—"my stomach, my head, reality, everything."

Only on the island, where the solitude and tranquility calm him, does he feel "complete balance."

You now have a sensory diet of grand meals and snacks: modulating touch, movement, sound, light, odors, temperature, colors, and spatial composition. Yet obstacles such as poor nutrition, inefficient breathing, poor posture, emotional blockages, and negative thoughts can dampen its effect. In Part 4, you will learn how to remove these obstacles to give your sensory diet the best chance to work.

Part Four

Removing Treatment Obstacles

Move from worry to action, and the action will absorb the anxiety.

—ROBERT ORNSTEIN AND D. S. SOBEL,
MENTAL MEDICINE UPDATE

13

Food for Your Nervous System

Let food be your medicine.

—HIPPOCRATES

Joshua has always had a nervous stomach. Jackie has a hiatal hernia. Nicole has a spastic colon. Serena is hypoglycemic. All suffer food allergies.

Over thirty gut hormones have been identified, many of which also act as neurotransmitters and directly "talk" with the central nervous system.[1] This makes the gut highly sensitive to the turbulence wrought by sensory defensiveness, and digestive problems and sensory defensiveness intensify each other.

Food is a drug. What you eat directly and significantly impacts your body's internal physiology and biochemistry. Certain foods and substances create additional stress and anxiety. Others calm the nervous system or have an antidepressant effect. It is essential that defensives nourish their already overtaxed systems; otherwise, digestive ailments will debilitate you further and interfere with your efforts to heal.

This goal is a challenge. The extreme effort needed to modulate arousal causes the sensory defensive to easily abuse food like chocolate, which has a calming effect, or substances such as caffeine, which boosts alertness.

Oral defensiveness affects food choice. If you can't tolerate mushy textures, you might eliminate many fruits, such as bananas, peaches, plums, blueberries, avocados, and tomatoes, all packed with nutrition. If you don't like crunchy, you might not munch on carrots, celery, broccoli, or cabbage. Because most foods felt irritating in her mouth, Serena mostly munched on chips and otherwise starved herself. Other sensory defensives overeat for oral input, which reduces tension, but leads to weight gain.

And the sensory defensive may eat all the right foods but be undernourished. During the flight-or-fight response, digestion and other bodily functions slow down to conserve energy, and this prevents adequate digestion. If you don't assimilate nutrition properly, food can pass through your system without being absorbed—a condition called *malabsorption*. The malabsorbed food putrifies and ferments, resulting in bloating, cramps, and gas.

Chronic stress uses up valuable vitamins and minerals and exhausts the system, making illness more likely. Overuse of drugs to combat illness, such as antibiotics, steroids, aspirin, or ibuprofen, eat up the gut and create problems like *leaky gut syndrome* and *Candida albicans*. And stress throws off your sugar level, which can eventually lead to problems like *hypoglycemia* (low blood sugar).

As your sensory diet becomes an integral part of your life, you will control some of the stress that interferes with good nutrition. In turn, learning which foods aggravate tension, destabilize sugar levels, upset the integrity of your gut, and compromise your immune system will remove the first major obstacle to treatment success.

FOOD AND THE JITTERS

If you have an overactive nervous system, you need to be cautious about food and substances that further hype arousal or destabilize your sugar level. These substances can keep you chronically tense and irritate the digestive tract.

Caffeine

One of the quickest ways to get hyped is by ingesting caffeine, in coffee, tea, colas, cocoa, chocolate, and some over-the-counter drugs. Caffeine releases adrenaline and raises the stress hormone cortisol, which causes the blood vessels to constrict and the heart to pump harder, provoking the same physiological arousal response triggered by stress. It interferes as well with adenosine, a brain chemical that normally has a calming effect, and it raises levels of lactate, a biochemical thought to produce panic attacks in vulnerable individuals. A single cup of tea or cola will cause some easily aroused sensory defensives to get jittery or spend a sleepless night. Caffeine increases the PMS symptoms that plague most sensory-defensive women, including irritability, anxiety, fatigue, and sleep disturbance. Heavy coffee consumption can lead to adrenal exhaustion (see Chapter 6), a common by-product of sensory defensiveness.

So why would the easily hyped sensory defensive have a caffeine problem? Caffeine increases levels of norepinephrine in the brain and causes you to feel alert and awake. While high-arousal sensory defensives generally wake up hyped, the nervous systems of other sufferers spike from low to high arousal and caffeine gets their system going. To feel alert enough to function, Serena relied on Coke and strong expresso coffee; Trish was a Pepsi addict. At the same time, the excessive caffeine use may have contributed to their wired state and unstable arousal.

The defensive need not eliminate all caffeine; even the highly sensitive can tolerate some caffeine a day. You need to test how much caffeine your system can tolerate. For those who can't get going in the morning, try drinking something with intense flavor, like pure cranberry juice or lemon juice. Heavy work to the jaw from chomping and biting is energizing, and munching on an apple provide you the needed early-morning boost.

Hypoglycemia

When under stress, your body burns up sugar very rapidly and can quickly deplete it. When this happens, your brain does not get enough sugar, and you feel trembly, confused, spacey, and anxious, similar to how you might respond to sensory overstimulation. You feel more nervous and aroused as well because your adrenal glands release adrenaline and cortisol to prompt your liver to release stored sugar and stabilize your sugar level.

When you experience chronic periodic drops of blood sugar below normal, you have a condition called hypoglycemia. As the symptoms are similar to sensory defensiveness, it's hard to know if you feel agitated from sensory overload, a sugar imbalance, or both. Until your blood sugar returns to normal, interventions for sensory defensiveness, like brushing or heavy work, won't be as effective. Moreover, hypoglycemia weakens and exhausts you. You may lack the stamina to do activity, the foundation of your sensory diet. Discouraged, you may discontinue your daily push-ups and further destabilize your system.

How can you establish if you suffer from low blood sugar? If you are hypoglycemic, you will feel anxious, light-headed, weak, irritable, and you may have a rapid heartbeat 2 to 3 hours after a meal, in the middle of the night, or early in the morning, when your blood sugar is lowest, since you've fasted all night. These symptoms disappear soon after eating. After eating sugar, your mood will elevate and then rapidly drop to depression, irritability, or spaciness 20 to 30 minutes later.

If you suspect hypoglycemia, it's important to control your sugar level. This isn't easy. Sweet taste from mother's milk is sugar in its natural form, and the very substance that provides the energy to sustain life. As you walk through the mall and catch a whiff of chocolate ice cream, you make a bee-line for the Häagen Dazs counter because your hypothalamus is signaling "energy!" before your cerebrum reminds you that sugar is not on your diet. And if you had to hunt for your food, as did our early ancestors, high-calorie foods had higher survival value.

Fortunately, hypoglycemia can be overcome. Your diet should avoid foods that are quickly absorbed, as this results in rapid changes of glucose levels in the blood. Stay away from:

- *Simple sugars:* candy, cookies, cakes, colas, ice cream, honey, corn syrup, molasses, high fructose
- *Simple starches:* pasta, refined cereals, potato chips, white bread
- *High glycemic foods that quickly raise blood sugar levels, thus raising insulin:* white bread, puffed rice, puffed wheat, instant rice, instant potatoes, corn chips, raisins

Some healthy food, such as carrots, corn, flax seeds, bananas, apricots, papaya, watermelon, and mangoes, have a high glycemic level. Some authorities suggest moderation, while others claim that, as long as you don't mix them with other high glycemic foods, you can't eat enough at one sitting to destabilize your sugar level.

A daily chromium supplement will help to stabilize your sugar level by aiding the process by which insulin carries sugar to your cells. Vitamin B complex, which helps regulate the metabolic process that converts carbohydrates to sugar, and vitamin C, a powerful antioxidant, increase your resiliency to stress.

A snack between meals helps to maintain a steadier blood sugar level. Some nutritionists recommend a complex carbohydrate or protein snack, like nuts, a whole-grain bagle and cheese, or a glass of orange juice. Others, like Barry Sears, author of *The Zone*, recommend that every meal, including snacks, consist of 30 percent protein, 30 percent fat, and 40 percent carbohydrates.[2]

What if you feel jittery and spacey following a meal but your symptoms don't fit into a hypoglycemic profile? The pancreas is subject to stimulation through the vagus nerve, which goes through the hypothalamus, the seat of emotions. Stress alone can force the pancreas to secrete insulin and thereby determine how much glucose is converted to energy.

If you do suspect you may be hypoglycemic, your doctor can give you a glucose tolerance test.

EATING UP THE GUT

As a vulnerable nervous system makes for a vulnerable gut, the sensory defensive often suffer from food allergies, leaky gut syndrome, candida overgrowth, and acidity. These problems are enormously destabilizing. Eliminating them and restoring balance to the gut is paramount for modulating the nervous system and controlling sensory defensiveness.

Food Allergies

The relationship between allergies and sensory defensiveness is well established. If you are sensory defensive, you likely have food sensitivities of which you may be unaware.

When you eat something to which you are allergic, your body acts immediately and intensely—for example, you eat peanuts and break out in hives. More common are food sensitivities or food intolerance, which are delayed immune reactions to food that can occur from a few hours to a few days after exposure. The day after eating pizza, you feel dizzy, irritable, confused, tired, depressed, anxious, and even panicky. As you are unlikely to connect this delayed response to the wheat, cheese, or other ingredients in the long-digested pizza, you assume you feel this way in response to sensory overload or other stresses in your life. Stressed out, you eat more pizza!

What causes food sensitivities? They appear to result when foods, particularly their protein component, are not completely digested and some of it putrefies. When absorbed by your body, your immune system recognizes these components as foreign bodies and goes on the defense. Once in the bloodstream, this foreign matter causes havoc. It can go anywhere in the body and cause problems. In the brain, it causes headaches, confusion, dizziness, fatigue, anger, irritability, anxiety, or mood swings. In the joints, tissues, or bones, it causes stiffness or arthritis. In the skin, it cause rashes. In the kidneys, it causes fluid retention. Binge eating, diarrhea or constipation, and craving for a particular food all indicate food intolerance.

If you are unsure what foods cause you to react, start by removing all sugar, alcohol, wheat, dairy products, and corn from your diet, the foods to which most people react. The casein and gluten in wheat especially tend to cause problems. Milk allergies appear to be the culprit in many cases of ear infections in children, and as we learned, both milk and wheat are implicated in some cases of autism. By eliminating these foods, you might find that symptoms like fatigue, bloating, gas and constipation, and aches abate.

To test for food allergies and intolerance, you can have a formal allergy test from your physician or consult a qualified nutritionist. You can also use your body as a laboratory and systematically monitor your own reaction to foods. One way is to take your pulse after eating a particular food. Elevation above 10 beats of your normal rate is a likely sign of an allergic reaction. A simple home urine test is also available.

Unlike food allergies, food sensitivities are generally temporary and typically disappear when you eliminate the reactive food for 60 to 90 days. Quite often you can reintroduce the foods back into your diet without recurrence of symptoms. The most effective way of preventing food sensitivities from recurring is to rotate, combine, and cook foods properly.

Leaky Gut

The most frequent cause of allergies is leaky gut syndrome—excessive permeability of the digestive tract, which allows food allergens as well as undigested food or bacteria to slip into the bloodstream. The body thinks it's sick, and the immune system reacts in a number of ways, with rash, diarrhea, joint pain, migraines, even psychological symptoms such as anxiety and depression. Alcohol consumption, the use of nonsteroidal anti-inflammatory drugs (NSTAIDs, such as aspirin, ibuprofen, and acetaminophen), and assorted viral, bacterial, parasitic, and yeast infections can all bring on leaky gut syndrome. Leaky gut is linked to an untold number of disorders that the sensory defensive complain of, such as irritable bowel syndrome and chronic fatigue syndrome, and is prevalent in populations that suffer sensory defensiveness, such as the autistic and people with attention deficit disorder.

If you have leaky gut

- Avoid any foods to which you are allergic
- Take a digestive enzyme at all meals and snacks to help the intestinal tract break down food more completely and minimize small fragments (peptides) leaking into the blood undigested
- Take a probiotic supplement that contains acidophilis, bifidus, and other friendly bacteria or eat yogurt daily
- Take L-glutamine daily, an amino acid shown to help heal leaky gut

Candida Overgrowth

Often associated with leaky gut syndrome and a potential hidden link between what you eat and how you feel is another food-related problem that can make you feel hyped and in a fog: *Candida albicans*, or yeast overgrowth.

Bacteria and yeast, including *Candida albicans*, are present on your skin and in your mouth, nose, and digestive tract. Normally, the microorganisms living in your lower digestive tract assist in digestion of food and in synthesizing essential vitamins.

But certain conditions, among them long-term use of antibiotics and steroids, allow *Candida albicans* to overgrow in your lower intestinal tract. As stress depletes the immune system, sensory defensives are more prone to infection and likely to take frequent courses of long-term antibiotics or steroidal drugs. Other conditions include the hormonal changes that occur with the use of oral contraceptives or changes that accompany pregnancy; anything that depresses immune function like autoimmune disease, such as Crohn's disease; and diets high in sugars and other refined simple carbohydrates, which are the nutrients in which yeast thrive.

This upset of the balance of bacteria usually results in an infection that can manifest as cravings for sugar or breads, chronic bloating and cramps, aching joints and muscles, ear infections, chronic congestion, coughing, frequent infections, itching or discharge. Depression, irritability, inability to concentrate, and frequent mood swings are also common, as are PMS, headaches, rashes, and food allergies. Sufferers experience increased sensitivity to tobacco smoke, perfumes, fabrics, and chemical odors, creating sensory defensiveness.

As stress makes the sensory defensive crave sugar, and sugar feeds the candida, it's a hard condition to eliminate.

To control yeast overgrowth:

- Eliminate yeast, sugars, wheat, oat, barley and rye, dairy products, and peanuts.
- Limit carbohydrates.
- Limit fruit to Granny Smith apples, lemons, and limes.
- Take grapefuit seed extract to kill the yeast.
- Take cranberry extract to kill bacteria and yeast and as a powerful antioxidant.
- Take scFOS, a product from Japan that feeds good bacteria and reduces unwanted yeast.
- Take probiotics (acidophilus and other friendly bacteria) or eat yogurt daily to introduce friendly bacteria.

Some physicians prescribe antifungal medication. Length of treatment varies by how closely you follow dietary restrictions. As treatment progresses and the yeast die off, you may experience headaches, fatigue, gastrointestinal problems, and sugar cravings. These discomforts will pass. Most people begin to experience relief from their symptoms within two weeks of initiating treatment.

258   Too Loud, Too Bright, Too Fast, Too Tight

Acid-Alkaline Balance

The systems of the sensory defensive are in a state of imbalance. Unless you are a strict vegetarian and very health conscious, this likely includes the acid-alkaline balance of your biological terrain, or the state of the body's tissues and functions.

People with acute and chronic inflammatory and pain syndromes, congestive disorders that include recurrent infections and allergies, and degenerative diseases such as cancer, cardiovascular problems, and diabetes are all overly acidic. As such, some nutritionists believe that correcting this imbalance is more important even than getting rid of parasitic, fungal, and other infections.[3] This could mean major dietary changes.

Meat, poultry, dairy and cheese products, eggs, refined foods such as sugar and flour, and nuts and seeds are more acidic in composition and leave an acid residue in the body after they are metabolized. This can increase the transit time of food through the digestive tract, and vitamins and minerals might not be adequately assimilated. The resulting underabsorption of vitamins, especially B vitamins, vitamin C, and minerals, further stresses the body and eventually leads to low-grade malnutrition. Nor will taking supplements necessarily correct this condition, as you might not adequately absorb them.

Over time, an animal product–based diet creates a metabolic breakdown in the body. This is especially likely when you are already stressed and not properly digesting protein foods. You feel increasingly sluggish, tired, and congested with excess mucous or sinus problems, all of which further stresses the body and aggravates tension and anxiety. Medications as well as foods can have an acid reaction in the body and create similar problems.

To maintain a proper acid-alkaline balance in the body:

- Decrease consumption of acid-forming foods: animal-based foods, sugar, refined flour products, nuts, and seeds.

- Consume about 70 percent of calories as alkaline-forming foods: vegetables; most fruits, except plums and prunes; whole grains such as brown rice, millet, and buckwheat; and bean sprouts.

To eat for the most nutritional benefit, follow these basic guidelines:

- Eat organic raw fruits and vegetables when possible (the more color, the higher in important phytonutrients—red pepper versus green pepper; butternut squash versus zucchini; red cabbage versus white; pink grapefruit versus white).
- Eliminate highly processed foods and refined sugars.
- Use extra virgin olive oil (cold pressed) primarily.
- Drink 8 glasses of water daily.
- Chew your food well.
- Make sure you have essential fatty acids, both omega 3 and omega 6, by eating deep sea fish, lake trout, and raw seeds (flaxseeds, sunflower seeds, and walnuts).

Eating Habits

The constantly keyed-up sensory defensive are prone to eating quickly and chomping away tension until they feel stuffed. These eating habits can strain your stomach and intestines and interfere with proper digestion. This can create indigestion, bloating, or cramps and increase your level of stress.

Eating is a parasympathetic activity. When possible, try to eat meals in a relaxed atmosphere, with calming background music. Food must be partially predigested in your mouth for adequate digestion later; savor your food by chewing it slowly, at least 15 to 20 times per mouthful, which is a lot. And limit drinking during meals to 1 cup of fluid; drinking too much with your meals can dilute stomach acid and digestive enzymes.

NUTRITIONAL ANXIETY BUSTERS

If you are stressed, anxious, or depressed, your adrenal glands work overtime, and your body has an enormously increased need for particular vitamins and minerals. It is important that the sensory defensive refurbish their nervous system with the necessary vitamins and minerals.[4]

The B vitamins and vitamin C, which are rapidly depleted under stress, should be replenished daily. Vitamin B_1, B_2, B_6, and B_{12} deficiencies, in particular, can lead to anxiety, irritability, restlessness, fatigue, and emotional instability. You need sufficient amounts of the minerals calcium and magnesium. Calcium acts as a tranquilizer, which is why having a glass of milk before bedtime helps you sleep. Take it in combination with magnesium, since these two minerals work synergistically. Chromium, critical in lowering insulin requirements, is another important mineral. Lower insulin levels aid healthy function of many body systems, including the serotonin system.

A daily multivitamin, particularly one for stress, will probably include most if not all of these vitamins and minerals, as well as vitamin E, selenium, zinc, copper, manganese, and iron—also essential for the proper functioning of the nervous system. If not, you can supplement as needed. And try raw adrenal extract, preferably under the supervision of a doctor or nutritionist experienced in using glandular extracts.

Natural Serotonin Boosters

The extreme stress that results from sensory defensiveness depletes the neurotransmitter serotonin. Food can help maintain healthy levels of serotonin in your brain and stabilize your mood, which is why it is literally a drug.[5] We need vitamin C to make serotonin, along with sufficient quantities of vitamin E and the minerals magnesium, zinc, copper, manganese, and iron. And we need the amino acid tryptophan—the building block of serotonin contained in pineapple, bananas, turkey, chicken, tuna, eggs, yogurt, and milk. A form of tryptophan, 5-hydroxytryptophan (5-HTP), is sold over the counter in health food stores. Take it with food, as it can cause digestive problems.

Mother Nature's Tranquilizers

Within nature's pharmacy exists a plethora of harmless nerve tonics to help balance the functions of the body of the sensory defensive and to make it more resistant to stress.

Kava is a popular natural tranquilizer. Relaxing both muscles and emotions, kava calms without sedating, as prescription tranquilizers often do.[6] Some fifteen different chemical compounds known as *pyrones* account for kava's anxiety-easing and muscle-relaxing effects. These appear to reduce activity at the spinal part of the nervous system. Kava also acts upon the limbic system, specifically the amygdala, where it dampens fear and anger, thereby perking up pleasant feelings. These effects are felt within 30 minutes to 2 hours. When you're restless, kava in somewhat larger doses will help ease you into sleep.

Kava can help menopausal sensory-defensive women better cope with their symptoms. In two placebo-controlled, double-blind studies of 80 women with menopause-related symptoms, the kava group reported reductions in anxiety symptoms, hot flashes, and other menopausal symptoms, along with improvements in sleep, mood, and a sense of well-being.

Though safer to take than anti-anxiety drugs, kava does have warnings. Do not use if pregnant, nursing, being treated for depression, or if you have Parkinson's disease. Do not mix with anti-anxiety or antidepressant medications.

Here are other popular stress-reducing herbs from nature's pharmacy:[7]

- *Valerian root:* A natural relaxant useful for gut-related problems, it seems to block the transmission of stressful nerve impulses to the bowel. Together with kava, it can enhance the action of gamma amino butyric acid (GABA), a neurotransmitter that is low in many high-strung people.

- *Passionflower:* A popular herb that has a mild, relaxing effect.
- *Gotu kola:* It mildly relaxes and revitalizes the nervous system, as well as decreasing fatigue and depression while increasing memory and intelligence.
- *St. John's wort:* Apparently raising serotonin level, numerous studies have documented it to relieve mild to moderate depression.
- *SAMe:* S-adenosylmethionine is a naturally occurring enzyme in the body that in supplement form elevates serotonin levels and balances other neurotransmitters to work as an antidepressant. Studies show that 70 percent of depressed patients who try SAMe notice improvement in mood within days.
- *Ginkgo biloba:* It improves brain function by increasing cerebral blood flow and oxygenation, helping ease depression, anxiety, headaches, memory loss, tinnitus, vertigo, headache, and poor concentration.
- *Asian ginseng (panax):* It enhances and revitalizes the power of the mind and body, helping to protect against chronic stress and debilitating fatigue and improve vitality, alertness, concentration, coordination, memory, and mood. It stimulates the immune system as well.
- *Siberian ginseng:* It promotes adaptation of climactic extremes of heat, cold, and altitude; improves visual and hearing acuity; restores homeostasis to stressed adrenals and pituitary glands; enhances immune function; and increases stamina, endurance, and general health.
- *Reishi:* A relaxing medicinal mushroom, it reduces anxiety and insomnia.
- *Milk thistle:* It enhance the liver's adaptation to stress.
- *Licorice root:* Glycyrrhizic acid, an important active component of licorice root, is a natural corticosteroid with activity resembling cortisone that can raise blood pressure. It relieves symptoms of some chronic fatigue syndrome patients with neurally

mediated hypotension, a disorder that causes the blood pressure
to drop swiftly when a person stands.
* *Grapeseed:* It helps reduce light sensitivity.

A word of caution: If you are taking any medication, check with your
physician to see if it interacts with herbal supplements. St. John's wort, for
instance, is counterindicated when taking SSRIs or other antidepressants.
It interacts as well with Coumadin, theophylline, digoxin, triptan drugs for
migraines, oral contraceptives, several AIDS medications, and transplant
antirejection drugs. Nor is taking kava recommended while taking prescription drugs. The sensory defensive are in general unusually sensitive to
drugs, natural and synthetic.

A toxic gut can both trigger and exacerbate illness, weakness, stress and
anxiety, and sensory defensiveness. It may be the core cause of more illness
and anxiety than we realize, and its cure is the sine qua non for handling
sensory defensiveness. Yet, even with a squeaky-clean gut, you cannot
hope to benefit from treatment until you normalize your breathing patterns. Let's now look at how to enhance proper breathing.

14

Breathing Lessons

> Conscious breathing, the technique employed by both the yogi
> and the woman in labor, is extremely powerful. There is a
> wealth of data showing that changes in the rate and depth of
> breathing produce changes in the quality and kind of neuro-
> transmitters.
>
> —CANDACE PERT, *MOLECULES OF EMOTION*

Breath is the essence of being. In the relaxed body, you breathe slowly and
deeply, filling your body with energy and vitality. In the chronically tense
body that most defensive inhabit, you breathe fast and shallow, have a tendency to hold your breath and feel rushed, depleted, and worn. This disordered breathing keeps you constantly overaroused and hyperalert and
perpetuates your tension and defensiveness. To achieve a relaxed state
requires that you change the rhythm, rate, and depth of your breathing.
It's the only way you will begin to feel more centered: at home in your
body and open to the world.

As breathing is largely unconscious, this is hard to do in a state of
chronic stress. Nor is achieving this state the same as learning to control
your breath through mechanical exercises that are often employed to control panic. Deep breathing is a result of deep relaxation. To achieve this, a
fundamental shift in your essential breathing must take place. Generally

this takes a whole-body approach, including the sensory diet outlined in the previous chapters, the yogic pranayama breathing exercises described in this chapter, and the bodywork and mind-body activities outlined in subsequent chapters. It helps also to have a relaxed partner to whom you can entrain your breathing rhythm.

CHEST BREATHING

In a relaxed state, you breathe from your abdomen: as you inhale, the abdomen and rib cage expand; as you exhale they contract. Breathing is three-dimensional and, if you pay attention, you will feel the breath expand out in the front of your body, in your back, and in your rib cage. If you watch a sleeping baby, you will see this natural, whole-body breathing rhythm. When you are relaxed and grounded, you can feel your breathing as a wave: on the inhale it starts deep in the abdominal cavity and flows upward to the head, and on the exhale it moves from head to feet.

At the first sign of stress or anxiety, breathing instantly changes. To ready your body for quick flight, you gasp, suck in your abdomen, and breathe high into your chest with short, shallow spurts. Once the stress has passed, the parasympathetic nervous system kicks in. In the normal nervous system the body calms, returning to a baseline of relaxed, regular breathing.

If you are sensory-defensive, you don't easily recover from distress and may never return to a baseline of normal diaphragmatic "belly breathing." Instead, you routinely breathe quick, shallow breaths from your chest. In this restricted chest-breathing pattern, your upper chest projects forward, the surface muscles tighten, and the length of exhalation is reduced. This prevents the diaphragm, the muscle that separates the lung cavity from the abdominal cavity, from descending completely in order to inhale. You are unable to get the air you need and may struggle on the next breath to suck the air in, setting up a vicious cycle: The harder you try, the less air you get. Breathing primarily in your upper chest also reduces oxygenation of the blood and starves your body of energy. As this is the way one breathes under stress, many sensory defensives live with chronic, free-floating anxiety and fatigue.

Once habitual, chest breathing affects your whole body. You learn to rely almost entirely on your upper-body muscles to breathe, which are weaker than the primary muscles that make up your diaphragm. This reliance results in chronic tension in the neck, shoulders, and upper back and chronically tightened abdominal muscles from not expanding your abdomen. This tension prevents the organs in your lower body from getting sufficient circulation, and that affects your digestion, assimilation, and elimination. Tension affects sexuality as well, as sexual feelings of warmth and melting in the pelvis are missing, and sexual excitement may be confined to the genitals.[1] There is also reduced blood flow to the heart, since during chest breathing the diaphragm is prevented from descending completely. In fact, chest breathing directly correlates with heart disease and hypertension.

The accumulated tension of chest breathing will prevent therapy such as massage or bodywork from relaxing you fully because the tension returns as soon as you resume chest breathing. Bad breathing is why many sensory defensives never know total relaxation: anxiety leaves you breathless.

HYPERVENTILATION

If you are unable to breathe in fully, you can't breathe out fully. To compensate, you start breathing more quickly: you hyperventilate; that is, you breathe out too much carbon dioxide relative to the amount of oxygen in your bloodstream.

Though most people know that we need oxygen to survive, they might be unaware that we need carbon dioxide to help the body maintain the right combination of acid and alkaline on which cell metabolism depends. Even slight alterations of this balance changes the rates of chemical reactions in the cells, slowing down some and speeding up others. This imbalance can unleash a whole chain of adverse events.[2]

- Less oxygen is released to the tissues, causing dizziness and breathlessness.
- Diminished blood flow to the brain and other parts of the body causes headaches, lack of concentration.
- An increase in alkalinity creates excess calcium in muscles and nerves, that makes them hyperactive and causes muscle tension.
- Reduced blood flow to the extremities causes cold hands and feet.
- Overexcitability of the nervous system causes irritability, overreaction, rushed reactions, inappropriate responses.

The hyperventilation associated with panic attacks causes heart palpitations, chest pain, rapid pulse, faintness, tingling in the limbs, and shortness of breath that has sent more than one sensory-defensive person to the emergency room thinking that he was having a heart attack.

There seems no end to the repercussions of hyperventilation. Other symptoms can include exhaustion, distorted vision, ringing in the ears, yawning, a feeling of a lump in the throat, burping, difficulty swallowing, stomach irritation, allergies. People may experience insomnia, nightmares, and feelings of unreality and depersonalization. Also associated with hyperventilation is increased sensitivity to light and sound, setting off or exacerbating sensory defensiveness.

Most people think of hyperventilation as acute and obvious. Your breaths are erratic, noisy, and rapid; your chest is heaving; and your abdomen is barely moving. You may feel the need to take an occasional deep breath, you may find it difficult to breathe out and may sigh at intervals to relieve this, and you may feel dizzy.

But hyperventilation can be chronic and subtle, and may go unrecognized. It is chronic if you are an upper-chest breather, breathe through the mouth rather than the nose, or breathe heavily, or if you breathe 18 or more breaths per minute (normal breathing is 12 to 14 BPM for men and 14 to 15 BPM for women), frequently sigh, gasp, yawn, cough, clear the throat, or if you moisten the lips.

You are probably unaware of breathing poorly. For example, most people brace with their upper bodies the moment their fingers rest on a computer keyboard, and chest-breathe and breathe quickly while typing.[3]

To catch how you routinely breathe, put something eye-catching on the refrigerator, the bathroom mirror, a reading lamp, and at your computer monitor. When you see the pink or green sticky dot, notice your breathing pattern. Is it too fast? Are you chest-breathing? Mouth breathing? If so, stop a moment and breathe slowly and deeply into your abdomen and through your nose. As you breathe, notice if the air coming into your nostrils and touching your upper lip is cold or warm. Observe if you breathe in and out through both nostrils, or in one and out the other. When you notice your breathing, you change it. After several breaths, has each breath become easier or more labored? Are you calmer or more anxious? Has your heartbeat slowed down or speeded up? Noticing these changes begins breath awareness.

DEEP BREATHING

Breath control is the ultimate means of body control and becoming present in the moment. If you do deep breathing for 3 to 10 minutes a day (ten to forty breathing cycles), twice a day, you will strengthen the muscles that support breathing and gradually enhance their flexibility and resilience. This will reset the rhythm and rate of your breathing, and with regular deep-breathing practice, increase your lung capacity to enable you to breathe more deeply. From the back of a large room, you can hear my yoga teacher's lungs fill like a surge of wind. If you've ever been in the mountains, where there's less oxygen in the air, you may recall spontaneously breathing more deeply and getting a "Rocky Mountain high." When you breathe deeply, you blow off more carbon dioxide than you inhale, allowing more oxygen to get to the brain. Along with increases in levels of natural opiates, this helps to explain the heightened states that climbers experience.

As your lung capacity increases, you will be able to train yourself to breathe slower and deeper, even as slow as 8 to 12 times per minute. This will increase the amount of oxygen getting to your brain and muscles, nourish essential body organs, heighten energy levels, and increase metabolic rate. It will stimulate your parasympathetic nervous system to override your sympathetic nervous system, thereby inviting the relaxation response to take over.

Whatever breathing exercise you do, try to get the breath deep into the belly and extending enough into the pelvis to feel the pelvic floor. By doing so, explains Alexander Lowen, originator of bioenergetics (see Chapter 15), you will activate suppressed sadness and sexuality.

Pranayama Breathing

Pranayama, the ancient yogic means of breath control, offers formal breathing techniques. Many focus on slowing breathing and breathing from the diaphragm. The potential of yogic breath control to revitalize the nervous system is enormous. Psychologist David Shannahoff-Khalsa of the University of California in San Diego has demonstrated that yoga breathing techniques significantly decrease the symptoms of obsessive-compulsive disorder.[4] Of eight adults who completed a one-year course of yogic breathing techniques, five were able to discontinue their medication (fluoxetine) and two others drastically reduced the dosage. Another study showed that slow, deep breathing alone resulted in a significant reduction in menopausal hot flashes.[5]

Ujjayi Breathing

Start out lying down, so you're not fighting gravity. Close your eyes and note the tension you feel and your breathing pattern. If you are defensive, you are chronically stressed and take feeling overanxious for granted.

Become aware of how your breathing pattern reflects your level of tension.

Place one hand on the upper abdomen just below the base of the sternum, your power spot. Place the other hand on your chest. Place the tip of your tongue against the back of your top front teeth. Inhale slowly and deeply through your nose to the count of 4 (one one thousand, two one thousand, etc.), creating a yawning sensation in the back of your nose and throat and expanding your abdomen like a balloon. Your hand should rise as you feel your navel rise to the ceiling. You should hear your breath filling your lungs—a "dragon" breath—and rising up to where your throat and the back of your nose meet, and you should feel your throat vibrating. Your chest should move only slightly while your abdomen expands. If you feel your belly expand without the sensation of air rising up to where your throat and the back of your nose meet, you are breathing incorrectly.

To start the exhale, place the tip of your tongue behind your bottom front teeth. With slightly pursed lips, breathe out through your nose, slowly pushing the stale air out of your lungs to the count of 4. Feel your navel collapse toward the floor, minimizing your upper-chest motion. The hand on your chest should stay as still as possible. Be sure to squeeze all the air out of your lungs and allow your whole body to just let go. You can also breathe out through your mouth, emphasizing the exhalation by making a "hah" sound with your mouth open and relaxed. Though intuitively we take in a deep breath to breathe more fully, in fact it is by exhaling fully that we prepare for deeper, spontaneous inhalations. The longer your exhalation, the more you will feel your eyes relax and your facial muscles soften.

Pause briefly at the end of the exhalation and let your next inhalation begin on its own, without "grabbing" for it. Pausing following exhalation extends parasympathetic arousal, which will prolong a feeling of calm, while holding the breath on the inhale, as some yogic breathing exercises do, extends sympathetic nervous system arousal—which the overly anxious sensory defensive don't want to do. As you learn to relax into the breath, you may find that the pause lengthens on its own accord. When you feel yourself going into overload, deep breathing with a pause at the end of the exhalation will help you rest and replenish.

Do at least ten full abdominal breaths slowly and smoothly, prolonging your exhale. Slowly increase the amount to forty cycles a session. Take a few regular breaths between each ten-breath cycle.

Though most recommend doing deep breathing while lying flat on your back, other yogic positions will better help open up your rib cage to allow for deeper breathing. One is the extended-child position. Start by kneeling and then gently fold forward until your head is resting on the floor in front of your knees. Open your knees like frog legs. Extend your arms forward over your head, palms down, as if reaching for the wall in front. Can you feel your chest open and your breath deepen? Another way to open up the rib cage is to lie on the floor on your back with a rolled-up blanket under the small of the back, with your knees bent, your arms down by your sides, and your backside pressing the floor.

Alternate Nostril Breathing

Another excellent breathing exercise to help soothe and calm the sensory defensive is alternate nostril breathing (ANB). In one research study, ANB increased spatial memory in 10- to 17-year-olds.[6] Increased spatial awareness relates to field independence, the ability to be relatively independent of the physical environment and still accurately orient and maneuver in space. As the field independent are more centered and grounded in space, this exercise offers the sensory defensive an important opportunity for better body awareness. Many researchers hypothesize that right-nostril dominance stimulates the arousal-producing sympathetic nervous system and left-nostril dominance elicits the relaxation-producing parasympathetic system.

Here's how to do ANB. Sit comfortably in a chair or cross-legged on a cushion on the floor. Clear your nostrils by blowing each separately. Even better, clear your sinuses first by sniffing water through one nostril and expelling it from the other with a Neti Pot (ayurvedic sinus relief), a nasal-irrigation device shaped like a miniature Aladdin's lamp that can be purchased in most well-stocked health food stores.

The ANB cycle is as follows:

1. Close the right nostril with your right thumb. Exhale completely through the left nostril.
2. Inhale slowly and evenly through the left nostril.
3. Close the left nostril with the left thumb and hold the air for a few seconds.
4. Release the right nostril and exhale slowly through it.
5. Inhale through the right nostril.

This completes one cycle. Try to continue for up to 20 cycles. Always finish by exhaling through the left nostril. If you can hold your breath without discomfort, inhale, retain, and exhale in a 1 to 3 to 2 ratio, and then graduate to a 1 to 4 to 2 ratio. For example, you would inhale for a count of 3, hold for 9, and then release for 6. Doubling the exhale creates a slight oxygen deficiency so that the body readily delivers the oxygen to the far reaches of the body. Regular practice will enhance the ability of the defensive to shut out sensation. In some cases, people go into a deep meditative, almost trancelike state.

Body-Breath Synchrony

Here are some exercises where simple hand and arm movements synchronize with your breathing and eye contractions to quickly effect deeper breathing. Doing these breathing exercises will help the sensory defensive entrain to a slower and more concordant internal rhythm, as well as provide an eye massage to help reduce light sensitivity.

Lens Flexor

The exercise will open your breathing, increase circulation, and exercise your eyes.[7] With eyes shut, sit comfortably with both feet flat on the floor. Hold your hands cupped in your lap, one resting on top of the other.

As you inhale, breathe fully through your nose, maintain your hands in the round cupped-hand position; as you exhale, flatten out your hands so your palms become parallel to each other. Also, let your stomach round out as you inhale and contract your abdominal muscles as you exhale. As your hands open and close, can you feel how the movement coordinates with a flexing sensation in your eyes?

Sea Anemone

This similar exercise enables you to experience a deepening expansion of your breath and contraction of the eyes.[8] Sit comfortably in a chair so you can feel your pelvic bones in contact with the chair. Close your eyes so they don't entrain to distracting outside movement. Place your hands on your thighs with the palms facing upward and fingers softly extended. Then relax the hands and let the fingers curl so your palms form a slight hollow. Continue to rhythmically fold and unfold the hands for a few minutes in this way. Notice the relationship between the movement of your hands and eyes when you inhale and exhale and how the movement of your eyes deepens from one flex to the next.

Now let the movement expand into your chest, opening it up as you gently extend the arms and letting it settle as you turn the arms inward. Let your whole body open and close like a sea anemone. Let the movement grow larger and more expansive and then gradually smaller until you are quiet and still. Can you feel the movement pulse inside you like an echo? Do you feel a change in your breathing? Can you feel how the movement of the hands and arms stimulates the movement of the breath, determining its rhythm and speed? This exercise will help you to kickstart fuller breathing. As it can be done subtly, you can do it almost anywhere without drawing attention.

If at First You Don't Succeed

As it's hard to breathe properly when overly anxious, breath control might not come easy for the sensory defensive. Shifting the center of your breathing from your chest to your abdomen will take time and effort. Remember, you haven't used these muscles in a long time. They need to be developed again. But don't despair. You were once an infant in your mother's arms, breathing deeply and peacefully. The memory can be restored, and you can train yourself to breathe normally.

During deep, breathing exercises, you may need to catch your breath. This will subside. You want to breathe in quickly because your brain is telling you that you are suffocating. As the symptoms associated with hyperventilating take a few minutes to subside, the pause after the exhalation again triggers a perception of suffocating. Try to breathe slowly and deeply, but gently. Vigorous or forced breathing may create light-headedness—an indication of a rapid lowering of carbon dioxide levels. If this happens, stop briefly and then start again.

Also, try to bring your breathing under control first by relaxing with other means, such as skin brushing (if you know the Wilbarger protocol), heavy work, vestibular input, light therapy, or listening therapy. Progressive relaxation before you get out of bed in the morning, which I'll describe in Chapter 16, helps slow the breath and sets you up for deep breathing exercises. Or take a daily yoga class, where you will learn to breathe deeply throughout the class. Imagine the transformational power of all that oxygen!

If light-headedness continues, it's likely that the muscles involved in breathing, namely the chest, diaphragm, throat muscles, and jaw, remain tense, which is why the sensory defensive don't like anything tight around their neck. Bodywork presented in Chapter 15, together with the following exercises, will help relax your chest, diaphragm, and throat muscles.

Chest Muscles

1. Square your shoulders and bend your elbows so your forearms are straight out in a 90-degree angle, like a puppy begging for food.
2. Try to touch your shoulder blades together and hold for 3 seconds.
3. Release the tension and relax your chest. Repeat three to five more times until your chest relaxes.

Diaphragm Muscles

1. Suck your stomach in and up under your rib cage.
2. Hold the tension for 5 seconds.
3. Release the tension and relax your stomach.
4. Repeat until your light-headedness subsides.

Throat Muscles

1. Point your chin toward the ceiling, fully stretching the throat muscles.
2. Place your tongue in the roof of your mouth and push with your tongue as hard as you can.
3. Hold the tension for 5 seconds.
4. Release the tension and relax your throat.
5. Repeat three to five times, or until you feel the tension in your throat muscles dissipate.

Suck, Swallow, Breathe

There are other ways to slow down breathing and regulate the level of arousal: sucking, biting, blowing, crunching, chewing, and licking.

Stick out your tongue as far as you can and hold it there for a second.

Now bring it back in your mouth. Did you start to take in a deep breath? Suck and swallow, which depend on the tongue—try swallowing without using your tongue—are our first organizers. Straight out of the womb, some newborns will find their fist and suck. If you put your finger in a newborn's mouth, you feel the strength and coordination of the suck. The infant will use the suck for feeding, to calm and self-regulate, to learn and explore the environment, and to learn to distinguish self from not-self—to know that his thumb is part of his body and not his mother's. If a newborn doesn't breathe well, sucking and swallowing will increase respiratory effort and help him organize. This reliance on oral input as our first line of defense never changes. When nervous, we chomp.

Suck, swallow, breathe (SSB) lays the foundation for attending, focus, and arousal.[9] Did you know, for instance, that sucking helps you perk up when lethargic and calm down when excited. Patricia Oetter, director of the Ayres Clinic, explains that "sucking or mouthing causes the eyes to come together and focus. This sharpens our alertness. When you suck, your eyes pull in; when you blow, your eyes go out." To concentrate, we bite our lip, our fingernail, or a pencil. To sustain attention, children learning to cut with a scissors often move their mouths in rhythm with the cutting. Gum chewing during classtime actually helps children concentrate. And then there's Michael Jordan's famous tonguing during a slamdunk; baseball players' tobacco chewing; and tennis players who cannot go on the court without a stick of gum.

Many functions depend on rhythmical coordination of the SSB. Even opening our mouths to greet someone with a hello means intricately coordinating the muscles of the lips, jaw, tongue, palate, pharynx, larynx, and respiratory system. Digestion is another example. The vagus nerve goes from the inner ear down the larynx, heart, and lungs to the stomach and is critical to swallowing, regulating respiration, and visceral control. If you feel tense, your breathing will throw off your digestion and you get a nervous stomach. The vagus nerve influences the hyoid bone, which supports the larynx and trachea, the jaw pulling open, and the protrusion of the tongue. Stress and the attendant stiffness it creates in your shoulders and neck can throw off muscle coordination of the hyoid, as when food seems to go down the wrong pipe and you get into a coughing fit. It may even contribute to choking or aspirating. Chronic stress leads to stiff neck, throat, and jaw muscles. This in turn makes it hard to take in a deep breath.

We may not always suck, munch, crunch, or chew foods that are good for us, but the jaw action is. It influences breathing and increases alertness when we're feeling low and calmness when we feel wired. Though nutritional needs may vary and should be strictly adhered to (see Chapter 13), here are some general suggestions for heavy work to the jaw.

For sucking, try fresh orange and grapefruit wedges, jello cubes and peanut, almond, cashew, or sunflower butter. Sucking on anything tart, like a lemon, or spicy like cloves, drinking smoothies through a straw, or tart juices like cranberry, lemonade, apple, or grapefruit, adds extra exercise to the mouth muscles.

For munching and crunching, try apples, bread sticks, chips, granola, nuts, pickles, pretzels, popcorn, rice cakes, raw veggies, and toast. For chewing, indulge in chewing gum, cheese, dried fruits, fruit rollups, licorice, and oranges. Dr. Barry Jacobs of Princeton University discovered that repetitive movement, like chewing or licking, boosts the level of the mood regulating neurotransmitter serotonin. He suggests that the repetitive motion involved in much of the ritualistic behavior in obsessive-compulsive disorder may be a form of self-medication via the serotonin system.[10]

To really wake up your mouth, try carbonated beverages, hot tamales, ice chips, sour-fruit gumballs or Popsicles, cloves, lemon, pure cranberry juice, or sour pickles. An electric toothbrush, toothpick, floss, and sparkling water provide direct stimulation of the mouth.

Blowing also increases exhalation and stimulates the mouth. Blowing through or into a straw, a wind instrument (flute, recorder, clarinet, saxophone, etc.), a whistle, a respiratory breathing "whistle,"* or a balloon are all good activities to deepen the breath. Whistling, chanting, humming, and singing all increase exhalation. And be sure to laugh, cry, and giggle— all change respiration, helping bring the nervous system into balance, and organize other systems in the body. Nervous people often giggle a lot as self-therapy.

Directly related to proper breathing is proper posture. If your posture is poor, proper breathing is impossible and you will need to do body work to unlock your breathing. In the next chapter we explore how to get your body straightened out.

*Breathing whistles can be purchased at medical supply stores. Be sure to get one that you exhale, rather than inhale, into.

15

Posturing for Inner Peace

The body does not, I would almost say cannot, lie.
—MARY WHITEHOUSE

Your posture reflects your level of tension, fear, anger, depression: slumped, stooped, ramrod straight, or walking with short, jerky steps, nose to ground.

Imagine walking down a dark street and suddenly hearing footsteps. The whole body begins to flex and crouch, as if readying to fall and curl into the fetal position. This folding is a primitive startle or "red light" reflex wired into our system to help evade a threat. Originating in the lower-level brain stem, a cascade of neural impulses unfolds from head to toes: eyes narrow, jaw and face tense, head juts forward, shoulders lift, elbows flex, abdominal muscles contract, crotch muscles tighten, knees bend and point inward, ankles roll in, toes lift upward.[1]

When sensory defensiveness has been present for years, muscles never get a chance to relax, and the body freezes in this primitive survival stance. Muscles can get so tight and tangled that they pull the bones out of alignment and create back and neck problems. Poor posture prevents you from breathing three-dimensionally (expanding the abdomen, rib cage, and back) and relaxing into your body. When you are under stress, your muscles tighten for another reason. If you make your muscles work hard, the tightness gives you proprioceptive input that cancels out some of the anxiety.

Such rigidity makes it harder to feel the body as a relaxed container that is good to be in. When this distortion has been present for years, you may not even sense it. Bodywork provides a new sense of the body.

Energy in your body flows like water through a hose. If the hose gets twisted, the energy gets blocked wherever your body holds tension. Bodywork provides sensory feedback to make you aware of your body's tightness and to help retrain your muscles and change stiff constricting posture; blockages unleash and energy flows more freely. This enhances circulation and the efficiency of your nervous system and muscles so that energy, biochemicals, blood, and nutrients can get to and better nourish every cell. As your posture aligns correctly and your body's rhythms free up, your whole body works more efficiently. You move with greater grace and lightness. Sex feels more pleasurable, as hips and pelvis free up to allow for spontaneous pleasurable thrusting during intercourse. Your breath automatically expands and you feel a more solid presence in the world.

Bodywork also frees healthy emotional expression that has been restricted by distorted posture. For instance, if facial muscles are tight, your face does not light up with a smile or show clear sadness. Consequently, you actually feel less joy or sadness and you fail to convey accurate signals about your emotional state to others. Trish, the defensive woman who experienced depersonalization, was told that her facial expressions varied little: "I could be perfectly happy, or I could be ready to explode, and still look the same. Learning to smile has been hard. And without the appropriate facial expressions, as well as difficulty making eye contact, people tend to think you are not interested or don't care."

Your life history is etched in your body. If the approach of the mother or father felt threatening, either because of tactile defensiveness, emotional issues, or both, the body learned to respond self-protectively and freezes in a startle position. As physical blocks are loosened, you may feel lifelong tension let up in a specific part of the body—the crushed-in stomach, the hunched shoulders—and a release of pent-up emotions stored at a cellular level. As physician Christiane Northrup explains, "The body often tries to bring our attention back to the 'scene of the crime' to help us heal."

Because you relive memories somatically, rather than just mentally, the experience can feel more powerful than talk therapy. To use Carl Jung's words: "Often the hands will solve a mystery that the intellect has struggled with in vain." A combination of both bodywork and psychotherapy is most effective, however. Some memories can be overwhelming, and it is best to work with a supportive psychotherapist. If you do not experience emotional release during body work, the right conditions may not be present. You may not feel psychologically ready to face the memory or sufficiently comfortable with the therapist.

Hands On

Hands-on bodywork improves functioning of the body's systems by manipulating the soft tissues of the body. Most structural bodywork manipulates deep fascia. Though bodywork is essential for helping the sensory defensive make postural changes that enhance other treatment effects, many cannot tolerate a stranger's touch enough to permit it. But if you can learn to permit the contact, as many gradually do when they find a therapist with the right touch, bodywork can untie the knots, relieve some skin hunger, awaken pleasurable sensation, and teach you that touch can be safe. Before a session, set up your system first with skin brushing and heavy work. Explain to the therapist the need to avoid light strokes and to maintain skin contact.

Craniosacral Therapy

Although you can't feel it, your head expands and contracts every few seconds. If you look in the mirror you won't see this movement but a craniosacral therapist will *feel* it. If you suffer headaches, temporomandibular joint dysfunction (TMJ), ringing in the ears, dyslexia, or aches and pains, the fact that your head expands and contracts at a rate of 8 to 12 times a minute becomes relevant.

Craniosacral therapy, developed by osteopath John Upledger in the late 1970s, is a gentle, noninvasive, manipulative therapy that focuses on the membranes encasing the brain and spinal cord. It helps correct posture, relieve pain, free traumatic memories, and relax you.

The craniosacral system includes the bones of the skull, face, and mouth (the "cranium") and extends to the lower end of the spine (the "sacrum"). It is connected by dura matter, the body's deepest fascia, which houses the brain and central nervous system. Cerebrospinal fluid bathes the brain and spinal cord and gets pumped through the dura in a distinct craniosacral rhythm (CSR) that feeds the distant nerves all over the body. When stress overwhelms our coping capacities, it throws off this rhythm, and the craniosacral system cannot do its job effectively. Such stress can cause migraines, TMJ dysfunction, hyperactivity, chronic pain, depression, and a range of other conditions.

Picking up subtle cues from the pulsing movement of fluids, craniosacral therapists can detect discrepancies in the rate, amplitude, symmetry, and quality of the CSR. They use gentle compression to help realign the skull bones and stretch the underlying dura, thus removing the obstacles inhibiting the free flow of fluids and energies in the body. Your natural, self-adjusting system can then take over to help you heal; you may feel a tingling through to the fingertips from increased circulation.

Freed from restraint, the body may start to undulate in a sinewy dance, unfurling in its own direction and at its own pace. This natural, freeflowing, primitive energy resides within all living things. If you lay a newborn prone and lightly trace your finger along her spine, her body will wave like a sea anemone. This movement is called the incurvation reflex and harkens back to our amphibian roots. Though no longer needed by land dwellers, a swimming reflex remains deeply recorded within our brain and perhaps helps the baby swim through the birth tunnel to the outside world.

During therapy, often the part of the body that stores the trauma will begin to spasm, jerk, or gyrate. Stored-up emotions may be released and some will begin to shake, sweat, laugh, or cry. At the end of the session, many feel relaxed and grounded, with a greater ease of movement and sense of their bodies. For days, the body continues to shift and unwind.

Craniosacral therapy is especially helpful for TMJ, a debilitating condition that involves pain in the muscles of the jaw used for chewing and/or the temporomandibular joint, which connects the lower jaw with the skull. TMJ restricts use of the jaw and creates jaw and joint sounds (clicking, popping, or grating noises) when the jaw is used. This condition is rampant in defensives from constantly clenching their teeth and jaw. It can create a host of problems that extend throughout the body. The temporomandibular joint is the center of the balancing system of the body and acts as the reference point to the entire proprioceptive system. Neural receptivity between the TMJ and the neuroskeletal muscle system affects the pain of other parts of the body, such as the ears, nose, face, head, neck, upper back, and shoulders. More rarely, TMJ can cause disturbances of vision and balance. TMJ is a condition that must be corrected for neurocranial integrity. If your face is stiff, your body is stiff. If your face is relaxed, your body is relaxed.

In addition to a craniosacral therapy session, you can purchase from the Upledger Institute in West Palm Beach, Florida, a "still-point inducer." Made of two soft foam globes, you place the self-help device under your head, in the slight horizontal depression in your skull, about a third of the way up from the top of your neck. The gentle pressure of the inducer creates the "still point," a quiet pause in the rhythm of the craniosacral system. Used for around 15 minutes a day, this device is a good "shotgun" technique for relaxing fascia, enhancing tissue and fluid motion, and slowing breathing and heart rate. To jump-start your nervous system for the day, try using it before getting out of bed in the morning.

Neurocranial Restructuring

While a naturopathic medical student in 1980, Dean Howell observed J. R. Stober, D.C., N.D., peforming Bilateral Nasal Specific Therapy, a treatment dating from the 1930s. Dr. Stober inserted small balloons through the nose into the throat and inflated them briefly to move a patient's nasal and head bones.

Excited by Stober's work and hopeful that it might correct sinus problems and sports injuries that left him unable to breathe through his nose, Howell spent the next year working on himself. Howell's breathing was quickly restored and his right cheekbone, pushed a half-inch lower from a traumatic water-skiing accident, realigned. Chronic back and neck pain ceased.

Over nineteen years, Howell expanded, refined, and redefined BNS, which conceptually resembled auto bodywork—"banging out the bumps in a dented car from the inside"—into neurocranial restructuring. NCR now focuses on precise realignment of the deepest-positioned bone in the head, the sphenoid, to release the connective tissues of the skull to push the bones like a spring, creating permanent, cumulative changes in the skull alignment. As the head becomes symmetrical, tension patterns relax and the body's reflexes push the head straighter on the spine, which gradually optimize the functions of the nervous system, spine, and posture. Patients breathe deeper, feel calmer, and sleep more soundly.

Here are some of the symptoms of a misaligned skull, many of which are suffered by the sensory defensive:

- Chronic sinus problems
- Chronic pressure in the eyebrow area
- Pressure behind the eyes
- A choking, tight feeling at the base of the skull

- Chronic head pressure
- Temporomandibular dysfuncion (TMJ) (aching and/or clicking in the jaw joints)
- Vertigo and balance problems
- Recurrent ear infections
- Catarrhal deafness
- Low energy and fatigue
- Chronic fatigue syndrome
- Fibromyalgia

In his practice, Howell has observed anxiety and nervousness, aggression, OCD, learning disabilities, and hyperactivity to abate. As sensory defensiveness drives these symptoms, SD should decline as well.

Treatments are performed in a series of four daily treatments, generally repeated every six weeks to three months until treatment goals are achieved. Treatment can be started in the newborn period and continued into the late nineties without problems.

Trager

Born in Chicago in 1908, Milton Trager was a professional boxer. One day after massaging his achy trainer, he discovered that his golden hands worked better at healing than at creating pain. He intuitively worked with his hands on anyone in discomfort in the neighborhood. By age 19, he had cured his first polio victim, who walked after being paralyzed for more than four years. Trager studied medicine in Mexico, where he was called upon to work on a 4-year-old girl who had no function from the waist down. After Trager spent 40 minutes playing with her leg, the girl was able to move and twitch her leg, and within 3 weeks she was walking. The university organized a clinic for Trager, and in 1959 he opened a private clinic in Hawaii. In 1975, Trager demonstrated his approach at Esalen and eventually set up a practice in California. In 1980, he founded the Trager Institute.

When we are babies, our parents gently cradle and jiggle our bodies and rhythmically rock, wave, knead, swing, and stretch them. Tragerwork repeats these pleasurable and integrating sensations as clients lie stretched out on a padded table. These gentle movements elongate and soften the tight muscles of the sensory defensive, releasing deep-seated rigid physical and mental patterns that inhibit movement, cause pain, and disrupt normal function. The intent of the therapist is to reeducate the body's movements back to a preinjury or pretension state so the client can experience free, effortless physical movement that the body continues to remember. Throughout the 90-minute session clients report feeling tingling throughout the body and pleasant reverberations that relax and rejuvenate. The therapist also teaches some slow, easy, dancelike movements called Mentastics, which recall and reinforce the movements on the table and can be practiced at home.

Rolfing

Ida Rolf was born in 1896 and trained in biochemistry and physiology. After receiving osteopathic treatment for a displaced rib, she became interested in body manipulation and explored osteopathy, homeopathy, yoga, and other disciplines. Her research led her to develop a method of myofascial manipulation and structural integration that would eventually become known as Rolfing. The basis of Rolfing is the basis of sensory integration: the key to physical and emotional health rests on being in balance with gravity. A balanced body heals itself.

Imagine how it might feel to live in a fluid, light, balanced body, free of pain, stiffness, and chronic stress. Such are the goals of Rolfing. Painter Georgia O'Keeffe attributed nimbleness in her eighties to having been rolfed.

In a balanced body, gravity supports and holds connective tissue in place. But physical and emotional stress on the body causes fascia to shorten, twist, bunch, and harden, the characteristic patterns of strain and tightness. Over time gravity molds connective tissue into an unnatural shape—head too far forward, hypererect body bowed backward, knock knees or bowed legs, flat feet or high arches.

Rolfers realign the body so that it can work with, rather than against, gravity. Over a series of ten sessions, each focusing on a different part of the body with results building on each other, the rolfer applies firm pressure to different areas of the body to slowly stretch and soften the body's connective tissue, allowing the body to right itself effortlessly in gravity. The penetrating and powerful sensations can be painful. But once the head, shoulders, abdomen, pelvis, and legs are correctly aligned, aches and pains caused by muscular tension are alleviated. Afterward, the feeling is one of lightness and freedom of movement and the experience is therapeutic and restorative. Many discover greater self-awareness.

Massage

While not containing as much transformational power as therapies like craniosacral, Trager, and Rolfing, the deep pressure of massage is the most immediately pleasurable of bodywork therapies.

Massage stimulates circulation of the blood and lymph fluids and fuels the muscles with fresh oxygen and nutrients while flushing away metabolic waste products. It releases physical tension and soothes the nerves by lowering the stress hormones cortisol and norepinephrine and by releasing endorphins in the brain. Deep pressure stimulates the vagus cranial nerve, which in turn stimulates the gastrointestinal tract to produce glucose and insulin and aids in food absorption, thus enhancing digestion. It influences the immune system as well. For the sensory defensive especially, rhythmic pressure, stretching, and percussion stimulate sensory receptors, reducing tactile defensiveness, alleviating stress, and modulating arousal: applied slowly, massage sedates; applied vigorously, it activates.

At the Touch Research Institute at the University of Miami, Florida, developmental psychologist Tiffany Field conducts studies on the effects of massage on conditions from prematurity to AIDS and finds remarkable changes. Massaged premature infants often show greater weight gain, as much as 47 percent.[2] The massaged infants also show fewer postnatal complications, and decreased cortisol levels. They are more social, more alert, less fussy and restless; sleep better; and have smoother movements. After one month of 15-minute touch therapy sessions twice a week, autistic children were more willing to be touched, showed less autistic behavior, and were more focused.[3]

There are many different kinds of massage techniques, from the long sweeping strokes of Swedish massage (in the direction of the heart) to the firm finger pressure of Japanese shiatsu, designed to increase the circulation of vital energy. But studies have shown that all are remarkably effective in dispelling muscle tension and revitalizing the body.

Therapeutic Touch

If you can't tolerate getting a massage, consider relaxation, self-healing, and pain reduction through touch therapy (TT), a noncontact therapeutic touch in which a therapist's hands hover 2 to 4 inches from the skin in what some believe to be a bioenergetic field surrounding it. An ancient practice, touch therapy was popularized in the late 1960s by Dolores Krieger, professor of nursing at New York University, who learned the technique of laying on of hands from a healer, Dora Kunz.

During treatment, the practitioner centers herself to become clear, channeling her energy field with yours so that disturbances in your energy flow are balanced and your body's healing powers can work freely. When ready, she places her hands above your body and, holding one palm toward your back, the other at the front, gently moves her hands down your body from head to toe, assessing changes or blockages in your energy field. She may feel sensations of heat or cold, thickness or emptiness, heaviness, pulling, tingling, buzzing, or lack of movement. Using sweeping movements, she will try to clear imbalances by visualizing healing energy directed from her body to yours.

During the session, some feel a surge of energy in parts of their body and even feel connected to the therapist. Following a 10- to 15-minute session, many feel centered, peaceful, and calm. Is this sense of well-being in the client's mind, or does it have a scientific basis? Studies carried out in the 1960s by Krieger showed that levels of hemoglobin (the oxygen-carrying component of blood) increased in some patients receiving TT. Later studies in the 1980s showed that TT was more effective than simple touching in allaying anxiety and relieving tension headaches, and a 1997 study revealed that TT could reduce the effects of stress on the immune system.

Even if you're a skeptic, you can get a sense of your energy field. Sit comfortably with your eyes closed. Keep your elbows and forearms away from your body and hold your palms facing each other. Bring your palms close together but not touching and then back out again about 2 inches. Slowly move them back toward each other, and then separate them about 4 inches. Repeat the process, increasing the separation to 6 inches, then 8 inches. The last time, as you return to the original close-in position, stop every 2 inches and test the energy field between your hands. You may sense bounciness, resistance, elasticity, heat or cold, tingling, or pulsing.

To try touch healing on yourself, visualize the energy coming down from above and flowing through your body. Hold the palms of your hand a few inches from your body and sweep them slowly from head to toe or on specific areas that need healing. You might be amazed at the pull of your energy field and how it gets stuck in various places on your body where you feel imbalance, and how breathing coordinates with the slow rhythmic movement of your hands. Our bodies are rhythmic energy fields.

Touch therapy is powerful. In considering it, the sensory defensive must find a compassionate person with whom they feel comfortable. Though the therapist is generally not actually touching the person, personal space is invaded and can induce anxiety.

MOVEMENT THERAPY

For those sensory defensives who cannot adjust to another's touch or close physical presence, other kinds of body work provide sensory feedback, not from hands-on manipulation but through teaching movement awareness without contact or closeness. At the same time, movement therapy works best when combined with a structural approach like craniosacral therapy or Rolfing, as it both reinforces and maintains the changes gained through the hands-on work.

The Feldenkrais method and the Alexander technique teach "proprioceptive literacy," or the ability to read your body's sensations from within so you can move and live with greater ease and joy. You become intimately aware of physical states like feeling cold, tight, numb, heavy, or moist. With greater ability to detect the messages coming from your body, you can more easily recognize when your system is going into overload and stop to recharge.

Relaxation means moving at ease. "Relaxation does not mean going limp or collapsing. . . . [It] means moving efficiently. It means resting while you are moving," says therapist Anna Halprin. The ancient mind-body systems of yoga and qigong are movement meditations that coordinate with breathing and do much toward enhancing body awareness, nervous system organization, fluid movement, and relaxation.

Body and mind are one. Childhood experiences inhabit flesh and bone, and any bodywork, from the touch of the craniosacral therapist to holding a yoga posture, can unlock repressed emotions and memories. The focus on bodywork, however, is on body structure and function. And as bodywork therapists and yoga teachers are generally not trained in psychotherapy, they may not know how to handle emotional catharsis as it arises. But a form of body-oriented psychotherapy works through the body to access the mind. Bioenergetics is one of the most established approaches.

Feldenkrais

Moshe Feldenkrais, an Israeli nuclear physicist, judo black belt, and soccer player, began to study human movement when recovering from a serious knee injury that refused to heal. Observing the natural grace of children, along with anatomy, physiology, neurology, and psychology, he developed a method of encouraging ease of movement with "minimum effort and maximum efficiency." He was able to restore function in his knee and walk again without pain.

In the Feldenkrais method, you repeat a movement sequence correctly many times. This develops "awareness through movement," replacing old patterns of movement with new ones and leading to greater body awareness, increased mobility, and improved breathing and circulation. If you can tolerate contact, treatment also includes a gentle hands-on approach tailored to your individual needs.

Somatics

A student of Moshe Feldenkrais and the first to direct a Feldenkrais training program in the United States in 1975, Thomas Hanna (1928–1990) started out as a philosophy professor before turning to somatic education.

Basing his ideas on those of Hans Selye and Feldenkrais, Hanna noted that the body responds to the unending stresses and traumas of modern life with two specific muscular reflexes: the red light reflex described at the beginning of the chapter and the green light reflex. In the red light reflex, the body responds to a threat (you stub your toe) by withdrawing. In the green light reflex, the body prepares for action (the doorbell rings) by moving forward: eyes and jaw open, neck pulls back and shoulders down, elbows extend, hands open, chest lifts, and so on. When everyday life repeatedly triggers these reactions, habitual muscular contractions become deeply unconscious and you cannot voluntarily move freely: you suffer *sensory-motor amnesia*.

Hanna Somatic Education reprograms the nervous system through slowly executed specific movement sequences combined with conscious sensing of how your body reacts to each movement.

The Alexander Technique

In the late nineteenth century, Frederick Matthias Alexander, an Australian Shakespearean actor, repeatedly lost his voice during performances. The doctors couldn't cure him, but by speaking in front of a mirror, he became aware of how he pulled his head back and down, arched his back, and tensed his arms. He found that when he moved with an easy neck and lightly poised head, his torso expanded and cured him of throat and vocal troubles as well as respiratory and nasal difficulties he had suffered since birth. He eventually went on to develop the technique that bears his name.

How many times daily do we sit, bend, stand, reach, and walk without thinking about it? And yet Alexander discovered that unconscious habits of movement cause many of the posture limitations so many of us face. The Alexander technique educates followers to become aware of how they are misusing their body in everyday life. By repeatedly experiencing correct movement, clients learn to realign their bodies so that their heads are aligned on the tip of their spines, optimally lengthening the spine and resulting in more fluid movement in general.

Yoga

When it comes to learning to control the body and its experiences, few exercises can beat the over-3,000-year-old practice of yoga, which means "union of body and soul." It involves exercise (hatha yoga), breathing (pranayama), and meditation, all directed at controlling consciousness and focusing attention. To further this end, yoga classes generally take place in a dim, warm room with soft music playing and minimum distraction—the sensory defensive's dream workout. Practicing yoga postures, breathing, and meditation exercises regularly will help you feel more connected to the basic workings of your body.

Yoga postures, called asanas, comprise movement sequences executed standing, sitting, or upside down and coordinate with deep breathing. Performed slowly and meditatively, each asana is held at length without strain or fatigue to prepare the body for the endurance required for meditation. Generally, the routine is structured and each pose counterbalances the preceding one, stretching and strengthening. Some exercises are easy, and you barely sweat; others are designed to build strength and endurance, and you drip from start to finish.

At once calming and energizing, the postures properly practiced lubricate joints, release muscle tension, stretch and tone muscles, facilitate good posture, improve circulation and digestion, and massage internal organs. Pranayama, or breath control, slows the breath, expands lung capacity, and relaxes the body.

Standing postures enhance concentration and create emotional stability. In the mountain pose, you stand straight, feet together and weight evenly distributed, head slightly tilted forward and hands in prayer position. If you place one hand on your lower abdomen and the back side of the other hand on the base of your spine, you will feel your sacrum tilt under, your pelvic bone lift up and slightly forward, and your knees bend slightly, lengthening your spine as your whole body unfolds in perfect posture. You will automatically take in a full, three-dimensional breath and feel your whole torso expand. This is a good stance to assume under stress. Forward-bending postures with the head down lengthen the spine, stretch the back muscles, increase the supply of oxygen to the brain, and stimulate the vestibular system, which has a calming effect. Inverted postures (shoulder stands and headstands) relax the heart by allowing blood to flow to the upper body, improving circulation, stimulating the brain, and enhancing energy. Back bends elevate mood but create anxiety in those with vestibular issues. As waking up the vestibular system is one of the main ingredients in a sensory diet, you should continue the posture slowly. Over time, the anxiety should dissipate.

Also oiling the vestibular system is the continual head change—upright, forward, backward, rotated—as you move through the postures. Postures in which you balance on one leg, such as the "dancer's pose" or the "eagle," provide much joint compression. Such vestibular and proprioceptive nourishment relaxes you and makes you feel more grounded, profoundly altering energy level, concentration, defensive behavior, and anxiety.

This is not just hearsay from yogis in loincloths and twisted into pretzels. Studies document that yoga increases body awareness, which, as sensory integration theory would predict, enhances mental abilities.[4] Following ten months of regular yoga practice, college students in a 1995 study shifted toward field independence, meaning they had greater spatial awareness and ability to maneuver in space.[5] With their generally shaky vestibular systems, sensory defensives typically have poor spatial awareness. Another 1995 study reported that after 10 days of yoga training, a group of college students had improved visual discrimination—they were better able to focus and process visual information.[6]

Comparing mood following a yoga class and a swimming class, a 1992 study at Brooklyn College found both to decrease anger, confusion, tension, and depression.[7] Men reported far greater reduction in tension, anger, and fatigue after yoga than after swimming, while women showed a similar reduction in negative mood following both types of exercise. Yoga met seven of the eight stress-reducing criteria, excepting only aerobic exercise. Swimming, on the other hand, met all eight of the requirements. The authors concluded that the abdominal breathing, not the aerobic component, was beneficial.

There are a wide variety of yoga styles to choose from. Although the basic asanas and breathing exercises remain the same, the order in which you do them and the central focus varies. Here are some popular styles.

- *Iyengar yoga* uses props such as straps, blocks, blankets, and sandbags and focuses in great detail on only a few asanas so you can refine the movements. The props allow anyone, including the elderly, to get into a pose.
- *Ashtanga yoga*, or "power yoga," is a vigorous workout that consists of a fast-paced series of vinyasas (flowing asanas linked by the breath) to purify and strengthen the body.
- *Kundalini yoga* uses asanas, pranayama, and meditation to arouse

the kundalini energy, a powerful energy believed to lie at the base of the spine.

- *Bikram yoga* focuses on repeating twenty-six specific postures, repeated twice and held up to 1 minute, to stretch and tone the whole body, and two breathing techniques. The room is over-heated, so muscles warm up quickly and stretch more easily, enabling you to prevent injuries and get into postures more eas-ily. Working up a good sweat also eliminates waste products through your skin.

Qi Gong

Translated as "working with life energy," the Chinese movement called qigong (chee gung) is the art and science of using breath, slow movement, visualization, and meditation to cleanse and open energy—chi—channels for healing. In Chinese parks you can witness millions of people practicing some form of qigong. Daily practice lowers blood pressure, pulse rate, metabolic rate, and oxygen need. The basic postures are easy to learn and suitable for anyone, including the aged and infirm. Many can be per-formed anywhere, even in a wheelchair or a bed.

Bioenergetics

Developed in the 1960s by American psychotherapist Alexander Lowen, bioenergetics is a body-oriented form of psychotherapy that seeks to release the stress or trauma programmed into the muscles and linked with buried memories.

Lowen was a student and patient of Wilhelm Reich, an Austrian-born protégé of Sigmund Freud who believed that the body, mind, and emo-tions are closely intertwined. Believing we *are* our bodies, Reich used his hands to try and break down tense muscle tissue—"body armor"—and free restricted emotions. Lowen's first therapeutic session with Reich was a moment of truth.

> I lay on a bed wearing just a pair of shorts so that he could observe my breathing. Reich's only instruction was to breathe. It seemed to me that I was, but after ten minutes Reich said, 'Lowen, you're not breathing. . . . Your chest isn't moving.' Then he asked me to put my hand on his chest to feel how it moved in and out with his inspiration. I saw that my chest wasn't moving as much as his and decided to mobilize mine so that it would move with my breathing. I did that for a number of minutes, breathing through my mouth. Then Reich asked me to open my eyes wide. As I did, a scream broke from me. . . . When I left his office, I realized that I had some deep problem of which I was completely unaware. I also realized that deep and free breathing had the power to reach and release suppressed feelings.[8]

Adapted from many of Reich's ideas, Lowen's bioenergetics employs physical exercises, breathing techniques, psychotherapy, and other forms of emotional-release work to help liberate sufferers from their "character armor" and restore a sense of well-being. Exercises focus on tense areas, such as a "frozen" chest, a "locked" pelvis, and tension in the jaw and, similar to occupational therapy, on "grounding" you. For instance, as you inhale, you might be asked to put a little pressure on your feet to feel the support of the floor.

Activities might include wringing a towel, venting emotion by hitting a bed with a bat, or stretching backward over a stool to open up breathing constrictions and release a "primal" scream. Vigorous outpouring of emotions and reliving of long-forgotten memories is not uncommon.

Some caution is advised. If the client is not ready for such cathartic release or the psychotherapist is not sufficiently empathic, the experience can be overwhelming. Some newer body-based therapies have a softer touch and less provocation.

Bodywork helps correct postural restrictions, relaxes us, and can help free traumatic memories. Let's now further explore the body-mind, mind-body connection and healing.

16

Mind/Body—Only Connect!

> When the mind thinks, the body listens.
>
> —JOHN MADDEN

Each of our lives is a story played out in acts—infancy, childhood, adolescence, adulthood—in which we play different roles in relation to a few main characters that occasionally change. At times dramatic or comedic, surreal or absurd, the narrative we spin is governed by our "mind." What eludes awareness is what takes place behind the scenes—the story played out in the sinews of our bodies, under the direction of the primitive brain. Yet the mind can greatly influence that story as well.

The mind and body are in intimate and continual dialogue. The abstract entity we call the mind influences the brain, the tangible part of the mind, to produce physiological and chemical reactions in the body. An example is the placebo effect, when people experience changes because they *believe* changes will occur. The brain releases pleasure-producing endorphins and the body heals itself. Like the placebo effect, practices such as deep relaxation, meditation, visualization, hypnosis, and, for some, prayer also fool the body into producing endorphins, while cognitive-behavioral therapy teaches a person how to change negative thought processes.

Unfortunately, sensory defensiveness, by its nature, defies mind control. How do you talk yourself out of an automatic response when the body just *reacts*? True, you can give yourself a pep talk ahead of time for a situation that will stress your senses. *But sensations are everywhere and all the time.* There's no predicting when you'll get walloped. Mind control presents another problem. Mind-altering techniques such as meditation and hypnosis require the person to block out external sensation, specifically what the defensive cannot do.

But there is hope. As the sensory diet outlined in previous chapters helps to rewrite the tale told in limb and gut, the mind *can* start to take center stage and mind-body techniques become a powerful tool for modulation.

Fair warning: The power of mind over body can also backfire. As you get defensiveness more under control, your mind may remain protectively in a defensive mind-set of "I can't," "I shouldn't," "I'll fail" and impede progress. Changing this mind-set is the other half of your battle.

DEEP RELAXATION

Mind-body practices have the potential to create a state of deep relaxation. This distinct physiological state is different from what you feel unwinding at the end of the day in front of the TV or soaking in a hot bath. It is an altered state of consciousness, similar to how you feel after sex: in a state of deep relaxation, heart rate lowers, your breathing rate and blood pressure drop, and you experience slower alpha brain waves. You are in a different place.

To prepare for deep relaxation, retreat to your rejuvenation room where noise, lights, bothersome odors, and other distractions are minimal. To jump-start your day, practice deep relaxation as you wake and before going to bed. Ideally you want to practice at least 20 to 30 minutes per day, and preferably twice a day. If you continue your routine for at least 21 days, it will become a habit.

If you are sensory defensive, it's unlikely your body will easily relax. Don't force it. As your sensory diet helps to retrain your senses not to falsely signal alarm, and as you correct breathing, posture, and nutritional deficiencies, your body should slowly ease out of its tense, hyperalert state. It takes patience and perseverance, but it can happen. Try deep pressure and heavy work first to set up your system. Once you learn deep relaxation, you return to the world with a different consciousness and sense of self. It becomes addictive and the day will seem incomplete without it.

Tense to Calm: Progressive Relaxation

It is physically impossible for the body to be relaxed and tense at the same time. One quick way to loosen up those taut, knotted muscles, especially in your shoulders and neck, is progressive relaxation, a short exercise in which you tense and then release or relax each muscle group. Though the exercise offers little deep joint compression, this quick and intense workout provides enough calming proprioceptive input to make you feel immediately less uptight. Like the pendulum's swing, the more you pull your muscles into one direction, the farther they will swing to the other. So, during the exercise, it's okay to really tense up. With practice, body awareness of the sensation of tension and the sensation of relaxation will increase.

To do progressive relaxation, start by closing your eyes and lying still with your head resting on a small pillow for comfort. Take in a few deep abdominal breaths. Tense and relax each muscle group: feet (clench and pull your toes in as if grasping something with your foot); calves (squeeze); thighs (tighten down to knees); buttocks (pull them together); abdomen (pull toward your spine); back (arch up); hands (clench); biceps (draw forearms up toward your shoulders and make a muscle with both arms); triceps (extend arms out straight and lock your muscles); shoulders (shrug up to your ears); shoulder blades (tighten as if trying to touch them together);

neck (pull your head way back); head (push into the surface); jaw (clench tightly); tongue (push against roof of mouth); mouth (open wide); eyes (squint); forehead (furrow).

Hold the tension for 5 to 10 seconds and then release abruptly, feeling the muscle group go limp. Relax for 10 seconds or so and breathe deeply. Concentrate on the heaviness of the muscle groups. You might need to repeat some especially tight muscle groups, like the shoulders or neck. If your muscles are very tense, tensing your muscles may create spasms. If so, try tensing only those muscle groups that do not spasm or avoid the protocol until bodily tension subsides.

You can work feet to face or you can vary the order. For instance, you might start with hands and arms, work down to your feet and then up to your face. You can tense and release each muscle group individually or a whole muscle group at once, like making an ugly face, thereby engaging jaw, mouth, nose, eyes, and forehead at the same time. If you suffer from TMJ, try this exercise. Extend your lower jaw as far forward as possible and hold for five seconds. Release and relax. Repeat three to five times.

When you finish, lie still and comfortable for a few minutes and focus on your breath, which should be more regular and smooth. This is an ideal time for Ujjayi breathing (see Chapter 14). Free your mind of thoughts. Feel your body heavy, sinking into the ground. Imagine a white, warm light traveling up your body, from your toes to the top of your head, enveloping you. Try to stay in this state of calm for at least 5 minutes. As your heart rate and blood pressure have probably dropped, sit up slowly.

Those in a chronic state of stress will still feel some tension following progressive relaxation, as your body returns to your overaroused baseline state. This is to be expected. As you repeat the protocol, and especially if it becomes a daily ritual and you learn to breathe fully, you will lower your baseline arousal level and feel greater and longer-lasting relief from immediate tension. Over time, you should experience a more relaxed state and feel less bothered by tension headaches, backaches, tightness in the jaw, muscle spasms, and insomnia. As your body relaxes, so will your mind; your thoughts will race less and your concentration should improve.

As you feel tension build during the day, slow down your breathing for a few minutes and focus on each muscle group in turn, remembering how it feels when it is relaxed. To bring about an alpha state, concentrate on the sensation of heaviness, warmth, or a floating feeling. Or, starting at your toes, scan your body and tell each body part, "Relax."

That Still Place: Meditation

A deeper level of relaxation comes from meditation. Meditation is a means of concentrating our attention away from thoughts, which are primarily on the left side of our brain, and onto images and sensations, primarily on the right side of our brain. The ancient Egyptians gazed upon an oil-burning lamp. The yogis stare at a mandala, a pattern on a vase. The Islamic mystics of Turkey—whirling dervishes—concentrate on their body movements and the rhythms of their breathing. These methods bring you to a place of deep peace and quiet, where you can "just be," free of thoughts and worries—a place where you are resting deeply, as in sleep, but still be wide awake. Some report feeling oneness, rapture, great insight, nirvana, a state the yogis define as transcending pain, suffering, and individual consciousness.

Scientists can't measure "oneness." But they can measure stress-shielding body changes. Herbert Benson of Harvard Medical School found meditation to produce a "relaxation response": lowered heart rate, blood pressure, and breathing rate; less need for oxygen consumption; lower concentration of lactic acid in the blood; and increased circulation and alpha brain wave activity, the brain waves associated with relaxation.[1] Those who meditate consistently generally feel more relaxed, alert, patient, energetic, and productive, more open to experiences, and a greater sense of identity and self-worth. They are less prey to illness, as meditation enhances immune function.

Unfortunately, the very nature of meditation eludes the sensory defensive. To get inside your mind requires shutting out external stimulation. This is precisely what sensory defensives cannot do. As it takes effort to slip into the natural state of sleep, it takes far greater effort to slip into an altered state of consciousness.

This inability to shut out sensation doesn't make meditation unachievable. While those with normal nervous systems may close their eyes and almost instantly enter into stillness, the sensory defensive will have to work harder to do so. You may require a half-hour or more before achieving a meditative state and, as outside sensations impinge on your consciousness, find it harder to stay down under.

To help minimize outside distraction, find the quietest spot you can. Surround yourself with anything that contributes to peace and tranquility—calming colors (blues, greens, lavender), a tranquil panorama, aromatherapy, and soft music or meditation tapes.

Close your eyes and sit comfortably in a straight-backed chair, feet on the floor, legs uncrossed, and hands on your thighs. Or sit yogi style, cross-legged on the floor, back straight, leaning slightly forward, with a pillow supporting your buttocks. Meditation seats work well. Try not to lie down, which invites sleep.

Many different paths lead to inner stillness. Following the path of transcendental meditation (TM), introduced to the West from India in the 1950s by the Maharishi Mahesh Yogi, select a mantra (a word or sound such as *om* or *ieng*) and utter it silently or out loud as you exhale. Or you may select your own mantra, preferably a single-syllable word. Repeat the sound mentally, concentrating completely on the mantra and letting distractions just pass through your mind. Repetition, as you recall, appears to boost the mood-altering neurotransmitter serotonin in the brain.

If you get too easily distracted to concentrate on a mantra, there are other ways to a meditative state. One is visualizing a scene. To appreciate the power of imagination, close your eyes and visualize biting into a lemon. The easily overaroused will immediately begin to salivate. To develop imaging skills, try to focus on details. The more detail you visualize, the more the image will absorb your attention and free you from anxious thoughts, thereby deepening relaxation.

An alternative to repeating a word or visualization is to concentrate on the inflow and outflow of your breath, counting as you inhale and exhale. Or try chanting and rocking side to side, or staring at a physical object like a candle. Any sensation that shoos thoughts away and focuses you will get you there.

Start by meditating for 5 minutes daily and build up to 20 minutes or more twice a day. If you have a family to care for, try to get up earlier than others to have that quiet time to meditate.

To get inside your head may take persistent and disciplined effort over a period of several months, especially for beginners. With enough persistence, it will eventually come—even for those initially too tense to let go of the world. As you enter into an altered state of consciousness, you lose awareness of your breathing and your body, and feel as though you're floating in serenity. There's some resistance in returning to the mundane world. When you do, you feel more at peace.

Soul Food

There is another ancient form of meditation to counteract stressful thoughts, lower heart rate and breathing, slow brain waves, and relax muscles: prayer. Through spirituality and prayer, more and more people are finding hope, a way to cope, a sense of peace, and greater well-being.

Blessed are those who believe in something larger than self to give life meaning and lower blood pressure. For some it is God, for others nature, for others the creation of something that we throw our whole being into—a poem, a song, a dance, a painting. Whatever gets you to transcend self and merge with a larger entity, pursue it with a vengeance. As mythologist Joseph Campbell said, "Follow your bliss." Doing so offers distraction from an overwhelming world, reduces tension and discomfort, and is an important way for the sensory defensive to feel less alienated.

Hypnotherapy

Another means of achieving an altered state is hypnotherapy. For centuries, different cultures have experimented with inducing trancelike states by hypnosis to promote healing. The ancient Egyptians and Greeks are said to have used healing trances, and tribal cultures in Africa and the Americas have long used dancing and drumming to hypnotic effect.

The founder of modern hypnosis was Franz Anton Mesmer, who treated patients in the eighteenth century with hypnosis, or "mesmerism." Practitioners induce a state of consciousness akin to deep daydreaming, in which the patient is deeply relaxed and open to suggestion and can be desensitized to fears, phobias, or pain. Sigmund Freud used hypnosis in his early work, but later preferred to use free association, with the patient fully conscious.

Practitioners believe that the mind has different levels of consciousness. Under hypnosis, the conscious, rational part of the brain is temporarily bypassed, making the subconscious part, which influences mental and physical functions, extremely receptive to suggestion. This makes it a powerful therapy for the sensory defensive. Like light therapy and some bodywork like craniosacral and Rolfing, hypnotherapy too can unleash traumatic memory. Like meditation, though, hypnosis requires easily tuning out the world, and not all defensive may succumb.

There are different approaches to hypnotherapy. The sensory defensive should look for someone trained in analytical hypnotherapy. A practitioner trained in this approach will "regress" you by asking you to recall any buried memories or emotions that might be at the root of your problem. By focusing attention on the sensory details, cues, emotions, and circumstances of special life events, the person under light or medium hypnosis can discuss and therapeutically reframe the memory.[2]

Less Is More: Quiet Therapy

What if you can't block out sensation enough to be hypnotized or to meditate? Try lying in a sensory deprivation chamber.

Imagine lying solitary for 24 hours in a soundproof tomb. Do you see yourself coming out screaming? In fact, most people who are prepared for this experience want to stay longer. Without external distractions, people feel less stressed and are better able to tune into inner space, similar to meditation.[3]

At the University of British Columbia, Peter Suedfeld uses restricted environmental stimulation therapy (REST) to help dieters and smokers modify their behavior. In one experiment, smokers listened to antismoking messages while spending 24 hours lying on beds in quiet, dark rooms (rising only to drink a liquid diet available through tubes or to use toilets next to the beds).[4] In the week that followed, none relapsed to smoking. A year later, two-thirds were still abstaining. Similar positive results have been shown with REST and hard-drinking college students.

"Quiet therapy," as they call it in Japan, achieves the same goal as meditation but rather than having to work to shut out sensation, the job is done for you—the sensory defensive's panacea. In morita, a therapy for depression or anxiety, the Japanese sometimes begin with a week of bedrest and meditation, progressing gradually to light tasks.

BANISH THE THOUGHT!

It took you a long time to learn coping styles and habits that protected you from sensory overstimulation or at times to seek out stimulation. Once the primary symptoms of sensory defensiveness have abated, you may remain stuck in old patterns of behaving and interacting that continue to generate stress and anxiety. Psychotherapy can help.

Psychotherapy can help you connect to an empathic listener, feel less alone, gain self-confidence, and deal with the emotional and day-to-day issues that emerge, while cognitive-behavioral therapy can help you work on your belief system. Psychotropic medication helps take off the edge for many. Look for a therapist specializing in post-traumatic stress disorder. Symptom relief is half the battle; the other half is cognition—the belief that life *can* be different. Go and be purposeful and happy.

Appendix A

Sensory Defensiveness
Survival Kit

Set up your day by starting it with a nutritious sensory meal. Ideally, you would like to do some form of deep relaxation, like progressive relaxation, visualization or meditation, and deep breathing. Deep pressure touch (your choice, but the Wilbarger protocol will give you the most bang for your buck) is a must for the tactile defensive, as well as heavy work (even if only 5 minutes of play wrestling). Do exercise daily for modulation and to slough off excess adrenaline. You should work up a sweat. Try to get in a few minutes of swinging, rocking, or jumping on a trampoline as often as possible. Do all activity to healing music and aromatherapy. If your activity isn't doing the trick and you still can't relax, try adding more proprioception.

Be aware of your breathing and posture, which reciprocally influence each other. Without proper breathing or body alignment, you cannot work your way out of chronic tension, and tactile, vestibular, and proprioceptive input offer only temporary solutions.

End your day with some form of tactile stimulation, healing music, and aromatherapy.

Here are some general suggestions for a well-rounded sensory diet:

- Treat yourself to scuba or deep-sea diving, horseback riding, a backyard trampoline.
- Do deep breathing exercises daily.
- Chomp, chew, and suck on foods that fit into your dietary needs.
- Come prepared with fidget objects for overstimulating environments.
- Stare at the sunset, a fish tank, a lava light.
- Use full-spectrum lighting, an Ott light at your computer terminal, and colored bulbs.
- Explore light filters, color-therapy eyewear, and, if affordable, light therapy devices, or find a practitioner of syntonic light therapy.
- Infuse (with cool air, not heat), douse, bathe in essential oils.
- Listen to relaxing music, wind chimes, a waterfall fountain.
- Find a practitioner who knows auditory listening, either Tomatis, Berard, or SAMONAS.
- In public, try earplugs under headphones that cover the whole ear and listen to calming music. The earplugs will block out some sounds and the music will mask other uncontrollable sounds.
- Make your car a sensory haven: infuse essential oils; play a relaxing CD (see Vital Sounds on p. 355) and sing, hum, chant, or sing loudly to fast music; use an electric back massager on your car seat and hand massagers for deep pressure; take a deep breath at a red light; blow a kazoo; chomp, chew, suck (fat-free, low-calorie food!); if it doesn't interfere with visual alertness, wear color-therapy eyewear.
- Try hypnotherapy, visualization, meditation, progressive relaxation.
- Try a massage once or twice a week and consider investing in a high-powered massager.
- Get bodywork as often as possible: craniosacral therapy, dental manipulation, myofascial release, Trager, Feldenkrais, Rolfing, somatics.

- Make yoga, tai chi, or martial arts a part of your life.
- Reduce indoor toxins.
- Substitute herbal tea for caffeinated beverages.
- Stop smoking, drinking alcohol, or using recreational drugs.
- Find out if you suffer from an excess of *Candida albicans* fungus and explore diets that eliminate this problem.
- Eat natural food, preferably organic, fresh vegetables and fresh fruits, protein in the form of beans and grains, organic poultry or fish.
- Take daily vitamin B complex, vitamin C, calcium, magnesium, and chromium.
- Get plenty of fresh air and sunshine.
- Simplify your lifestyle.
- Structure your day to help stay on track.
- Give yourself permission to take on less responsibility.
- Get as much sleep as you need to feel alert and productive.
- Try to avoid feeling rushed and pressured.
- Plan vacations very carefully to control your surroundings and minimize unexpected events.

Appendix B

Defensive Reactions
to Sensation

Touch / Tactile

- Reacts excessively to light, unseen, or sudden touch, especially of strangers, exhibiting anxiety, hostility, or aggression and spontaneously flinching, withdrawing, or lashing out
- Tenses at friendly or affectionate pats and caresses even from loved ones, but at times accepts same
- Dislikes hugs or craves deep pressure of hug but irritated by light touch of a kiss
- Scratching or rubbing the spot that has been touched
- Irritated and anxious standing in line, taking an elevator, people standing too close, or weaving through a crowd
- As infant, not calmed by cuddling or stroking
- Prefers to touch rather than be touched
- Fussy about clothing, such as stiff new clothes, rough or synthetic textures, shirt collars, tags, turtlenecks, belts, elasticized

waists or cuffs, hats, scarves, and pantyhose, or clothing tight in certain places

- Frequently adjusts clothes, as if uncomfortable
- Irritated by clothes that touch certain places, such as skirts that brush the legs, and to movement of clothes against skin during clothing changes
- Overdresses to minimize skin exposure, regardless of weather
- Wears minimal clothes, regardless of weather
- Avoids touching certain textures or surfaces, like some fabrics, blankets, rugs
- Bothered by footwear, particularly sock seams, and may prefer to go without socks or pantyhose and wear shoes loosely tied or untied
- Avoids walking barefoot, especially in sand or grass
- Bothered by touching certain textures or material with hands such as sand, clay, fingerpaint, paste, or food, or getting hands dirty
- Chooses bedding and sleepwear to create pressure against the skin and minimize light touch and displacement by body movements
- Dislikes touch of certain animals—dogs, horses, cats
- Certain parts of the body especially sensitive to touch
- Excessively ticklish
- Irritated by hair displacement, as when brushing hair, receiving a haircut, shampoo, or pat on the head
- Dislikes nail trims
- Bothered by creams or lotions, make-up, lipstick, chapstick
- Avoids jewelry, even wedding band
- Dislikes baths or showers, and especially being splashed
- Seeks tight spaces, especially during sleep

ORAL/TACTILE

- Picky about food, preferring or avoiding certain textures, like mushy, crunchy, or chewy, or taste, such as sharp, bitter, or spicy
- Dislikes objects in mouth, like a toothbrush, dentist's fingers, or drill
- Dislikes taste of toothpaste
- Mouths objects, like pens

TEMPERATURE/TACTILE

- Easily cold
- Easily hot
- Fussy about food temperature
- Fussy about bath or shower temperature
- Irritated by quick change in temperature (hot shower to cold air)

PAIN/TACTILE

- Overreacts to pain
- Underreacts to pain
- Excessive reaction to inoculations

VIBRATION/TACTILE AND AUDITORY

- Dislikes touching vibrating objects
- Annoyed by vibration in vehicles
- Annoyed by vibration in buildings from heating or cooling, elevators, or trucks going by
- Unnerved by loud bass of music, especially in cars

Sounds

- Dislikes loud, high-pitched, high-frequency sound
- Vigilant to and easily distracted by ambient noise
- Overreacts to unexpected or loud noises (sirens, fire alarms, landscaping or construction equipment)
- Picks up sounds before anyone else, or sounds others can't hear
- Excessively irritated by and unable to tune out sounds in the environment, like air conditioners, vacuum cleaners, noisy appliances, toilet flush, running water, alarms, or lots of different kinds of sounds at once
- Unable to tune out ticking clock, dripping water, etc.
- Irritated by volume and pitch of certain voices
- Difficulty listening against background noise, such as whispering, eating, sneezing, or coughing, in a movie theater or at a concert or large gathering

Visual Sensation

- Irritated by bright light—sunlight, fluorescent lights, car lights
- Annoyed by objects close to face, like a car sun visor
- Easily distracted by visual stimulation
- Annoyed by moving visual field
- Overexcited by busy or complex visual field
- Overstimulated by eye contact
- Fears visual cliffs (i.e., stairs, balconies, inclined theaters)
- Hypervigilant of environment

Vestibular/Movement and Balance

- Feels threatened when tipping head backward, tilted, or upside down as when having hair shampooed over the sink
- Feels uncomfortable surge in stomach, and even panic, on

swing, jumping off diving board, roller coaster, or carnival rides that spin
- Fearful or hesitant when climbing or descending stairs and holds tightly to banister or walls
- Uncomfortable in elevators, especially when open, and on escalators
- Experiences motion sickness in car or airplanes
- Fears heights, even slightly raised surfaces, such as stairs or curbs
- Fearful of visual cliffs (i.e., stairs, balconies, inclined theatres)
- Fearful of activities moving through space
- Avoids activities that challenge balance or center of gravity
- Uncomfortable maintaining balance on uneven terrain, like grass
- Fear of falling when no real danger exists—primal terror
- Fears flying

SMELLS

- Dislikes sharp odors that don't seem to bother other people
- Smells odors before others, or faint odors unnoticed by others
- Hypersensitive to body odors such as breath, underarms, skin or hair, scents of soap, perfume, etc.
- Easily light-headed or nauseous from chemical smells: paint, carpet, gasoline, cleaning supplies, dry cleaning, laundry soaps, certain perfumes
- Dislikes certain food smells
- Dislikes certain shampoos, lotions, or perfumes

Notes

Introduction: Too Sensitive for Your Own Good

1. Patricia Wilbarger and Julia Wilbarger, *Sensory Defensiveness in Children Aged 2–12: An Intervention Guide for Parents and Other Caretakers.* Santa Barbara, Calif.: Avanti Educational Programs, 1991.

2. A learned defensive response might manifest differently from one that is inborn. For instance, someone who was physically abused might flinch if he is tapped on the shoulder but wear any texture clothing on his body. Neuropsychologist Steven Cool of Pacific University suggests that the two responses may be biochemically different.

3. Moya Kinnealey, Barbara Oliver, and Patricia Wilbarger, "A Phenomenological Study of Sensory Defensiveness in Adults," *American Journal of Occupational Therapy* 49, no. 5 (1995): 444–51.

4. Carol Stock Kranowitz, *The Out of Sync Child. Recognizing and Coping with Sensory Interpretation Dysfunction.* New York: Skylight/Perigee, 1988.

5. Patricia Wilbarger and Julia Wilbarger, Sensory Defensiveness and Related Social/Emotional and Neurological Problems. Seminar presented in multiple locations. Denver, Avanti Educational Programs, 1992, rev. 1997.

6. Ibid.

7. See: J. D. Bremner, P. Randall, T. M. Scott et al., "MRI-Based Measurement of Hippocampal Volume in Combat-related Posttraumatic Stress Disorder. *American Journal of Psychiatry* 152 (1995): 973–81. J. D. Bremner, P. Randall, E. Vermetten et al., "MRI-Based Measurement of Hippocampal Volume in Posttraumatic Stress Disorder Related to Childhood Physical and Sexual Abuse: A Preliminary Report. *Biological Psychiatry* 41 (1997): 23–32.

8. P. W. Gold, F. K. Goodwin, and G. P. Chrousos, "Clinical and Biochemical Manifestation of Depression: Relations to the Neurobiology of Stress," *New England Journal of Medicine* (August 18, 1988). G. L. Wilcox, "Excitatory Neurotransmitters of Pain." In M. R. Bond, J. E. Charlton, and C. J. Woolf, eds., *Proceedings on the Vth World Congress on Pain*. New York: Elsevier Science Publishers BV, 1991. Glutamate fed to infant rats produces lesions in brain areas unprotected by the blood-brain barrier, specifically the hypothalamus.

9. From a study headed by National Institute of Mental Health psychiatrist Frank Putnam, and reported in *Clinical Psychiatry News* 19, no. 12 (1991): Bff.

10. Sharon Cermak, "Romanian Children Demonstrate Sensory Defensiveness," *Attachments* (Spring 1994).

11. Sharon Heller, *The Vital Touch: How Intimate Contact with Your Baby Leads to Happier, Healthier Development*. New York: Owl/Henry Holt, 1997.

12. Gary Evans, Staffan Hygge, and Monika Bullinger, "Chronic Noise and Psychological Stress," *Psychological Science* 6 (1995): 333–38.

13. Patricia Wilbarger and Julie Wilbarger, Sensory Defensiveness and Related Social/Emotional and Neurological Problems.

14. Moya Kinnealey and M. Fuiek, "The Relationship Between Sensory Defensiveness, Anxiety, Depression and Perception of Pain in Adults," *Occupational Therapy International* 6, no. 3 (1999): 195–206.

15. Patricia Oetter, Combining Approaches for Treating Children with Autism: The Art and Science. Paper presented at the 20th Symposium on Intervention for Persons with Mild to Severe Dysfunction, February 2000, Minneapolis, Minn.

16. A. Jean Ayers, *Sensory Integration and Learning Disorders*. Los Angeles: Western Psychological Services, 1972, p. 35.

17. Patricia Wilbarger and Julie Wilbarger, *Sensory Defensiveness in Children Aged 2–12*.

18. Patricia Wilbarger and Julie Wilbarger, Sensory Defensiveness and Related Social/Emotional and Neurological Problems.

19. A. Jean Ayres, *Sensory Integration and Learning Disorders*.

Chapter 1: Senses on the Defense

1. Patricia Wilbarger and Julia Wilbarger, *Sensory Defensiveness in Children Aged 2–12*.

2. A. Jean Ayres, *Sensory Integration and the Child*. Los Angeles: Western Psychological Services, 1998.

3. Sandra Weiss, "The Language of Touch," *Nursing Research* 28, no. 2 (1979): 76–80.

4. Frank A. Geldard, "Body English." *Psychology Today*, December 1968, p. 44.

5. R. Heslin and T. Alper, "Touch: A Bonding Gesture," in *Nonverbal Interaction*, J. M. Wiemann and R. P. Harrison, eds. (Beverly Hills, Calif.: Sage, 1985), pp. 47–75

6. T. Morgan, *Somerset Maugham*. London: Jonathan Cape, 1980.

7. Barbara Oliver, "The Social and Emotional Issues of Adults with Sensory Defensiveness," *Sensory Integration Special Interest Section Newsletter* 13, no. 3 (1990): 1–3.

8. E. Borg and S. A. Counter, "The Middle Ear Muscles," *Scientific American*, August 1978, pp. 74–80.

9. Don Campbell, *The Mozart Effect*. New York: Avon Books, 1997, p. 35.

10. Sheila Frick, Colleen Hacker, and Genevieve Jereb, "Hands-on Treatment Options to Enhance Modulation in Individuals with Autistic Spectrum, Attention Deficit and Related Sensorimotor Disorders," 20th Symposium on Intervention for Persons with Mild to Severe Dysfunction, February 24–27, 2000, Minneapolis, Minn.

11. Jerome Kagan, *Galen's Prophecy*. New York: Basic Books, 1994.

12. Patricia Wilbarger and Julia Wilbarger, Sensory Defensiveness and Related Social/Emotional and Neurological Problems.

13. A. M. Widström, A. B. Ransjö-Arvidson, K. Christensson et al., "Gastric Suction in Healthy Newborn Infants: Effects on Circulation and Developing Feeding Behavior," *ACTA Paediatrica Scandinavica* 76 (1987): 566–72.

14. R. H. Vallardi, J. Porter, and J. Winberg, "Does the Newborn Find the Nipple by Smell?" *Lancet* 344 (1994): 989–90.

Chapter 2: Sensory Processing: The Touchy Nervous System

1. E. Galanter, "Contemporary Psychophysics." In R. Brown, E. Galanter, E. H. Hess, and G. Mandler, eds., *New Directions in Psychology*. New York: Holt, Rinehart & Winston, 1962, p. 153.

2. A. Jean Ayres, *Sensory Integration and Learning Disorders*.

3. Ibid.

4. Nancy K. Dess, "Music on the Mind," *Psychology Today*, September-October 2000, p. 28.

5. Ashley Montagu, *Touching: The Human Significance of the Skin*. New York: Harper & Row, 1985, p. 5.

6. A. B. Roberts, D. Lille, and S. Campbell, "Twenty-four-Hour-Studies of Fetal Movements and Fetal Body Movements in Normal and Abnormal Pregnancies." In R. W. Beard and S. Campbell, *The Current Status of Fetal Heart Rate Monitoring and Ultrasound in Obstetrics*. London: Royal College of Obstetricians and Gynaecologists, 1977.

7. A. F. Korner, C. Guilleminault, J. Vanden Hoed, et al., "Reduction of Sleep Apnea and Bradycardia in Preterm Infants on Oscillation Waterbeds: A Controlled Polygraphic Study," *Pediatrics* 61, no. 4 (1978): 528–33.

8. D. Clark, J. Kreutzberg, and F. Chee, "Vestibular Stimulation's Influence on Motor Development," *Science* 196 (1977): 1228–1229.

9. W. A. Mason and G. Berkson, "Effects of Maternal Mobility on the Development of Rocking and Other Behaviors in Rhesus Monkeys: A Study

with Artificial Mothers," *Developmental Psychobiology* 8, no. 3 (1975): 197–211.

10. Sharon Heller, *The Vital Touch: How Intimate Contact with Your Baby Leads to Happier, Healthier Development*.

11. Steven Cool, "A View from the 'Outside': Sensory Integration and Developmental Neurobiology," *Sensory Integration Special-Interest Section Newsletter* 10, no. 2 (1987): 2–3.

12. Helen Colton, *The Gift of Touch*. New York: Putnam, 1983.

13. D. Sinclair, *Mechanisms of Cutaneous Stimulation*. London: Oxford University Press, 1981.

14. R. Bandler and J. Grinder, *Frogs into Princes*. Moab, Utah: Real People Press, 1979.

15. Jeffrey Meyers (ed.), *D. H. Lawrence and Tradition*. Boston: University of Massachusetts Press, 1984.

16. Andrew N. Meltzoff and R. W. Borton, "Intermodal Matching by Human Neonates,"*Nature* 282 (1979): 403–404.

17. Paul D. Maclean, *A Triune Concept of the Brain and Behavior*. Toronto: University of Toronto Press, 1973.

18. A. J. Ayres, *Sensory Integration and Learning Disorders*.

19. Hans Selye, *The Stress of Life*. New York: McGraw-Hill, 1976.

20. D. A. Werntz, R. G. Bickford et al., "Alternating Cerebral Hemispheric Activity and the Lateralization of Autonomic Nervous Function," *Human Neurobiology* 2 (1983): 39–43.

21. Marvin Zuckerman, *Behavioral Expressions and Biosocial Bases of Sensation Seeking*. New York: Cambridge University Press, 1994.

22. If you sever the amygdala, people become essentially autistic, without feelings or empathy for another.

23. For a detailed analysis of arousal and alertness, see Georgia DeGangi and Steven W. Porges, "Attention/Alertness/Arousal." In C. B. Royeen, ed., *AOTA Self Study Series*. Rockville, Md.: American Occupational Therapy Association, 1990.

24. Patricia Wilbarger and Julia Wilbarger, Sensory Defensiveness and Related Social/Emotional and Neurological Problems.

25. Sharon Cermak, "The Relationship Between Attention Deficits and

Sensory Integration Disorders," *Sensory Integration Special-Interest Section Newsletter* 11, no. 2 (1988): 1–4.

26. C. B. Royeen and S. J. Lane, "Tactile Processing and Sensory Defensiveness." In A. G. Fischer, E. A. Murray, and A. G. Bundy, eds., *Sensory Integration: Theory and Practice*. Philadelphia: F. A. Davis, 1991.

27. Patricia Wilbarger and Julia Wilbarger, Sensory Defensiveness and Related Social/Emotional and Neurological Problems.

28. Ibid.

29. Cited in Robert B. Melmo, *On Emotions, Needs, and Our Archaic Brain*. New York: Holt, Rinehart & Winston, 1975.

30. Joseph LeDoux, *The Emotional Brain*. New York: Touchstone/Simon & Schuster, 1996.

31. Stages adapted from Pat Holbrook, moderator of Adultsid@ yahoogroups.com.

Chapter 3: Levels of Defensiveness: From Mild to Maddening

1. Patricia Wilbarger and Julia Wilbarger, *Sensory Defensiveness in Children Aged 2–12*.

2. Patricia Wilbarger and Julia Wilbarger, Sensory Defensiveness and Related Social/Emotional and Neurological Problems.

3. Ibid.

4. Ibid.

5. Mary Main, "Parental Aversion to Infant-Initiated Contact Is Correlated with the Parent's Own Rejection During Childhood: The Effects of Experience on Signals of Security with Respect to Attachment." In K. E. Barnard and T. B. Brazelton, eds., *Touch: The Foundation of Experience*, Clinical Infant Reports, #4. Madison, Conn.: International Universities Press, 1989.

6. Patricia Wilbarger and Julie Wilbarger, Sensory Defensiveness and Related Social/Emotional and Neurological Problems.

7. Alice Gerard, "The Story of Me," *Sensory Integration Quarterly* (Spring/Summer 2000): 4.

8. Patricia Wilbarger and Julia Wilbarger, Sensory Defensiveness and Related Social/Emotional and Neurological Problems.

9. Ibid.

10. James Hardison, *Let's Touch*. Englewood Cliffs, N.J.: Prentice-Hall, 1980.

11. Temple Grandin and Margaret M. Scariano, *Emergence: Labeled Autistic*. New York: Warner Books, 1986.

12. Ibid., pp. 18–19.

13. Ibid., p. 50.

Chapter 4: Weaving a Web of Fear: Sensory Defensiveness Across the Lifespan

1. T. Berry Brazelton, *Neonatal Behavioral Assessment Scale*. Philadelphia: J. B. Lippincott, 1984.

2. Jerome Kagan, *Galen's Prophecy*.

3. Steven Suomi, "Uptight and Laid-back Monkeys: Individual Differences in the Response to Social Challenges." In S. Branch, W. Hall, and E. Dooling, eds., *Plasticity of Development*. Cambridge, Mass.: M.I.T. Press, 1991, pp. 27–55.

4. G. A. DeGangi and S. I. Greenspan, "The Development of Sensory Functions in Infants," *Physical and Occupational Therapy in Pediatrics* 8, no. 4 (1988): 21–33.

5. Patricia Oetter, Eileen Richter, and Sheila M. Frick, *M.O.R.E.: Integrating the Mouth with Sensory and Postural Functions*, 2d ed. Hugo, Minn.: PDP Press, 1995, p. 42.

6. D. Weiss-Salinas and N. Williams, "Insights in Practice. Sensory Defensiveness: A Theory of Its Effect on Breastfeeding," *Journal of Human Lactation* 17, no. 2 (2001): 145–51.

7. Patricia Wilbarger and Julia Wilbarger, Sensory Defensiveness and Related Social/Emotional and Neurological Problems.

8. Marie Anzalone, "Sensory Integration and Self-regulation in the Infant and Young Child: Strategies for Assessment and Intervention." 20th

Symposium on Intervention for Persons with Mild to Severe Dysfunction, Minneapolis, Minn., February 24–27, 2000.

9. Patricia Wilbarger and Julie Wilbarger, Sensory Defensiveness and Related Social/Emotional and Neurological Problems.

10. Susan Ludington-Hoe, A. Hadeed, and Gene C. Anderson, "Maternal-Neonatal Thermal Synchrony During Skin-to-Skin Contact," *Abstracts of Individual Papers*. Research Conference of the Council of Nurse Researchers, Chicago, September 1989, p. 286.

11. Tiffany Field, "Attachment as Psychobiological Attunement: Being on the Same Wavelength." In M. Reite and T. Field, eds., *The Psychobiology of Attachment and Separation*. New York: Academic Press, 1985.

12. E. W. Ingersoll and E. B. Thoman, "The Breathing Bear: Effects on Respiration in Premature Infants," *Physiology and Behavior* 56, no. 3 (1994): 855–59.

13. Currents Interview, "In Our Wild: Studies from a Rhesus Colony." Interview with Steven J. Suomi, *Currents in Affective Illness* 11 (1992): 5–14.

14. Thomas Lewis, Fari Amini, and Richard Lannon, *A General Theory of Love*. New York: Random House, 2000, p. 86.

15. Patricia M. Crittenden, "Compulsive Compliance: The Development of an Inhibitory Coping Strategy in Infancy," *Journal of Abnormal Child Psychology* 16, no. 5 (1988): 585–99.

16. Patricia Crittenden, "Quality of Attachment in the Preschool Years," *Development and Psychopathology* 4 (1992): 209–41.

17. Ibid.

18. Candace Pert, *Molecules of Emotion*. New York: Scribner, 1997.

19. Partricia Wilbarger and Julia Wilbarger, *Sensory Defensiveness in Children Aged 2–12*.

20. J. Case-Smith, L. Butcher, and D. Reed, "Parents' Report of Sensory Responsiveness and Temperament in Preterm Infants," *American Journal of Occupational Therapy* 52, no. 7 (1998): 547–55.

21. S. Wapner, *The Body Percept*. New York: Random House, 1965.

22. Ackerman, Diane, *A Natural History of the Senses*. New York: Random House, 1990, p. 96.

23. Rod McKuen, *Alone*. New York: Pocket Books, 1975.

24. Alice Gerard, "The Story of Me."

25. S.D. Hotz and C.B. Royeen, "Perception of Behaviors Associated with Tactile Defensiveness: An Exploration of the Differences Between Mothers and Their Children," *Occupational Therapy International* 5, no. 4 (1998): 2281–2292.

Chapter 5: From Anxiety to Addiction

1. For a review of sensation seeking and psychopathology, see Martin Zuckerman, *Behavioral Expressions and Biosocial Bases of Sensation Seeking*.

2. Moya Kinnealey and M. Fuiek, "The Relationship Between Sensory Defensiveness, Anxiety, Depression and Perception of Pain in Adults, *Occupational Therapy International* 6, no. 3 (1999): 195–206.

3. Barbara Oliver, "The Social and Emotional Issues of Adults with Sensory Defensiveness," *Sensory Integration Special Interest Section Newsletter* 13, no. 3 (1990): 1–3.

4. Temple Grandin and Margaret M. Scariano, *Emergence: Labeled Autistic*.

5. Moya Kinnealey and M. Fuiek, "The Relationship Between Sensory Defensiveness, Anxiety, Depression and Perception of Pain in Adults."

6. Harold Levinson, *Phobia Free*. New York: M. Evans, 1986.

7. Ibid., p. 53.

8. Moya Kinnealey, Barbara Oliver, and Patricia Wilbarger, "A Phenomenological Study of Sensory Defensiveness in Adults," *American Journal of Occupational Therapy* 49, no. 5 (1995): 444–51.

9. Ibid.

10. Patricia Oetter, Eileen Richter, and Sheila M. Frick, *M.O.R.E.: Integrating the Mouth with Sensory and Postural Functions*.

11. Judith J. Wurtman and Susan Suffes, *The Serotonin Solution*. New York: Fawcett Columbine, 1996.

12. A. Jean Ayres, "The Development of Perceptual-Motor Abilities: A Theoretical Basis for Treatment of Dysfunction," *American Journal of Occupational Therapy* 17, no. 6 (1963): 221–25.

Chapter 6: The Body Erupts: The Psychosomatic Side of Sensory Defensiveness

1. For a review of stress, stress-related disease, and coping, see Robert Sapolsky, *Why Zebras Don't Get Ulcers*. New York: W. H. Freeman, 1998.
2. Hans Selye, *The Stress of Life*. New York: McGraw-Hill, 1976.
3. Charles B. Nemeroff, K. Ranga, R. Krishnan et al., "Adrenal Gland Enlargement in Major Depression: A Computed Tomographic Study," *Archives of General Psychiatry* 19 (1992): 384–87.
4. Caroline S Koblenzer, "Cutaneous Manifestations of Psychiatric Disease That Commonly Present to the Dermatologist: Diagnosis and Treatment," *International Journal of Psychiatry in Medicine* 22, no. 1 (1992): 47–63.
5. Karyn Seroussi, *Unraveling the Mystery of Autism and Pervasive Developmental Disorder: A Mother's Story of Research and Recovery*. New York: Simon & Schuster, 2000.

Chapter 7: Getting Started

1. Patricia Wilbarger and Julia Wilbarger, *Sensory Defensiveness in Children Aged 2–12*.
2. Patricia Wilbarger and Julia Wilbarger, Sensory Defensiveness and Related Social/Emotional and Neurological Problems.
3. Ibid.
4. Ibid.
5. Ibid.

Chapter 8: Priming the Pump

1. Patricia Wilbarger and Julia Wilbarger, Sensory Defensiveness and Related Social/Emotional and Neurological Problems
2. D. R. Kenshalo, ed., *The Skin Senses*. Springfield, Ill.: Charles C. Thomas, 1968.
3. Patricia Wilbarger, *Sensory Defensiveness*. PDP Press Inc. A videotape.

4. Patricia Wilbarger and Julia Wilbarger, Sensory Defensiveness and Related Social/Emotional and Neurological Problems.

5. Sandra David, "A Case Study of Sensory Affective Disorder in Adult Psychiatry," *Sensory Integration Special-Interest Section Newsletter* 13, no. 4 (1990): 1–4.

6. Judith Reisman and Anny Yockey Gross, "Psychophysiological Measurement of Treatment Effects in an Adult with Sensory Defensiveness," *Canada Journal of Occupational Therapy* 59, no. 5 (1992): 248–57.

7. Patricia Wilbarger and Julia Wilbarger, Sensory Defensiveness and Related Social/Emotional and Neurological Problems.

8. Nancy Lawton-Shirley, "The Sensory Integrative Value of Horseback Riding Therapy," *Sensory Integration Special-Interest Section Newsletter* 13, no. 2 (1990): 3–4.

9. Michael Babyak, James A. Blumenthal, Steve Herman et al., "Exercise Treatment for Major Depression: Maintenance of Therapeutic Effect at 10 Months," *Psychosomatic Medicine* 62, no. 5 (2000): 633–38.

10. Mihaly Czikszentmihalyi, *Flow: The Psychology of Optimal Experience*. New York: Harper & Row, 1990.

11. Hans Eysenck, *Eysenck on Extraversion*. New York: John Wiley, 1973.

12. Patricia Wilbarger and Julia Wilbarger, Sensory Defensiveness and Related Social/Emotional and Neurological Problems.

13. Ibid.

14. V. Tibbetts and E. Pepper, "Effects of Imagery and Position on Breathing Patterns, *Proceedings of the Twenty-Seventh Annual Meeting of the Association for Applied Psychophysiology and Biofeedback*. Wheat Ridge, Colo.: AAPB, 1996. These researchers found as well that bracing and respiration patterns could also be altered by imagining walking on a hard or soft surface. Thus, one could increase or reduce arousal by imagining walking on a soft meadow or walking on a hard concrete road.

15. Patricia Wilbarger and Julia Wilbarger, Sensory Defensiveness and Related Social/Emotional and Neurological Problems.

16. Barbara Oliver, "The Social and Emotional Issues of Adults with Sensory Defensiveness," *Sensory Integration Special-Interest Section Newsletter*.

Chapter 9: Sound Health

1. Nietzsche, quoted in Jacques Barzun, ed., *Pleasures of Music*. Chicago: University of Chicago Press, 1977, p. 312.

2. Johns Hopkins study cited in Don G. Campbell, ed., *Music: Physician for Times to Come*. Wheaton, Ill.: Quest Books, 1991, p. 246.

3. W. S. Condon and L. Sander, "Synchrony Demonstrated Between Movements of the Neonate and Adult Speech," *Child Development* 45 (1974): 456–62.

4. C. Douglas, "The Beat Goes On," *Psychology Today*, November 1987, pp. 37–42.

5. Murray R. Shafer, *The Tuning of the World*. New York: Knopf, 1977.

6. T. Berry Brazelton, "Precursors for the Development of Emotions in Early Infancy." In R. Plutchik and H. Kellerman, eds., *Emotion, Theory, Research, and Experience*, vol. 2. New York: Academic Press, 1981.

7. Dale Bartlett, Donald Kaufman, and Roger Smeltekop, "The Effects of Music Listening and Perceived Sensory Experiences on the Immune System As Measured by Interleukin-1 and Cortisol," *Journal of Music Therapy* 30 (1993): 194–209.

8. Steven Halpern, *Sound Health*. San Francisco: Harper & Row, 1985.

9. Olav Skille, "Vibroacoustic Research 1980–1991." In Ralph Spintge and R. Droh, eds., *Music Medicine*. St. Louis: MMB Music, 1991, p. 249.

10. Steven Halpern, *Sound Health*, p. 138.

11. John Diamond, *Your Body Doesn't Lie*. New York: Warner Books, 1979.

12. For detailed information on the effect of different kinds of music on the body and emotions, see Don Campbell, *The Mozart Effect*. New York: Avon, 1997.

13. Liesi-Vivoni Ramos, "The Effects of On-Hold Telephone Music on the Number of Premature Disconnections to a Statewide Protective Services Abuse Hot Line," *Journal of Music Therapy* 30 (1993): 119–29.

14. To help her clients feel more in touch with their bodies, occupational therapist Sheila Frick, who lectures extensively on the therapeutic use of

music, will often use *Sacred Earth Drums and Sacred Spirit Drums* by David Gordon and Steve Gordon.

15. Tom Wilson, "Chat: the Healing Power of Voice and Ear. Interview with Alfred Tomatis." In Don Campbell, ed., *Music—Physician for Times to Come*. Wheaton, Ill.: Quest Books, 1991, pp. 11–28.

16. Sheila Frick and Nancy Lawton-Shirley, "Auditory Integrative Training from a Sensory Integrative Perspective," *Sensory Integration Special-Interest Section Newsletter*, 17, no. 4 (1994): 1–3.

17. In the 1950s, Alfred Tomatis discovered that the fetus is able to hear and recognizes its mother's voice at birth.

Chapter 10: Seeing the Whole Picture

1. John Ott, "Color and Light: Their Effects on Plants, Animals, and People," *Journal of Biosocial Research* 7, part 1 (1985).

2. John Ott, *Exploring the Spectrum* (a film by John Ott).

3. John Ott, "Color and Light."

4. See John Ott, *Health and Light: The Effects of Natural and Artificial Light on Man and Other Living Things*. New York: Pocket Books, 1973.

5. I. M. Sharon, R. P. Feller, and S. W. Burney, "The Effects of Lights of Different Spectra on Caries Incidence in the Golden Hamster," *Archives of Oral Biology* 16, no. 12 (1971): 1427–1431.

6. Cited in David Olszewski and Brian Breiling, "Getting into Light: The Use of Phototherapy in Everyday Life." In *Light Years Ahead: The Illustrated Guide to Full Spectrum and Colored Light in Mind-Body Healing*. Berkeley, Calif.: Celestial Arts, 1996, p. 263.

7. Mark D. Anderson and Jean M. Williams, "Seeing Too Straight: Stress and Vision," *Longevity* (August 1989); studies by Anderson and Williams confirm the effect of stress on vision.

8. Jacob Liberman, *Light: Medicine of the Future*. Santa Fe, N. M.: Bear and Co., 1991, p. 82.

9. F. Hollwich, *The Influence of Ocular Light Perception on Metabolism in Man and in Animal*. New York: Springer-Verlag, 1979.

10. Norman Shealy, "The Reality of EEG and Neurochemical Responses to Photostimulation: Part 1," In *Light Years Ahead*, pp. 165–84.

11. Reported in Jacob Liberman, *Light: Medicine of the Future*.

12. B. Weiss, "Dyslexics Read Better with the Blues," *Science News* (September 29, 1990): 196.

13. John Downing, "Clinical EEG and Neurophysiological Case Studies in Ocular Light Therapy," In *Light Years Ahead*, pp. 133–65.

14. J.J. Plack and J. Schick, "The Effects of Color on Human Behavior," *Journal of the Association for Study in Perception* 9 (1974): 4–16.

15. G. Legwold, "Color-Boosted Energy: How Lights Affect Muscle Action," *American Health* (May 1988).

16. Cited in Diane Ackerman, *The Natural History of the Senses*. New York: Random House, 1990.

17. John Downing, "Clinical EEG and Neurophysiological Case Studies in Ocular Light Therapy."

18. See Norman E. Rosenthal, *Winter Blues*. New York: Guilford, 1998.

19. Mary Bolles, "Learning Abilities' Dramatic Response to Light, Sound and Motion." In *Light Years Ahead*, pp. 297–320.

Chapter 11: Air Control

1. For a good review of chemical sensitivity, see Peter Radetsky, *Allergic to the Twentieth Century*. New York: Little, Brown and Company, 1997.

2. Sandra Blakeslee, "Buildings That Make You Sick," *San Francisco Chronicle*, June 15, 1980, p. 3.

3. See www.atlanticinstitute.com.

Chapter 12: A Harmonious Space

1. For a review of the effects of environment on behavior, see Carol Venolia, *Healing Environments*. Berkeley, Calif.: Celestial Arts, 1988. See also Winifred Gallagher, *The Power of Place*. New York: HarperPerennial, 1994.

2. A. G. Schauss, "Tranquilizing Effect of Color Reduces Aggressive Behavior and Potential Violence," *The Journal of Orthomolecular Psychiatry* 8, no. 4 (1979): 218–21.

3. Ashley Montagu, *Touching: The Human Significance of the Skin*. New York: Simon and Schuster, 1984, p. 357.

4. Edward T. Hall, *The Hidden Dimension*. New York: Anchor Books, 1966.

5. Barbara Oliver, "The Social and Emotional Issues of Adults with Sensory Defensiveness."

Chapter 13: Food for Your Nervous System

1. See Michael Gershon, *The Second Brain*. New York: HarperCollins, 1998.

2. Barry Sears, *The Zone*. New York: Harper Collins, 1995.

3. Elson M. Haas, *Staying Healthy with Nutrition*. Berkeley, Calif.: Celestial Arts, 1992.

4. For information on natural healing for a multitude of physical conditions, see James E. Balch and Phyllis A. Balch, *Prescription for Nutritional Healing*, 3d ed. Garden City Park, N.Y.: Avery Publishing, 2000.

5. See Michael J. Norden, *Beyond Prozac*. New York: Regan Books/HarperCollins, 1995.

6. Hyla Cass and Terrence McNally, *Kava: Nature's Answer to Stress, Anxiety and Insomnia*. Rocklin, Calif.: Prima Publishing, 1998.

7. See Harold H. Bloomfield, *Healing Anxiety with Herbs*. New York: HarperCollins, 1998. Also Mark Mayell, *Natural Energy*. New York: Three Rivers Press, 1998.

Chapter 14: Breathing Lessons

1. Alexander Lowen, *Bioenergetic*. New York: Penguin, 1976.

2. Robert Fried, *The Breath Connection*. New York: Plenum Press, 1990. Fried researched the chain of physiological events that follow hyperventilation.

3. E. Peper et al., "Repetitive Strain Injury: Prevent Computer User Injury with Biofeedback: Assessment and Training Protocol," *Electromyography Thought Technology* (1994).

4. David S. Shannahoff-Khalsa and Liana R. Beckett, "Clinical Case Report: Efficacy of Yogic Techniques in the Treatment of Obsessive-Compulsive Disorders," *International Journal of Neuroscience* 85 (1996): 1–17.

5. R. R. Freedman and S. Woodward, "Behavioral Treatment of Menopausal Hot Flashes: Evaluation by Ambulatory Monitoring," *American Journal of Obstetrics and Gynecology* 167, no. 2 (1992): 257–78.

6. K. V. Naveen, R. Nagarathna, H. R. Nagendra, and Shirley Telles, "Yoga Breathing Through a Particular Nostril Increases Spatial Memory Scores Without Lateralized Effects," *Psychological Reports* 8, no. 2 (1997): 555–61.

7. From Lisette Scholl, *28 Days to Reading Without Glasses*. Secaucus, N.J.: Citadel Press, 1998.

8. This exercise is adapted from one described by Donna Farhi in *The Breathing Book*. New York: Owl/Henry Holt, 1996.

9. Patricia Oetter, Eileen Richter, and Sheila M. Frick, *M.O.R.E.*

10. Cited in Michael J. Norden, *Beyond Prozac*.

Chapter 15: Posturing for Inner Peace

1. Thomas Hanna, *Somatics*. Reading, Mass.: Addison-Wesley, 1988.

2. Frank Scafidi, Tiffany Field, Saul Schanberg, et al., "Effects of Tactile/Kinesthetic Stimulation on the Clinical Course and Sleep/Wake Behavior of Preterm Neonates," *Infant Behavior and Development* 9 (1986): 91–105.

3. Angela Escalona, Tiffany Field, Ruth Singer-Strunck et al., "Brief Report: Improvements in the Behavior of Children with Autism Following Massage Therapy," *Journal of Autism and Developmental Disorders* 31, no. 5 (2001): 513–16.

4. N. Jhansi Rani and P. V. Krishna Rao, "Body Awareness and Yoga Training," *Perceptual and Motor Skills* 79 (1994): 1103–1106.

5. K. Sridevi, M. Sitamma, and P. V. Krishna Rao, "Perceptual Organization and Yoga Training," *Journal of Indian Psychology* 13, no. 2 (1995): 21–27.

6. Shirley Telles, R. Nagarathna, and H. R. Nagendra, "Improvement in Visual Perception Following Yoga Training," *Journal of Indian Psychology* 13, no. 1 (1995): 30–32.

7. Bonnie G. Berger and David R. Owen, "Mood Alternation with Yoga and Swimming: Aerobic Exercise May Not Be Necessary," *Perceptual and Motor Skills* 75 (1992): 1331–43.

8. Alexander Lowen, *Bioenergetics*, pp. 17–18.

Chapter 16: Mind/Body—Only Connect!

1. Herbert Benson, *The Relaxation Response*. New York: Morrow, 1975.

2. Ernest L. Rossi and David B. Cheek, *Mind-Body Therapy*. New York: W.W. Norton, 1988.

3. See Peter Suedfeld, *Restricted Environmental Stimulation: Research and Clinical Applications*. New York: Wiley, 1980.

4. Peter Suedfeld and J. L. Kristeller, "Stimulus Reduction as a Technique in Health Psychology," *Health Psychology* 1 (1982): 337–57.

Glossary

Agoraphobia: Fear of open places and of being in places or situations from which escape might be difficult or embarrassing and help might not be available.

Amygdala: Two almond-shaped neural centers in the limbic system of the brain structure that are linked to emotion.

Anxiety: A vague feeling of fear and apprehension that creates unease.

Arousal: A state that ranges from sleep to wakefulness; regulated by the reticular formation in conjunction with limbic input.

Attention deficit hyperactivity disorder (ADHD): A condition characterized by persistent inattention to tasks, hyperactivity, and impulsive behavior. Symptoms are manifested before age 7.

Audition: The ability to receive and apprehend sounds; hearing.

Auditory defensiveness: Oversensitivity to certain sounds that produces a startle response or avoidance behavior.

Autism: A developmental disorder usually appearing during the first three years of life; characterized by severe impairment in social relationships, communication, and development.

Autonomic nervous system: The division of the nervous system concerned with visceral activities, smooth muscles, and endocrine glands. It controls automatic, unconscious bodily functions, such as breathing, sweating, shivering, and digestion.

Bilateral integration: The neurological process of integrating sensations from both body sides, of knowing right from left, and the foundation for bilateral coordination.

Body awareness, body image, body perception, or body schema: The person's perception of his or her own body parts, where they are, how they interrelate, how they move, and how they appear in size and shape.

Brain stem: The most primitive portion of the brain; regulates elementary sensorimotor processes, such as breathing, swallowing, arousal, and calming.

Central nervous system: The part of the nervous system, consisting of the brain and spinal cord, that coordinates the activity of the entire nervous system.

Cerebellum: The brain part that is wrapped around the brain stem; processes proprioceptive and vestibular sensations to help coordinate body movements and maintain balance.

Cerebral cortex: The convoluted outer layer of the cerebrum that coordinates higher nervous activity; neocortex.

Cerebrum: The "thinking brain," where detailed processing of sensations occurs; composed of two cerebral hemispheres.

Cranial nerves: The set of nerves running from the head and face directly to the brain without passing through the spinal cord and from the brain back to the head and face.

Defensive (or protective) system: The component of a sensory system that alerts one to real or potential danger and causes a self-protective response. This system is innate.

Depersonalization: Feelings of unreality or a loss of personal identity.

Discriminative (or epicritic) system: The component of a sensory system that allows one to distinguish among stimuli; this system is not innate but develops with time and practice.

Generalized anxiety disorder: Prolonged, vague, unexplained, but intense fears that are chronic and felt in many different situations. The person is continually tense, apprehensive, and in a state of autonomic nervous system arousal.

Gravitational insecurity: An extreme fear of falling produced by change in movement or head position.

Habituation: The neurological process of tuning out familiar sensations.

Hippocampus: The brain structure that compares familiar and novel sensory stimuli and is involved with memory.

Hormones: Substances like cortisol, estrogen, testosterone, or growth hormone that travel through our bloodstream to act on our tissues and organs.

Hypersensitivity (also hyperreactivity, hyperresponsiveness): Oversensitivity to sensory stimuli, characterized by a tendency to be either fearful and cautious or negative and defiant.

Hyposensitivity (also hyporeactivity, hyporesponsiveness): Undersensitivity to sensory stimuli, characterized by a tendency either to crave intense sensations or to withdraw and be difficult to engage.

Hyperventilation: Involuntary rapid, shallow breathing that sometimes results in diminished carbon dioxide in the bloodstream, lightheadedness, dizziness, a feeling of unreality, shortness of breath, and numbness; not unlike having a panic attack.

Hypoglycemia: A condition in which blood sugar levels fall too low as a result of improper diet or stress.

Hypothalamus: The brain structure that regulates unconscious bodily processes such as body temperature and metabolic functions.

Inner ear: The organ that receives sensations of the pull of gravity and of changes in balance and head position.

Limbic system: The section of the brain that processes messages from all the senses and is involved primarily with one's emotions and inner drive.

Modulation: The brain's regulation of its own activity.

Neurotransmitters: Chemical messengers of the nervous system that makes possible the movement of the nerve impulse across the synapse.

Occupational therapy (OT): A health profession that helps people improve the functioning of their nervous system in order to develop skills leading to independence in personal, social, academic, and vocational pursuits.

Olfactory sense: The far sense that perceives odor, smell.

Optimal range of arousal: The midpoint between boredom and anxiety; a state of being alert and calm.

Oral defensiveness: The feeling of unpleasantness caused by certain food textures or combinations and some taste sensations; a desire to avoid eating these foods.

Overload: A dual state of physical exhaustion and sympathetic overarousal.

Panic: A sudden surge of acute terror accompanied by severe agitation.

Parasympathetic nervous system: The division of the autonomic nervous system that calms the body, conserving its energy.

Phobia: A disrupting and persistent fear aroused by a specific type of situations (e.g., heights), animals (e.g., snakes), or objects (e.g., open drawers) that is out of proportion to any proposed danger.

Proprioceptive sense: The unconscious awareness of sensations coming from one's joints, muscles, and ligaments; sense of body position in space.

Receptors: Special cells, located throughout one's body, that receive specific sensory messages and send them for processing to the central nervous system.

Reticular core: A network of neurons in the brain stem that receives impulses from every sensory system and that is the center for arousal and for calming down.

Self-regulation: One's ability to control activity level and state of alertness, as well as one's emotional, mental, or physical responses to sensations; self-organization.

Sensorimotor: Pertaining to the brain-behavior process of taking in sensory messages and reacting with a physical response.

Sensory defensiveness: A constellation of symptoms that are the result of aversive or defensive reactions to nonnoxious stimuli across one or more sensory modalities. The sensory-defensive person tends to react negatively or with alarm to sensory input that other people generally consider harmless or nonirritating.

Sensory sensitivity (or acuity): Keen awareness of a sensation and possible distraction by it, without discomfort.

Sensory diet: The optimum sensorimotor input one seeks on a daily basis to integrate mind, body, and emotion so that you feel alert, control is effortless, and you perform at your peak. A planned and scheduled activity program that an occupational therapist develops to help a person become more self-regulated.

Sensory integration (SI): The normal neurological process of taking in information from one's body and environment through the senses, organizing and unifying this information, and using it to plan and execute adaptive responses to different challenges in order to learn and function smoothly in daily life.

Sensory integration dysfunction (DSI): The inefficient neurological processing of information received through the senses, causing problems with learning, development, and behavior.

Sensory modulation: The ability of the nervous system to regulate, organize, and prioritize incoming sensory information, inhibiting or suppressing irrelevant information and enabling one to focus on relevant information.

Serotonin: One of a group of chemical neurotransmitters that implement neural transmission across the synapses; thought to be involved in some types of depression and anxiety.

Shutdown: The self-protective state in which energy is expended only for sheer survival, and sensation processing ceases or almost ceases.

Social phobia: A persistent fear of one of more situations in which the person is exposed to possible scrutiny by others and worries about doing something or acting in a way that will be humiliating or embarrassing.

Somatosensory: Tactile-proprioceptive perception of touch sensations and body position; body sensing.

Sympathetic nervous system: The division of the autonomic nervous system that arouses the body, mobilizing its energy in stressful situations.

Tactile defensiveness: Certain touch sensations, such as light or unexpected touch, feel aversive and create a strong emotional response.

Tactile sense: The sensory system that receives sensations of pressure, vibration, movement, temperature, and pain, primarily through receptors in the skin; the sense of touch, both touching and being touched.

Vagus nerve: The tenth cranial nerve, which supplies motor nerve fibers to the muscles of swallowing and parasympathetic fibers to the heart and organs of the chest cavity and abdomen.

Vestibular sense: The body's gyroscope, located in the inner ear, and responding to changes in head position and to body movement through space.

Visual defensiveness: Oversensitivity to light that may involve visual distractibility.

Resource Guide

Sensory Defensiveness

You will find most of these books and articles available through Sensory Integration International (SII), Professional Development Products (PDP), Southpaw Enterprise, or Avanti Educational Programs (see Practitioners, Supplies, and Information).

Books

Wilbarger, Patricia, and Julia Wilbarger. *Sensory Defensiveness in Children Aged 2–12: An Intervention Guide for Parents and Other Caretakers.* Santa Barbara, Calif.: Avanti Educational Programs, 1991.

Articles

Cool, Steven J. "The Use of a Surgical Brush in Treatment of Sensory Defensiveness: Commentary and Exploration," *Sensory Integration Special-Interest Section Newsletter* 13, no. 4 (1990): 4–5.

David, Sandra. "A Case Study of Sensory Affective Disorder in Adult Psychiatry," *Sensory Integration Special-Interest Section Newsletter* 13, no. 4 (1990): 1–6.

Frick, Sheila. "Sensory Defensiveness: A Case Study," *Sensory Integration Special-Interest Section Newsletter* 12, no. 2 (1989): 2–4.

Kinnealey, Moya, Barbara Oliver, and Patricia Wilbarger. "A Phenomenological Study of Sensory Defensiveness in Adults," *American Journal of Occupational Therapy* 49, no. 5 (1995): 444–51.

Kinnealey, Moya, and M. Fuiek. "The Relationship Between Sensory Defensiveness, Anxiety, Depression and Perception of Pain in Adults," *Occupational Therapy International* 6, no. 3 (1999): 195–206.

Oliver, Barbara. "The Social and Emotional Issues of Adults with Sensory Defensiveness," *Sensory Integration Special-Interest Section Newsletter* 13, no. 3 (1990): 1–3.

Reisman, Judith, and Anne Yockey Gross. "Psychophysiological Measurement of Treatment Effects in an Adult with Sensory Defensiveness," *Canada Journal of Occupational Therapy* 59, no. 5 (1992): 248–57.

Wilbarger, Patricia. "The Sensory Diet: Activity Programs Based on Sensory Processing Theory." *Sensory Integration Special-Interest Section Newsletter*, 18, no. 2 (1995).

Wilbarger, Patricia. "Planning an Adequate 'Sensory Diet'—Application of Sensory Processing Theory During the First Year of Life," *Zero to Three* 5, no. 1 (1984): 7–12.

Audio and Video

Wilbarger, Patricia, and Julia Wilbarger. *Introduction to Sensory Defensiveness.*

A 30-minute audiotape, abstracted from workshops presented nationally, that gives a brief overview of current perspectives on the diagnosis and treatment of sensory defensiveness. Available from Avanti and PDP.

Wilbarger, Patricia, *Sensory Defensiveness.*

A videotape for professionals and audiences (approximately 60 minutes). Using actual case studies, the tape describes the symptoms of sensory defensiveness, its social-emotional impact, and suggested intervention strategies for people of different ages. Available from Avanti and PDP.

Websites

www.sensorydefensiveness.com

Sensory Integration for Adults and Children

General Books

A Parent's Guide to Understanding Sensory Integration. Torrance, Calif.: Sensory Integration International, 1991.

Anderson, Elizabeth, and Pauline Emmons. *Unlocking the Mysteries of Sensory Integration*. Arlington, Tex.: Future Horizons, 1996.

Kranowitz, Carol Stock. *The Out-of-Sync Child: Recognizing and Coping with Sensory Integration Dysfunction*. New York: Skylight/Perigee, 1998.

Trott, M. C., M. Laurel, S. L. Windeck. *Sensibilities: Understanding Sensory Integration*. Tucson, Ariz.: Therapy Skill Builders, 1993.

Williams, Mary Sue, and Sherry Shellenberger. "Introduction," *How Does Your Engine Run? The Alert Program for Self-Regulation*. Albuquerque, N.M.: Therapy Works, 1992.

Professional Books and Articles

Ayres, A. Jean. *Sensory Integration and Learning Disorders*. Los Angeles: Western Psychological Services, 1972.

Ayres, A. Jean. *Sensory Integration and the Child*. Los Angeles: Western Psychological Services, 1998.

Fisher, Anne, Elizabeth A. Murray, and Anita Bundy. *Sensory Integration: Theory and Practice*. Philadelphia: F. A. Davis, 1991.

Kimball, Judith G. "Sensory Integration Frame of Reference." In Paula Kramer and Jim Hinojosa, eds., *Frames of Reference for Pediatric Occupational Therapy*, 2d ed. Baltimore: Lippincott Williams & Wilkins, 1999.

Websites

http://www.adultsid@yahoogroups.com
http://www.sinetwork.org
http://www.out-of-sync-child.com

Sound

Books About Music for Modulation

Campbell, Don. *The Mozart Effect*. New York: Avon Books, 1997.
Gardner, Kay. *Sounding the Inner Landscape*. Boston: Element Books, 1997.
Halpern, Steven. *Sound Health*. San Francisco: Harper & Row, 1985.

Books About Noise Control

Pearson, David. *The New Natural House Book*. New York: Fireside Press/ Simon & Schuster, 1998.

Books About Voice and Listening Therapy

Berard, Guy. *Hearing Equals Behaviors*. New Canaan, Conn.: Keats, 1993.
Campbell, Don. *The Roar of Silence: Healing Powers of Breath, Tone and Music*. Wheaton, Ill.: Theosophical Publishing House, 1989.
Newham, Paul. *The Healing Voice: How to Use the Power of Your Voice to Bring Harmony into Your Life*. New York: HarperCollins, 1999.
Tomatis, Alfred. *The Conscious Ear*. Rhinebeck, N.Y.: Station Hill Press, 1991.

Audio

Campbell, Don. *Healing Yourself with Your Own Voice*. Louisville, Colo.: Sounds True, 1994.

Light

Books

Darius, Dinshah. *Let There Be Light*. Malaga, N.J.: Dinshah Health Society, 1985.

Liberman, Jacob. *Light, Medicine of the Future*. Sante Fe, N.M.: Bear & Company, 1991.

Ott, John. *Health and Light: The Effects of Natural and Artificial Light on Man and Other living Things*. New York: Pocket Books, 1973.

Beiling, Brian, and Bethany Argisle (eds.). *Light Years Ahead: The Illustrated Guide to Full Spectrum and Colored Light in Mindbody Healing*. Berkeley, Calif.: Celestial Arts, 1996.

Audio and Video

Liberman, Jacob. *Healing with Light and Color: Medicine for the Coming Millennium*. An in-depth approach to using light and color for expanding consciousness and as a foundation for wellness. 120 minutes. Universal Light Technology, PO Box 520, Carbondale, Colo. 81623, 1-800-81-LIGHT.

Websites

www.ulight.com
www.syntonicphototherapy.com

Chemical Sensitivity

Dadd, Debra Lynn. *Home Safe Home: Protecting Yourself and Your Family from Everyday Toxics and Harmful Household Products in the Home*. Los Angeles: Jeremy P. Tarcher, 1997.

Krohn, Jacqueline. *The Whole Way to Allergy Relief and Prevention: A Doc-*

tor's Complete Guide to Treatment and Self-Care. Vancouver: Hartley and Marks, 1996.

Pearson, David. *The Natural House Book*. New York: Fireside Press/Simon & Schuster, 1998.

Radetsky, Peter. *Allergic to the Twentieth Century*. New York: Little, Brown, 1997.

Taylor, Renee R., Fred Friedberg, and A. Jason Leonard, *A Clinician's Guide to Controversial Illnesses: Chronic Fatigue Syndrome, Fibromyalgia, and Multiple Chemical Sensitivities*. Sarasota, Fla.: Professional Resource Exchange, 2001.

Aromatherapy

Cooksley, Valerie Gennari. *Aromatherapy*. Paramus, N.J.: Prentice-Hall, 1996.

Damian, Peter, and Kate Damian. *Aromatherapy Scent and Psyche*. Rochester, Vt.: Healing Arts Press, 1995.

Lawless, Julia. *The Illustrated Encyclopedia of Essential Oils: The Complete Guide to the Use of Oils in Aromatherapy and Herbalism*. Boston: Element Books, 1995.

Worwood, Valerie Ann. *The Complete Book of Essential Oils and Aromatherapy*. San Rafael, Calif.: New World Library, 1991.

Healing Space

Birren, Faber. *Color Psychology and Color Healing*. Secaucus, N.J.: Citadel Press, 1961.

Chiazzari, Suzy. *The Complete Book of Color*. Boston: Element Books, 1998.

Chiazzari, Suzy. *The Healing Home*. North Pomfret, Vt.: Trafalgar Square, 1998.

Gallagher, Winifred. *The Power of Place*. New York: Harper Perennial, 1994.

Morgenstern, Julie. *Organizing from Inside Out*. New York: Owl/Henry Holt, 1998.

Rossach, Sarah, and Lin Yun. *Interior Design with Feng Shui*. New York: E. P. Dutton, 1987.

Simons, T. Rafael. *Feng Shui Step by Step*. New York: Crown, 1996.

Venolia, Carol. *Healing Environments*. Berkeley, Calif.: Celestial Arts, 1988.

Nutrition

Balch, James E., and Phyllis A. Balch. *Prescription for Nutritional Healing: A Practical A-Z Reference to Drug-Free Remedies Using Vitamins, Minerals, Herbs, and Food Supplements*. Garden City Park, N.Y.: Avery Publishing, 2000.

Bloomfield, Harold H. *Healing Anxiety with Herbs*. New York: Harper-Collins, 1998.

Brostoff, Jonathan, and Linda Gamlin. *The Complete Guide to Food Allergy and Intolerance*. Rochester, Vt.: Inner Traditions International, 2000.

Cass, Hyla, and Terrence McNally. *Kava: Nature's Answer to Stress, Anxiety and Insomnia*. Rocklin, Calif.: Prima Publishing, 1998.

Crook, W. G. *The Yeast Connection Handbook*. Burr Ridge, Ill.: Professional Books, 1999.

Dufty, William. *Sugar Blues*. New York: Warner Books, 1974.

Mayell, Mark. *Natural Energy*. New York: Three Rivers Press, 1998.

Norden, Michael J. *Beyond Prozac*. New York: Regan Books/Harper-Collins, 1995.

Somer, Elizabeth. *Food and Mood*. New York: Owl/Henry Holt, 1995.

Breathing

Books

Bradley, Dinah. *Hyperventilation Syndrome: A Handbook for Bad Breathers*. Berkeley, Calif.: Celestial Arts, 1992.

Farhi, Donna. *The Breathing Book*. New York: Owl/Henry Holt, 1996.

Rama, Hymes, Alan, Swami Rama, Rudolph M. Ballentine. *Science of Breath*. Honesdale, Pa.: Himalayan Institute Press, 1998.

Zi, Nancy. *The Art of Breathing: Six Simple Lessons to Improve Performance, Health and Well-Being*. Glendale, Calif.: Vivi, 1997.

Audio and Video

Yee, Rodney. *The Art of Breath and Relaxation*, 1999. 120 minutes on two audiocassettes, with practice guide. Available from Living Arts, 1-800-254-8464.

Zi, Nancy. *The Art of Breathing Video: Six Simple Lessons to Improve Performance, Health and Well-Being*, 1997. Available from Vivi Company, 1-800-INHALE-8.

Bodywork

Cohen, Ken. *Qigong: Chinese Energy*. New York: Ballantine, 1997.

Feldenkrais, Moshe. *Awareness Through Movement*. New York: Harper & Row, 1991.

Hanna, Thomas. *Somatics*. Reading, Mass.: Addison-Wesley, 1988.

Howell, Dean. *NeuroCranial Restructuring: Unleash Your Structural Power*. 3d ed. Tonasket, Wash.: Howell Canyon Press, 2001.

Knaster, Mirka. *Discovering the Body's Wisdom*. New York: Bantam, 1996.

Kreiger, Dolores. *Accepting Your Power to Heal: The Personal Practice of Therapeutic Touch*. Santa Fe, N.M.: Bear & Company, 1993.

Lowen, Alexander. *Bioenergetics*. New York: Penguin, 1976.

Trager, Milton. *Movement as a Way to Agelessness*. Barrytown, N.Y.: Station Hill Press, 1995.

Upledger, John E. *Your Inner Physician and You: Craniosacral Therapy and Somatoemotional Release*. 2d ed. Berkeley, Calif.: North Atlantic Books, 1997.

Yee, Rodney, Nina Zolotow, and Michael Venera. *Yoga: The Poetry of the Body*. New York: St. Martin's Press, 2002.

Zake, Yamuna, and Stephanie Golden. *Body Rolling*. Rochester, Vt.: Healing Arts Press, 1997.

Mind-Body Healing

Books

Benson, Herbert. *Timeless Healing: The Power and Biology of Belief*. New York: Simon & Schuster, 1997.

Charlesworth, Edward A., and Ronald G. Nathan. *Stress Management*. New York: Atheneum, 1984.

Epstein, Gerald. *Healing Visualizations*. New York: Bantam Books, 1989.

Kabat-Zinn, Jon. *Wherever You Go, There You Are: Mindfulness Meditations for Everyday Life*. New York: Hyperion, 1994.

Audio and Video

Jon Kabat-Zinn. *Mindfulness Meditation*. 7 cassettes, $59.98. Order from Living Arts, 1-800-254-8464.

Practitioners, Supplies, and Information

Sensory Defensiveness

Sensory Integration International (SII)
1514 Cabrillo Avenue
Torrance, CA 90501-2817
Tel: (310) 787-8805
Fax: (310) 787-8130
E-mail: info@sensoryint.com

Website: www.home.earthlink.net/~sensoryint/

Provide lists of occupational therapists in your area experienced in SI therapy; courses, books, and materials to develop awareness, knowledge, skills, and services in sensory integration; members receive *Sensory Integration Quarterly.*

Avanti Educational Programs

PO Box 100400

Denver, CO 80210

Tel: (303) 733-8100

PDP Products and Professional Development Programs

14524 61st Street Ct. N.

Stillwater, MN 55082

Tel: (651) 439-8865

Fax: (651) 439-0421

E-mail: Products@pdppro.com

Website: www.pdppro.com

Toys and equipment that promote sensory processing, postural control, attention, self-regulation, and skills; books that support understanding, assessment, and treatment of clients with developmental and neurobehavioral problems, adults as well as children; workshops and continuing education on SI-related topics for professionals.

Southpaw Enterprise

PO Box 1047

Dayton, OH 45401-1047

Tel: 800-228-1698

Fax: (937) 252-8502

E-mail: therapy@southpawenterprises.com

Website: www.southpawenterprises.com

Provides sensory integration and special needs products.

Auditory Integration

Sound, Listening, and Learning Center
The Spectrum Center
4715 Cordell Avenue
Bethesda, MD 20814
Tel: (301) 657-0988
E-mail: spectrum@his.com
Website: www.tomatis.com

Auditory integration training, using the Tomatis method; information, brochures, and books; referrals to Tomatis centers in your area.

Vital Sounds
PO Box 46344
Madison, WI 53744
Tel: (608) 278-9330
Fax: (608) 278-9363
Website: www.vitalsounds.com or www.samonas.net

CDs and cassettes for auditory modulation and auditory integration training; U.S. outlet for SAMONAS CDs; brochures and books related to listening therapy.

Light Therapy

For general information about light treatments, national and international referrals to research volunteer programs, and a listing of manufacturers and suppliers, contact:

Society for Light Treatment and Biological Rhythms (SLTBR)
PO Box 478
Wilsonville, OR 97070
Tel: (503) 694-2404

College of Syntonic Optometry

15 Western Avenue

Augusta, ME 04330

Tel: (207) 622-5345

E-mail: dbilodo@aol.com

Dr. Betsy Hancock

21 E. 5th Street

Bloomsburg, PA 17815

Tel: (570) 784-3688

Dr. Hancock has devised an affordable home light-therapy device for syntonic light therapy.

Dinshah Health Society

PO Box 707-B

Malaga, NJ 08328-0707

Website: www.wj.net/dinshah

Information on how to utilize colored lights for medical problems. Spectro-Chrome color therapy is safe and inexpensive and can be used easily at home. Diseases from cancer and heart problems to arthritis and open sores have responded at some level to Spectro-Chrome. At the same time, Spectro-Chrome color therapy calms and organizes the nervous system.

Full-Spectrum Lighting

Lumiram

179 Westmoreland Avenue

White Plains, NY 10606

Tel: (800) 354-5596

E-mail: info@lumiram.com

Website: www.lumiram.com

Full Spectrum Solutions
4880 Brooklyn Road
Jackson, MI 49201
Tel: (888) 574-7014
Fax: (517) 764-4029
E-mail: fss@fullspectrumsolutions.com
Website: www.fullspectrumsolutions.com

Ott-Lite Technology Products
1214 West Cass Street
Tampa, FL 33606
Tel: (813) 621-0058
Fax: (813) 626-8790
Website: www.ott-lite.com

Tools for Wellness
9755 Independence Avenue
Chatsworth, CA 91311
Tel: (800) 456-9887
Website: www.toolsforwellness.com

Chemical Sensitivity

MCS Referral & Resources
501 Westgate Road
Baltimore, MD 21229
Tel: (410) 362-6400
E-mail: donnay@mcsrr.org
Website: www.mcsrr.org

Aromatherapy

Young Living Essential Oils
250 South Main Street
Payson, UT 84651

Tel: (800) 350-5042

Fax: (800) 763-9963

Website: www.younglivingessentialoils.com

Pacific Institute of Aromatherapy

Tammy Gilman

415 Orchard

Santa Fe, NM 87501

Tel: (505) 471-5920

Aromatherapy Accessory Shop

Driftwood Health

3687 Kingston Boulevard

Sarasota, FL 34238

Tel: (800) 268-1745 in the U.S. or

(941) 923-7291 outside the U.S.

Website: www.pureproducts.net

They carry a quiet essential oil diffuser.

Feng Shui

American Feng Shui Institute

108 North Ynez Avenue

Suite 202

Monterey Park, CA 91754

Tel: (818) 571-2757

E-mail: fsinfo@amfengshui.com

Website: www.amfengshui.com

Bodywork

The Upledger Institute

11211 Prosperity Farms Road

Suite D-325

Palm Beach Gardens, FL 33410

Tel: (561) 622-4334

E-mail: upledger@upledger.com

Website: www.upledger.com

NeuroCranial Restructuring

PO Box 448

Tonasket, WA 98855-0448

Tel: (888) 252-0411

E-mail: information@drdeanhowell.com

Website: www.ncrdoctors.com

Trager Institute

21 Locust Avenue

Mill Valley, CA 94942

Tel: (800) 726-2070

E-mail: admin@trager.com

Website:www.trager.com

Rolf Institute of Structural Integration

205 Canyon Boulevard

Boulder, CO 80302

Tel: (800) 530-8875

E-mail:info@boulderguide.com

Website:www.boulderguide.com

Nurse Healers Professional Associates (Touch Therapy)

1211 Locust Street

Philadelphia, PA 19107

Tel: (215) 545-8079

Feldenkrais Guild of North America

3611 SW Hood Avenue

Suite 100

Portland, OR 97217

Tel: (503) 221-6612 or

(800) 775-2118

E-mail: Media@feldendrais.com

Website: www.feldenkrais.com

International Somatic Movement Education and Therapy Association (ISMETA)

c/o 148 W. 23rd Street, 1H

New York, NY 10011

Tel: (212) 242-4962

North American Society of Teachers of the Alexander Technique

3010 Hennepin Avenue South

Suite 10

Minneapolis, MN 55408

Tel: (612) 824-5066 or

(800) 473-0620

American Yoga Association

PO Box 19986

Sarasota, FL 34236

Tel: (941) 927-4977

Website: www.americanyogaassociation.com

Qigong Institute

561 Berkeley Avenue

Menlo Park, CA 94025

Website: www.qigonginstitute.org

The International Institute for Bioenergetic Analysis

One Post Road

Fairfield, CT 06430

Tel: (203) 319-0521

E-mail: Iibanet@aol.com

Website:www.Bioenergetic-therapy.com

Most practitioners are already qualified in some form of psychotherapy before training as bioenergetic therapists.

Hypnotherapy

American Board of Hypnotherapy
2002 East McFadden
Suite 100
Santa Ana, CA 92705
Tel: (800) 872-9996
Fax: (714) 245-9881
E-mail:aih@hypnosis.com
Website:www.abh.cc

Index

abuse, 9, 121, 141
acidity, 254, 258–59
acoustic sound reflex, 32
Ackerman, Diane, 110
activities, 179–80, 185, 189
adaptation, diseases of, 151–54
adenosine, 251
addictions, 119–44, 149, 150
adjustment disorder, 119
adolescence, 114–15, 133
adrenal exhaustion, 150, 251
adrenal glands, 147, 148, 149, 252, 260
adrenaline (epinephrine), 10, 11, 60, 67,
    147, 149, 251, 252
adrenaline rush, 57, 172
adrenocorticotrophic hormone (ACTH),
    148
aggression, 121
agitation as diversion, 166–67
agoraphobia, 86, 120, 130
air, 221, 223–33, 244
alarm, 147
alarm response, 196
alcohol addiction, 137, 138
Alexander, Frederick Matthias, 294
Alexander technique, 292, 294
allergic reactions/allergies, 9, 95, 145, 148,
    149, 151, 152–53, 226, 254, 255
alternate nostril breathing (ANB), 58,
    272–73

American Medical Association, 225
Amini, Fari, 105
amygdala, 59, 60, 70, 96, 147, 223,
    261
analytical hypnotherapy, 306
anorexia, 133–37
anticipatory anxiety, 98, 125
anxiety, 2, 3, 7, 12, 18, 55, 154, 267
    and addictions, 119–44
    defined, 123
    letting go of, 166–67
    misdiagnosed, 13
    in moderate defensives, 80
    panic differs from, 130
anxiety busters, nutritional, 260–63
Anzalone, Marie, 100
approach/avoid, 59–61, 62, 66, 170
    behavior change, 67–68
    going to extremes, 63–64
    high arousal, 64–66
    low arousal, 64
    staying centered, 62–63
aromatherapy, 2, 228, 229–30
    transdermal, 231
aromatherapy massage, 231
arousability, 89, 182, 183
arousal, 56, 170, 277
    high, 64–66
    low, 64
    modulating, 249–50, 289

arousal (*continued*)
　optimal, 56, 59, 62, 67, 94, 101, 131,
　　182, 185
arousal curve, 56–57
arousal level, 61, 63, 186–87, 200–201
　baseline, 57–58, 65, 68, 302
　extremes, 63–64
　and food, 132
　rating, 187*f*
Ashtanga yoga, 296
Atlantic Institute of Aromatherapy, 229–30
attachment, 93, 101, 102, 107
attention deficit hyperactivity disorder
　(ADHD), 3, 135
Auden, W. H., 236–37
auditory defensiveness, 24, 32–35, 129–30,
　204
auditory discrimination, 46
auditory integration training (AIT), 205
auditory processing, 55, 66, 204
autism, 7, 35, 86, 88–89, 153
autonomic nervous system, 11, 48, 57
avoidance, 3, 7
　of objects, people, situations (list),
　　160–63
　see also approach/avoid
avoidant personalities, 120
Awakenings (film), 48–49
Ayres, A. Jean, 8, 16, 19, 127, 135

balance, 29, 30, 43, 47, 51, 128, 130, 204
Bates, William, 213
bear hug vest, 178
behavior, 14–15, 67, 80, 121
　changing, 53, 66–67, 105
　and defensiveness, 96–97
　light and, 220–21
　repetitive, 120–21
belonging
　feeling, 112
Benson, Herbert, 303
Berard, Guy, 205, 206
Bergman, Ingmar, 245–46
Bikram yoga, 297
Bilateral Nasal Specific Therapy (BNS),
　286
biochemistry, 62, 130, 132
　of infant, 95–96, 100
bioenergetics, 292, 297–98
biology, 208, 235, 236
blowing, 276, 278–79
body, 40, 158, 294
　aging, 151
　balanced, 288–89
　breakdown, 147–50
　connection to, 238

disconnection from, 110–12
energy and vibration, 208
healing itself, 299
life history etched in, 282–83
listening to, 164
memories in, 108, 109
scanning for tension (list), 165
in space and time, 236
undulating, 284–85
see also mind/body
body awareness, 47, 111, 179, 272
　through movement, 293
　music and, 201
　sense of self starts with, 110
　of tension and relaxation, 301
　therapeutic listening for, 204
　in yoga, 296
body-breath synchrony, 273–74
body functions, 208, 220–21, 292
body language, 28, 238
body rhythms, 58–59, 93, 194
　of mother, 103, 104
　and music, 200, 201–2
　odors and, 223
　and posture, 282
　and thermal environment, 245
body rolling, 178–79
Body Rolling (Zake and Golden), 179
body sensitivity, 26–27
bodywork, 219, 266, 267, 275, 279,
　282–83, 306
Bolles, Mary, 221
borderline personality, 86, 121, 139
bottom-up processing, 169–91
brain, 10–11, 13, 14, 15, 123
　approach/avoid, 59–61
　in balance, 30
　effect of essential oils on, 230–33
　emotional, 52–53
　influenced by mind, 299
　light in, 214–15
　memory stored as prototypes in, 108–9
　primitive, 50–51, 299
　resculpted, 170
　response to trauma, 69
　rewiring, 70
　right/left hemispheres, 17, 56, 58, 61,
　　96, 203, 303
　sensory integration, 38
　sensory processing, 39–41, 43
　of tactile defensive, 25, 26–27
　thinking, 53
　three parts of, 49, 53–56
brain chemistry, 9
brain stem, 50–51, 53, 56, 57, 59, 60, 168,
　169, 172, 281

brain waves, 199, 215
Brazelton Neonatal Behavioral Assessment
    Scale (NBAS), 94–95
breath, 265, 269, 305
breath control, 275–79
breathing, 17, 18, 246, 263, 265–79, 301
    deepening, 16
    in yoga, 294, 295, 302
breathing exercises, 16, 17, 276, 277

caffeine, 250, 251
Campbell, Don, 33, 199
Campbell, Joseph, 305
candida overgrowth, 250, 254, 256–57
carbon dioxide, 267–68, 269, 275
centered, staying, 62–63
cerebellum, 51, 170
cerebral cortex, 53, 61, 215, 219
cerebrum, 50, 51, 70, 252
Chakra Chants (Goldman), 109
chakras, 109–10
change, fear of, 158–59
chanting, 202–3
chemicals, 10, 223, 224–26, 229
chest breathing, 266–67, 269
children
    defensiveness, 102–3
    fear of dark, 129
    heavy work with (list), 171–72
    optimal arousal, 185
    movement, 180
    reactive inhibited, 95–96, 104–5
    sensory-defensive, 83, 112–15, 121, 166
    and sensory diet, 158
chronic fatigue syndrome (CFS), 9, 145,
    151, 255
circadian rhythms, 58, 208–9
claustrophobia, 125, 126
clothing, 7, 25, 78, 79, 135
cognitive-behavioral therapy, 123, 300,
    308
color, 207–8, 209–10, 216–18, 241–44
Colton, Helen, 47
Conscious Ear, The (Tomatis), 245
consciousness, 53, 189, 306
    altered state of, 300, 301, 304
control, 28, 73, 80, 158, 170
Cool, Steven, 45, 176
coordination, 128, 131, 204
cortisol, 60, 96, 106, 132, 147, 149, 252,
    289
    caffeine and, 251
craniosacral therapy, 16, 18, 284–86, 292,
    306
culture, and space, 237–38
Czikszentmihalyi, Mihaly, 181

daily routine, 183–84, 189
    heavy work (list), 171–72
danger, 61, 62, 63, 65, 196
deep breathing, 2, 265, 269–79
deep pressure, 27, 88, 111, 112, 172, 180,
    182, 301
    of massage, 289–90
deep-pressure interventions, 178–79
deep-pressure skin stimulation, 174–
    77
deep pressure touch, 169–70, 175, 180,
    186
deep relaxation, 299, 300–301
DeGangi, Georgia, 96
denial, 159–64, 167
depersonalization, 121, 133, 139–44
depression, 12, 13, 64, 107, 121, 139, 149,
    154, 164, 208
    exercise and, 181
development, 7, 86, 89, 98, 105, 117
    nervous mother and, 106
diagnoses, 86, 139
*Diagnostic and Statistical Manual of Mental
    Disorders, The* (DSM-IV), 119, 122
Diamond, John, 200
digestion, 249, 250, 259, 289
    SSB and, 277–78
digestive tract, 251, 255, 258
Dinshah, Darius, 218
disconnection
    from body, 110–12
    from feelings, 112–17
discriminatory sensory system, 61
dis-ease, 57, 144, 154
disease(s), 57, 144, 154
    of adaptation, 151–54
disruptions, sensory diet, 190
dissociation, 121, 139, 140, 142, 214
distal (far) senses, 41, 45
distress, 57, 106, 164–66
diversion, agitation as, 166–67
Donne, John, 32
dorsal horn, 109
Downing, John, 216, 218
drugs, 13, 19, 250, 308
    addiction to, 137–39
duration (activities), 185–86, 187
dyslexia, 126–27

ear, 45–46
eating, 131–33, 259
educating others, 190–91
electricity, 195, 235
emotional hijacking, 69–70
emotional issues/emotions, 7, 9, 18, 52,
    56, 63, 117, 246, 282, 283

emotional issues/emotions (*continued*)
  limbic system and, 50
  releasing, 285, 292, 298, 306
  seat of, 253
endocrine system, 147
endorphins, 69, 131, 167, 177, 181, 289,
    299, 300
  chant and, 203
  light therapy and, 215
energy, 207–8, 282
  healing, 290–91
energy field, 291
energy flow, 239–41
enjoyment
  in sensory diet, 188
entraining/entrainment, 104, 105, 194, 195,
    218
  of sound, 193, 198, 202–3
environment, 184, 236, 239–45
Environmental Protection Agency (EPA),
    225
essential oils, 227–30
  effect on brain, 230–33
eustress, 57
exercise, 180–82, 188, 294
exhaustion, 147, 149–50
eyes, 204, 214–19
Eysenck, Hans, 183

face, 51, 79
fatigue, 121, 149, 208
fear, 93–117, 129, 238
feelings
  disconnection from, 112–17
  suppression of, 167
  see also emotional issues/emotions
Feldenkrais, Moshe, 292–93
Feldenkrais method, 292–93
feng shui, 239–41
fetus, 43, 44, 112, 196
fibromyalgia, 9, 145, 151, 152
Field, Tiffany, 104, 289
field independence, 272, 296
flight-fight, 11, 34, 57, 61, 63, 66, 123,
    124, 132, 146, 147, 157, 175, 238
  and digestion, 250
fluorescent lighting, 210, 211, 212, 213
food, 28–29, 132, 249–50, 260
  and the jitters, 250–53
food sensitivities/intolerance, 254–55
Fox, Nathan, 96
free radicals, 148–49
frequency (activities), 185, 187
Freud, Sigmund, 166, 297, 306
Frick, Sheila, 35, 204
full-spectrum light, 221

gastrointestinal problems, 152
Gates, Bill, 31
general anxiety disorder (GAD), 122–25
General Theory of Love, A (Lewis, Amini,
    and Lannon), 105
genetic link, 9, 96
genital arousal, 124–25
Gerard, Alice, 87, 113
Gift of Touch, The (Colton), 47
glucose tolerance test, 253
glutamate, 9
Golden, Stephanie, 179
Goldman, Jonathan, 109
Goleman, Daniel, 69
Grandin, Temple, 88–89, 124
gravity, 43, 54, 172, 173, 204
  being in balance with, 288–89
gravity receptors, 46
green light reflex, 293
Gregorian chant, 200, 202, 205
Grossenbacher, Peter, 49
growth hormone, 42
Gulf War syndrome, 225
gut, 249, 250, 254–59, 263

habituation, 60, 63
Hall, Edward, 237
Halpern, Steven, 198
Halprin, Anna, 292
Hanna, Thomas, 293
Hanna Somatic Education, 293
Hardison, James, 88
Harlow, Harry, 44
headaches, 145, 151
head trauma, 9, 17
healing, 18, 203, 206, 221, 229
hearing, 34–35, 43, 45–46, 195, 223
  and other senses, 47, 48
heavy work, 170–72, 180, 181, 182, 186,
    252, 275, 283, 301
  to jaw, 278–79
high-touch cultures, 237–38
hippocampus, 9, 59
Holbrook, Pat, 168
hormonal fluctuations, 152, 153–54,
    256
hormones, 52, 249
Howell, Dean, 286, 287
Hubel, David, 39
hyoid bone, 277–78
hyperactivity, 8, 127, 135, 205
hyperreactivity, 13, 55
hypersensitivity, 3, 8, 9, 24, 152, 154
hyperventilation, 267–69, 275
hypnosis, 299–300, 306
hypnotherapy, 219, 306

hypoglycemia, 250, 252–53
hypothalamus, 59, 60, 209, 215, 252, 253

identity, 166
imipramine, 177
immune system, 147, 148–49, 208, 226, 255, 289
  and allergies, 152, 153, 254
  stress and, 151, 256
immunoglobulin E (IgE) system, 152
incurvation reflex, 285
infancy, 3
  effects of experience in, 107–10
infants
  allergies, 152
  body rhythms, 103
  inborn style, 94–98
  interaction with mother, 98–99, 100–107
  movement, 43–44
  premature, 109
  proprioception, 44–45
  sensory-defensive, 99–102
information processing, 63, 65
intensity (activities), 185, 187
intimacy issues, 82–83, 136, 237–38
intimate space, 237
introversion, 8, 182, 183
irritable bowel syndrome, 151, 255
Iyengar yoga, 296

Jacobs, Barry, 278
James, William, 225
jaw, heavy work to, 278–79
joint compressions, 175, 177, 186
Jung, Carl, 283

Kagan, Jerome, 36, 95, 96, 97, 104–5
kava, 261
Kennedy, John F., Jr., 29
Krieger, Dolores, 290, 291
Kundalini yoga, 296–97
Kunz, Dora, 290

lactate, 251
language, 65–66, 98
Lannon, Richard, 105
Lawrence, D. H., 48
leaky gut syndrome, 250, 254, 255–56
learned helplessness, 121, 164
learning, sensory processing in, 40–41, 215–16
learning disabilities, 7, 44, 55, 127
LeDoux, Joseph, 70
lemon-drop test, 183
lens flexor, 273–74
Let's Touch (Hardison), 88

Let There Be Light (Dinshah), 218
Levinson, Harold, 126–27
Lewis, Thomas, 105
Liberman, Jacob, 214, 215–16
life span, sensory defensiveness across, 93–117
lifestyle, sensory diet in, 187–88
light, 35–36, 120, 207–21, 242–43
  alarm response to, 196
  healing power of, 206
Light (Liberman), 214
lighting
  full-spectrum, 211–12, 213
  unnatural, 10, 209–10, 211
light therapy, 19, 215–19, 275, 306
  and memories, 219–20
limbic brain, 54, 60
limbic system, 50, 51, 52–53, 59, 147, 215, 223, 261
  light hitting, 219
  odors, 223, 228
  retraining, 170
listening, 199–201
  therapeutic, 19, 204–6, 275
Lowen, Alexander, 111, 270, 297–98
low-touch cultures, 237
Lumatron phototherapy device, 215, 216

McKuen, Rod, 111
MacLean, Paul, 49–50
Mahesh, Maharishi 304
Main, Mary, 82
malabsorption, 250
marasmus, 42
massage, 178, 267, 289–90
Maugham, Somerset, 28
medications, 123, 124, 127, 137, 308
meditation, 2, 16, 48, 195, 199, 299–300, 303–5
  in yoga, 294, 295
medulla, 51
melatonin, 209
memory(ies), 107–10, 283, 292, 306
  light and, 215–16, 219–20
menopause, 10, 151, 14, 221, 232, 270
menses, onset of, 209
mental experience, self-test, 6
Mentastics, 288
Mesmer, Franz Anton, 306
mild defensiveness, 7, 14, 73, 74–75, 89, 96
mind/body, 18, 225, 266, 292, 298, 299–308
mind control, 300
minerals, 258, 260
misdiagnosis, 13, 55
mistrust of authorities, 167

moderate defensiveness, 73, 75–83, 89, 96, 100, 102
Montagu, Ashley, 42, 107, 237
mood, 52, 121, 124, 149, 260
  color and, 241–42
  yoga and, 296
morita, 307
mother(s)
  body rhythms, 103, 104
  calm, 104–5
  nervous, 105–7, 109, 126
mother-baby relationship, 98–99, 100–107, 237
  calm mother, 104–5
  and child's tactile defensiveness, 113
  mother's rhythms in, 103
  nervous mother, 105–7
mouth, touchy, 28–29
movement, 10, 47, 48, 51, 130, 186
  awareness through, 293
  cerebellum and, 51
  in hearing, 45–46
  language of brain, 43–44
  is medication, 180
  rhythmic, 201–2, 203
  in seeing, 46
  unconscious habits of, 294
movement defensiveness, 24, 30–31, 123, 126, 128, 138
  and social phobia, 131
movement receptors, 33, 188
movement therapy, 291–92
Mozart, Wolfgang Amadeus, 34, 195, 196, 200, 205, 206
multiple chemical sensitivity (MCS), 225–26
multiple personality disorder, 121, 141
muscular reflexes, 293
music, 194
  choosing, 199–201
  effect on minds and bodies, 197–98
  fetal response to, 196
  and healing, 202–3
  loud, fast, 195
  moving to, 201–2
  processing, 40–41
  therapeutic listening, 204–6
myofascial manipulation, 288
myofascial pain syndrome, 152

Nabokov, Vladimir, 49
National Academy of Sciences, 224
Natural History of the Senses, The (Ackerman), 110
nature, escape to, 245–46
needs, evaluating, 182–84

negative thoughts, 246, 300
neocortex, 53
neocranial restructuring (NCR), 286–87
nervous system, 11, 26, 147, 154
  food for, 165, 249–63
  of infant, 94, 98–99, 104, 106
  modulating, 173, 178, 180, 185, 191, 254
  and noise, 32
  organization of, 14, 15, 18, 62, 164, 169–70
  organization of, in children, 105, 106
  senses mingle in, 47–49
  touchy, 39–71
  tripod of, 45–47
  yogic breath control and, 270
neuropeptides, 108–9
neurotransmitters, 52, 219, 249
Nietzsche, Friedrich, 194
night and day, 208–9
Nightingale, Florence, 225
noise, 10, 32–34, 195–97
  hearing sounds, 34–35
norepinephrine, 95, 147, 176, 251, 289
Northrup, Christiane, 283
nutrition, poor, 18, 246, 301
nutritional anxiety busters, 260–63

obsessive-compulsive disorder (OCD), 120–21, 270, 278
occupational therapists (OTs), 8, 16, 18–19, 43, 167, 174, 176
  pediatric, 15
occupational therapy, 102, 124
odor, 37–38, 120, 223, 224
Oetter, Patricia, 97, 168, 277
O'Keeffe, Georgia, 288
olfactory defensiveness, 224, 229
Oliver, Jim, 193
oppositional defiant disorder, 121
oral defensiveness, 24, 29, 97, 132–33, 134, 179, 250
otoliths, 30
Ott, John, 208, 211–12
Ott-Lite, 213, 221
out-of-control (stage), 71, 86
overarousal, 56, 93, 123, 124
  infants, 105–6
overload, 10, 67, 68–71, 86, 89, 200, 245
  infant, 106
  stage, 70
overreactivity, 2, 11, 12–13, 38, 147, 154
overstimulation, 8, 14, 147, 166
  genital arousal in, 124–25
  protection against, 11–12
oxygen, 267–68, 269, 270, 275
oxytocin, 52, 215

pain, 26, 33
pain threshold, 177
panic, 120, 121, 125–26, 149, 238
   space-related, 127–31
panic attacks, 97, 123, 125, 126, 128, 130, 154
   hormonal changes in, 153
   hyperventilation and, 268
panic disorder, 130, 139, 153
parasympathetic nervous system, 63, 217, 266, 270, 271, 272
parents/parenting
   acceptance of child's feelings, 112–13
   intimacy issues and, 82–83
partner(s), educating, 190–91
perception, 15, 47, 49
perfumes, 228–29
peripheral vision, 213–14
personal space, 237, 238
Pert, Candace, 108, 109
pheromones, 38
phobias, 125–26, 130
   space related, 127–31
photophobia, 35–36
pineal organ, 209
placebo effect, 299
plants, air-cleaning, 226–27
PMS, 151, 154, 209, 221, 232, 251
post-traumatic stress disorder, 9, 70, 139, 308
posture, 51, 279, 281–98, 301
   poor, 18, 246, 282
power spot, 16
prayer, 300, 305
pregnancy, 10, 30, 112, 141, 196
premenstrual sensitivity, 151
professional help, 15
progesterone, 153
progressive relaxation, 275, 301–3
"Prologue" (Auden), 236–37
proprioception, 110, 169–70, 173
   and vestibular input, 173–74
proprioceptive activities (list), 172
proprioceptive input, 51, 105, 112, 168, 175, 178, 179, 180, 186, 188, 282
   in relaxation, 301
proprioceptive literacy, 292
proprioceptive sense, 41, 44–45, 46
proprioceptive system, 285
protective sensory system, 61
Proust, Marcel, 225
proximal (near) senses, 41, 47
Prozac, 13, 19, 77, 136
psychological disorders, 121, 122–44
psychological treatment, 13
psychopathology, 15, 93–94, 119

psychosomatic complaints, 145–54
psychotherapy, 2, 13, 16, 220, 283, 307–8
   body-oriented, 292, 297
psychotropic drugs, 13, 19, 308
public space, 237, 238
push and pull, 170–71
pyrones, 261

qi gong, 297
quiet therapy, 307

receptor cells, 46
red light reflex, 281, 293
Reich, Wilhelm, 297–98
rejection by mother, 101–2
rejuvenation room, 245, 300
relationships, 121, 191
   moderate defensiveness, 77–78
   severe defensiveness, 85–86
   and touch, 27–28
relaxation, 157, 166, 292
   and breathing, 265, 266
   deep, 299–300
   in meditation, 303
relaxation response, 270, 303
repetition, 186, 278, 304, 305
reptilian brain, 50–52, 54, 70
resistance, 147, 148–49
restricted environmental stimulation therapy (REST), 307
reticular activating system, 170, 176, 204
reticular formation (RF), 50–51, 59, 60
rhythm(s), 48, 59, 185, 186, 187
   dissonant, 195
   internal, 209
   natural, 195, 198
   see also body rhythms
Rolf, Ida, 288
Rolfing, 288–89, 292, 306

Sacks, Oliver, 48
SAD (seasonal affective disorder), 220–21
sadomasochism, 88
SAMONAS method, 206
scaffolding, 104, 105
Schafer, R. Murray, 195
schedule, in sensory diet, 189
sea anemone (exercise), 274
Seitz, Philip, 107
self
   boundaries of, 236–37
   estrangement from, 116
   flawed perception of, 114, 133
   fragmented, 94
self-discovery, 158
self-efficacy, 99, 164

self-preservation, 14
    four Fs, 50
self-protection, 126
    children, 97–98
self-regulation, 50, 103, 131, 204
self-stimming, 62
Selye, Hans, 57, 147, 151, 293
sensation(s), 1–2, 7, 41
    appraising, 93
    bothered and distracted by, 3, 6–7
    in brain, 52
    defensive reactions to, 313–17
    modulation of, 15
    organizing, 94
sensation seekers, 64, 67, 195
sense of self, 93–94, 110, 117, 166
senses
    on defense, 23–38
    combining, 221
    near/far, 41, 45, 47
    proprioceptive, 44–45
    tactile, 41–43
    vestibular, 43–44
sensitivity, 3, 107, 153
sensorimotor activities, 124, 157
sensorimotor function, 9
sensorimotor input, 185, 187
sensorimotor processing problems, 142
sensory accuity, 166
sensory affective disorder, 12, 119
sensory defensiveness, 2–19, 24, 67, 225–26
    anorexia as response to, 133–37
    arousal level, 64–66
    begins at birth, 117
    central nervous system problem, 49
    effects of, 119
    emotions, 52
    interventions for, 252
    levels of, 73–89
    across life span, 93–117
    and meditations, 303–4
    and mind control, 300
    overreaction, 38
    problems of, 68–71
    in psychological disorders, 121, 122–44
    psychosomatic side of, 145–54
    self-test, 4–6
    stages of, 70–71
    survival kit, 309–11
    symptoms of, 3–4, 6
    understanding, 158
    see also mild defensiveness; moderate
        defensiveness; severe defensiveness
sensory defensives
    craving relief, 131–39
    social problems, 36

sensory deprivation, 9
sensory deprivation chamber, 307
sensory diet, 15, 17, 18, 102, 154, 165,
    167, 168, 169–91, 173, 246, 250, 252,
    295, 300, 301
    balancing with sound, 191, 193–206
    and breathing, 266
    evolution of, 180–82
    getting started, 157–68
    setting, 182–91
sensory discrimination, 54
sensory experience, self-test, 4–6
sensory integration, 8, 14–15, 19, 38,
    39–41, 49, 53–54, 105, 127, 296
    basis of, 288
    bottom-up, 49–50
    treatment in, 16–18
sensory integration dysfunction (DSI),
    54–56, 86, 127, 142, 188
sensory integration therapy, 47
sensory modulation, 54, 55, 56, 179–80
    eating for, 131–33
    problems with, 119
sensory-motor amnesia, 293
sensory organization, 53, 54
sensory processing, 17, 38, 39–71, 123
    in behavior, 14–15
    in learning, 40–41, 215–16
sensory processing problems, 51, 56,
    65–66
sensory reactivity, differences in, 94–95
sensory teamwork, 47–49
    bottom-up, 49–50
    emotional brain, 52–53
    primitive brain, 50–51
    thinking brain, 53
sensory threshold, 8, 57
serotonin, 13, 52, 62, 121, 132, 186, 188,
    203, 260, 278, 304
serotonin boosters, natural, 260–63
severe defensiveness, 7, 70, 73, 83–89,
    96–97, 102, 105, 120
sex/sexuality, 78, 88, 136, 176, 180, 282
    body awareness and, 111
    in moderate defensiveness, 81–
        82
Shannahoff-Khalsa, David, 270
Shealy, Norman, 215
shutdown, 66, 69, 71, 86, 89, 140, 165,
    166
    psychological, 107
    to smell, 152
shyness, 66, 67, 105
sick building syndrome, 225
sight, 43, 45, 223
    see also vision

singing, 202–3
skin, 25, 27, 28, 42, 79, 81
skin brushing, 8, 17, 124, 174–77, 275, 283
skin disorders, 151
skin hunger, 10, 111–12, 283
skin sensitivity, 151
skin stimulation, 174–77, 178–79
skull alignment, 286–87
sleep cycles, 209
sleep deprivation/problems, 33, 121, 151,
   209
smell, 24, 37–38, 153, 223
   sense of, 26, 47, 52–53
smoking, 166–67
snacks, sensory, 180, 182, 185
socially mediated anxiety, 123–24
social phobia, 120, 131
social space, 237, 238
solar radiation, 210–11
somatics, 293
somatosensory system, 44
sound, 10, 45, 193–206, 207
   balancing sensory diet with, 191
   interpreting, 46
   nourishing, 198–99
space, 47, 125–26, 233
   bubble of, 236–38
   grounded in, 201
   harmonious, 235–46
   place in, 46, 48, 51
   shaky place in, 127–31
spatial awareness, 272, 296
stapedius muscle, 32, 204
startle response, 68, 196, 281
starvation, 133, 134, 136
Steinback, Ingo, 206
still-faced paradigm, 100
still-point inducer, 285–86
stimulation, 10, 48
   see also overstimulation
Stober, J. R., 286
Streisand, Barbra, 34
stress, 2, 3, 6, 12, 18, 119, 121, 127, 289
   and breathing, 265, 266
   chronic, 12, 302
   controlling, 169
   and craniosacral system, 284
   and digestion, 250, 278
   effect on serotonin, 260
   effects of, 57
   and illness, 146–50, 151
   in infants, 95–96, 106–7
   misdiagnosed, 13
   in moderate defensiveness, 76, 78
   and muscle tightness, 282
   music's effect on, 199
   physical symptoms with, 164
   recuperating from, 115–16
   and sugar level, 252
   and tactile sensitivity, 124
   and visual field, 214
   yoga and, 296
stress chemicals
   purged by exercise, 180–81
stress chemistry, 68, 69
stressed (stage), 70
stress hormones, 11, 12, 60, 68, 95–96,
   147, 289
   in children, 105, 106–7
stress response, 146–47
suck, swallow, breathe (SSB), 276–79
sucking, 276, 277, 278
Suedfeld, Peter, 307
sugar level, 250, 251, 252–53
suicide, 121, 130
sun exposure
   optimize health, 212–13
sunlight, 208, 209–3, 226
Suomi, Steven, 96, 104
survival, 37, 69, 180
survival stance, 281–82
swallowing, 276, 277
sympathetic nervous system, 60, 63, 97,
   124, 148
   in breathing, 270, 271, 272
   color and, 217
synesthesia, 49
syntonic phototherapy, 215, 217, 218–19

tactile defensiveness, 8, 9, 12, 24–28, 30,
   49, 96, 122, 126, 134–35, 136, 140,
   144, 176, 179, 190, 283, 289
   and body awareness, 110–11
   in child, 112, 113, 121
   in infant, 101, 106, 109
   in moderate defensiveness, 78, 81, 82
   mouth, 28–29
   in severe defensiveness, 87, 88
tactile discrimination, 55
tactile input, 168, 179, 180
tactile processing problems, 127
tactile sense, 41–43, 45, 46
tactile sensitivity, 124, 153
Taos hum, 34–35, 146
temperament, 8–9, 67
temperature, 26, 244–45
temporomandibular joint (TMJ), 152, 284,
   285, 302
tension, 3, 164, 283
   body scanning for (list), 165
   breathing and, 267
   reducing with skin stimulation, 178

testosterone, 64
thalamus, 50–51
therapeutic listening, 204–6
therapeutic touch, 290–91
thermal environment, 244–45
thought, 123–24
threat, 62–63, 131
thyrotropic hormone, 148
timing (activities), 185, 186
Tomatis, Alfred, 202, 204, 205, 206, 245
Torii, Shizuo, 229
touch, 6, 12, 24–28, 42, 153, 223
  avoiding, 8
  can be safe, 283
  in development, 42–43
  educating others about, 190
  with extreme defensiveness, 87–88
  intensity of, 27–28
  in mothering, 98, 99
  organizing, 10
  and other senses, 47, 48, 49
  and sense of self, 110–11
  in sensory diet, 174–77
  and space, 237, 238
  touchy mouth, 28–29
touch-and-motion program, 47
Touching (Montagu), 42, 107
touch receptors, 25, 26, 51, 175
Touch Research Institute, 289–90
touchy mouth, 28–29
toxins, 9, 226–27
Trager, Milton, 287–88
Trager Institute, 287
Tragerwork, 288
tranquilizers, natural, 261–63
transcendental mmeditation (TM), 304
trauma, 9, 69, 146, 293
  memories stored as, 109
treatment, 3, 16, 18, 67, 125, 158, 177
  cause of defensiveness and, 19
  in sensory integration, 16–18
  for tactile defensiveness, 8
tryptophan, 260–61

Ujjayi breathing, 30, 270–71
ultraviolet (UV) light, 210–11, 213
Upledger, John, 284
Upledger Institute, 285

vagus nerve, 30, 204, 253, 277
vasopressin, 148

vertigo, 29, 120, 129
vestibular functioning, 120, 127, 153
vestibular input/stimulation, 105, 168, 169–70, 172–74, 179, 180, 182, 185, 202, 275
  activities for (list), 174
vestibular processing problems, 127, 130
vestibular receptors, 172–73
vestibular sense, 41, 43–44, 45, 46
  sound stimulates, 204
vestibular system, 29–31, 97
  anxiety-control system in, 127–28
  yoga and, 295, 296
vibration, 33–34, 178, 193–94, 201, 207–8
  in singing, 202–3, 204
violence, 3, 121
vision, 46–47, 204, 213
  new approach to, 213–14
  and other senses, 47, 48, 49
visual cliff, 36
visual defensiveness, 24, 35–36, 123
visual field, 36, 47, 213–14, 215, 217
visualization, 299–300, 304, 305
visual perception of space, 128–29, 130
visual processing, 140, 214
visual-spatial processing problems, 17, 55
vitamin D, 211, 212
vitamins, 258, 260
vocal power, 202–3

weight against body, 111, 112, 122
Weil, Andrew, 205
Weinberger, Norman M., 41
whole body action (list), 171
Wilbarger, Julia, 3, 61, 65, 73, 75, 177, 190
Wilbarger, Patricia, 2–3, 12, 15, 61, 73, 87–88, 99, 137, 158, 166, 174, 176, 177, 179, 190
Wilbarger protocol, 174–77, 178, 185, 186, 275
women, 9–10

yoga, 2, 16, 17, 275, 294–97
  breathing techniques, 266, 270, 271
  styles, 296–97
Yogananda, Paramahansa, 207
yoga postures (asanas), 294–95

Zake, Yamuna, 179
Zone, The (Sears), 253